Carotenoids

Carotenoids

Nutrition, Analysis and Technology

Edited by

Agnieszka Kaczor and Malgorzata Baranska

WILEY Blackwell

Registered Office
John Wiley & Sons, Ltd, The Atrium, Southern Gate, Chichester, West Sussex, PO19 8SQ, UK

Editorial Offices
9600 Garsington Road, Oxford, OX4 2DQ, UK
The Atrium, Southern Gate, Chichester, West Sussex, PO19 8SQ, UK
111 River Street, Hoboken, NJ 07030-5774, USA

For details of our global editorial offices, for customer services and for information about how to apply for permission to reuse the copyright material in this book please see our website at www.wiley.com/wiley-blackwell.

Library of Congress Cataloging-in-Publication Data

Carotenoids : nutrition, analysis and technology / [edited by] Agnieszka Kaczor, Malgorzata Baranska.
pages cm
Includes bibliographical references and index.
ISBN 978-1-118-62226-1 (cloth)
1. Carotenoids. I. Kaczor, Agnieszka, editor. II. Baranska, Malgorzata, editor.
QP671.C35C372 2016
612′.01528–dc23

2015020395

A catalogue record for this book is available from the British Library.

Wiley also publishes its books in a variety of electronic formats. Some content that appears in print may not be available in electronic books.

Cover image: Red Veldrif Salt Pans (Credit: Joseboy)
iStock / Getty Images Plus
Caption: Salt pans along the Berg River at Veldif, South Africa, shine red in the sunlight due to a micro-algae known as Dunaliella salina which has been used in dietary supplements due to its antioxidant capability.

Set in 9/11pt TimesTen by SPi Global, Pondicherry, India

1 2016

Contents

List of Contributors

Halina Abramczyk
Lodz University of Technology, Institute of Applied Radiation Chemistry, Laboratory of Laser Molecular Spectroscopy, Lodz, Poland

Malgorzata Baranska
Faculty of Chemistry, Jagiellonian University; and Jagiellonian Centre for Experimental Therapeutics (JCET), Jagiellonian University, Krakow, Poland

Rafal Baranski
Institute of Plant Biology and Biotechnology, Faculty of Biotechnology and Horticulture, University of Agriculture in Krakow, Krakow, Poland

Paul S. Bernstein
Moran Eye Center, University of Utah School of Medicine, Salt Lake City, Utah, USA

Fritz Boehm
Department of Dermatology, Photobiology Laboratory, Charité Universitätsmedizin Berlin, Berlin, Germany

Reinhold Carle
Institute of Food Science and Biotechnology, Hohenheim University, Stuttgart, Germany

Christopher I. Cazzonelli
Hawkesbury Institute for the Environment, University of Western Sydney, Hawkesbury Campus, Richmond, NSW, Australia

Krzysztof Czamara
Faculty of Chemistry, Jagiellonian University; and Jagiellonian Centre for Experimental Therapeutics (JCET), Jagiellonian University, Krakow, Poland

Maxim Evgen'evich Darvin
Charité Universitätsmedizin Berlin, Department of Dermatology, Venerology and Allergology, Center of Experimental and Applied Cutaneous Physiology (CCP), Berlin, Germany

Jan Cz. Dobrowolski
Institute of Chemistry and Nuclear Technology; and National Medicines Institute, Warsaw, Poland

Ruth Edge
Dalton Cumbrian Facility, The University of Manchester, Westlakes Science & Technology Park, Cumbria, UK

Aruna Gorusupudi
Moran Eye Center, University of Utah School of Medicine, Salt Lake City, Utah, USA

Wieslaw I. Gruszecki
Department of Biophysics, Institute of Physics, Maria Curie-Sklodowska University, Lublin, Poland

Sascha Jung
Charité Universitätsmedizin Berlin, Department of Dermatology, Venerology and Allergology, Center of Experimental and Applied Cutaneous Physiology (CCP), Berlin, Germany

Agnieszka Kaczor
Faculty of Chemistry, Jagiellonian University; and Jagiellonian Centre for Experimental Therapeutics (JCET), Jagiellonian University, Krakow, Poland

Fanny Knorr
Charité Universitätsmedizin Berlin, Department of Dermatology, Venerology and Allergology, Center of Experimental and Applied Cutaneous Physiology (CCP), Berlin, Germany

Jürgen Lademann
Charité Universitätsmedizin Berlin, Department of Dermatology, Venerology and Allergology, Center of Experimental and Applied Cutaneous Physiology (CCP), Berlin, Germany

Takashi Maoka
Research Institute for Production Development, Kyoto, Japan

Martina Claudia Meinke
Charité Universitätsmedizin Berlin, Department of Dermatology, Venerology and Allergology, Center of Experimental and Applied Cutaneous Physiology (CCP), Berlin, Germany

Marta Z. Pacia
Faculty of Chemistry, Jagiellonian University; and Jagiellonian Centre for Experimental Therapeutics (JCET), Jagiellonian University, Krakow, Poland

Vassilia Partali
Department of Chemistry, Norwegian University of Science and Technology, Trondheim, Norway

Hartwig Schulz
Julius Kühn Institute (JKI), Federal Research Centre for Cultivated Plants, Institute for Ecological Chemistry, Plant Analysis and Stored Product Protection, Berlin, Germany

Ralf Martin Schweiggert
Institute of Food Science and Biotechnology, Hohenheim University, Stuttgart, Germany

Hans-Richard Sliwka
Department of Chemistry, Norwegian University of Science and Technology, Trondheim, Norway

Jakub Surmacki
Lodz University of Technology, Institute of Applied Radiation Chemistry, Laboratory of Laser Molecular Spectroscopy, Lodz, Poland

Terence George Truscott
School of Physical and Geographical Sciences (Chemistry Section), Keele University, Staffordshire, UK

Christian Witt
Department of Pneumonology, Charité Universitätsmedizin Berlin, Berlin, Germany

Grzegorz Zajac
Faculty of Chemistry, Jagiellonian University; and Jagiellonian Centre for Experimental Therapeutics (JCET), Jagiellonian University, Krakow, Poland

Leonhard Zastrow
Charité Universitätsmedizin Berlin, Department of Dermatology, Venerology and Allergology, Center of Experimental and Applied Cutaneous Physiology (CCP), Berlin, Germany

1 Carotenoids: Overview of Nomenclature, Structures, Occurrence, and Functions

Agnieszka Kaczor[a,b], Malgorzata Baranska[a,b], and Krzysztof Czamara[a,b]

[a]*Faculty of Chemistry, Jagiellonian University, Krakow, Poland*

[b]*Jagiellonian Centre for Experimental Therapeutics (JCET), Jagiellonian University, Krakow, Poland*

Nature is painting for us, day after day, pictures of infinite beauty if only we have the eyes to see them.

John Ruskin (1819–1900)

1.1 Introduction

The beauty of nature never ceases to surprise: the countless number of shapes and forms, a large diversity of fragrances and sounds, the unlimited palette of colors. Every day, we perceive through the senses her breathtaking majesty. The reality seen with the eyes is a mixture, the collage of rays of visible light reflected by the objects. This incredible composition comes onto the retina where, thanks to the light-sensitive cells called *cones*, the perception of the color is achieved. After the numerous physical and biochemical processes that convert a light stimulus into nervous stimulus, an image of the world creates itself in the brain. However, the leaves on the trees would never be green and the ripe tomatoes would not be red without the presence of natural pigments. Plants are equipped with sophisticated chemical compounds that absorb a part of the vital sunlight energy for use in photosynthesis and to give them color. One of them, carotenoids, are the second most abundant (after chlorophylls) pigments in nature, currently comprising over 700 specimens [1, 2]. They are responsible for the yellow, orange, and red color of fruits [3], flowers [4], seeds [5], flamingos [6–8], shrimp [9], and various other higher animals [7, 10, 11]. The deep color of these pigments is also characteristic for various simple organisms, such as yeast [12, 13], fungi [14, 15], and algae [16, 17], being natural carotenoid producers.

Carotenoids: Nutrition, Analysis and Technology, First Edition. Edited by Agnieszka Kaczor and Malgorzata Baranska.

Carotenoids generally cannot be synthesized by animals, but they are necessary in their diets and involved in many purposes, for example, lutein and zeaxanthin accumulate in the human eye and serve as photoprotectants against damaging effects of free radicals [18, 19]. So, without these pigments, we cannot see the beauty painted by them. Carotenoids are ubiquitous in all kingdoms of living organisms and provide various pivotal functions resulting from their structural diversity.

This opening chapter is addressed to gathering the fundamental knowledge of carotenoids, concerning their nomenclature, structure with stereochemical features, occurrence, and functions. Throughout this introductory chapter, references are made to the topics that are discussed in this book in detail.

1.2 Nomenclature and structures

Carotenoids owe their name to carrots (*Daucus carota*) due to the fact that they constitute the major pigments in the carrot root [20]. According to the International Union of Pure and Applied Chemistry (IUPAC) definition [21], carotenoids belong to the class of organic, lipid-soluble compounds, tetraterpenoids, which are composed of eight isoprenoid units joined together in the polyene chain. The structure of isoprene and an example of carotenoid with marked segments are presented in Figure 1.1. The arrangement of units is not obvious. From the center of the molecule, they are reversed, and hence two central side-chain methyl groups are in the 1,6 positional relationship while the remaining nonterminal groups are in the 1,5 relative positions. All carotenoids are derivatives of lycopene (ψ,ψ-carotene), which is represented by the formula $C_{40}H_{56}$, having a long central chain of 11 conjugated double bonds in the E (*trans*) configuration. This base acyclic structure can be chemically altered by cyclization, hydrogenation and dehydrogenation, oxidation, or any combination of these processes, making a vast range of possible carotenoids and their derivatives [22].

The specific structure of the carotenoid backbone originates from its biosynthetic pathway [2, 23]. Carotenoids are synthesized by a large variety of phototrophic and non-phototrophic organisms, including fungi, bacteria, and algae. In higher plants, the first step of the synthesis is the condensation of two geranylgeranyl diphosphate molecules forming a linkage of two C_{20} hydrocarbon fragments. This tail-to-tail enzymatic reaction is catalyzed by the phytoene synthase. The resulting compound, 15-*cis*-phytoene, is the first carotenoid having three conjugated double bonds. In further steps, a series of desaturation reactions,

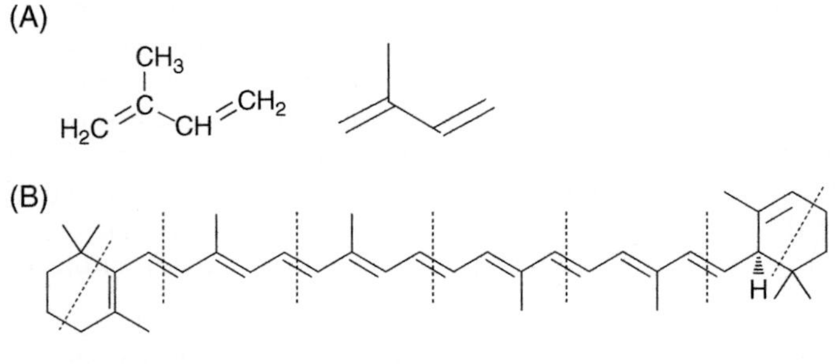

Figure 1.1 (A) The structure of isoprene; and (B) the arrangement of isoprenoid units in an exemplary carotenoid: α-carotene.

carried out by appropriate enzymes in the presence of light, introduce alternating double bonds in the 40-carbon basic skeleton leading to the lycopene structure. Thus, lycopene is the branching point of this pathway and starting point for synthesis of all other carotenoids. More information on the carotenoid biosynthesis and its regulation in plants is given in Chapter 10.

Carotenoids possess distinctive chemical reactivity and light-absorbing characteristics. One of their most remarkable features is the system of subsequent double and single bonds in the central part of the molecule. Due to the overlap of p-orbitals between adjacent carbon atoms, the delocalization of π-electrons over the entire length of the polyene chain occurs. The excited state of the molecule is accordingly of low energy, thus in general, absorption of the visible light is enough to give rise to the electronic transitions from π to π^* orbitals [24, 25]. Carotenoids possess 3–13 conjugated double bonds. Its number determines the color of the pigment from pale yellow (i.e., for ζ-carotene with 7 double bonds); through bright orange, characteristic for β-carotene (9 double bonds); to intense, deep red color (i.e., for canthaxanthin with 13 double bonds) [25]. Moreover, each double bond may exist in two configurations: as geometric isomers Z (*cis*) or E (*trans*), with *cis*-isomers being thermodynamically less stable, resulting in the all-*trans* isomers of carotenoids that are predominantly found in nature [24].

Carotenoids can be divided into two subgroups of hydrocarbons: carotens, composed only of carbon and hydrogen atoms (e.g., β-carotene), and their oxygen-containing derivatives, xanthophylls. In the latter, the additional oxygen atoms are found in various functional groups (i.e., hydroxy-, keto-, carboxy-, carbomethoxy-, epoxy-, and lactone), comprising a wide range of possible structures. Furthermore, the hydroxyl groups may also be esterified or glycosylated. Examples of some popular and structurally interesting carotenoids are shown in Figure 1.2.

To better understand the nature of studied compounds, it is essential to follow the nomenclature rules. Three naming conventions exist for carotenoids. The first one, the systematic nomenclature, is based strictly on the organic chemistry nomenclature. This method is not preferred for higher terpenoids and complex structures because their systematic names are long and awkward. The second naming system uses trivial names referring to plants or organisms from which they were originally extracted or to Latin words related to their properties. This approach is widely applied to natural products, but it can introduce ambiguity, as in the case of α-carotene that does not possess two α-ionone rings at the end of polyene chain but one α- and one β-ionone ring. Therefore, the IUPAC Commission on Nomenclature of Organic Chemistry and the IUPAC-IUB (International Union of Biochemistry) Commission on Biochemical Nomenclature have issued the *semi-systematic names*, based on both organic chemistry nomenclature and biological origin, to define precisely the structure of carotenoids [21]. A considerable advantage of this approach is the simplification in data searching in the literature and facilitation of communication between scientists from different science branches. Differences in the naming systems are presented in Figure 1.3 for lutein.

As was mentioned in this chapter, carotenoids' names originate from lycopene. Its hydrocarbon skeleton is a basic structure from which other names arise. The nomenclature consistent with the semisystematic rules starts from the correct numbering of the carbon atoms. The system is shown in Figure 1.4. However, the choice of locants of methyl groups at C1 atoms depends on the stereochemistry [21]. In acyclic terminal groups with a double bond between one and two carbon atoms (1′ and 2′ on the second end of the molecule), that methyl group is numbered as 1,6 which is in *trans* conformation to the main polyene chain. In β, γ, ε, and κ end groups, the 16 and 17 (16′ and 17′) are distinguished by the position of the R substituent denoting the rest of the molecule. If this moiety is on the right

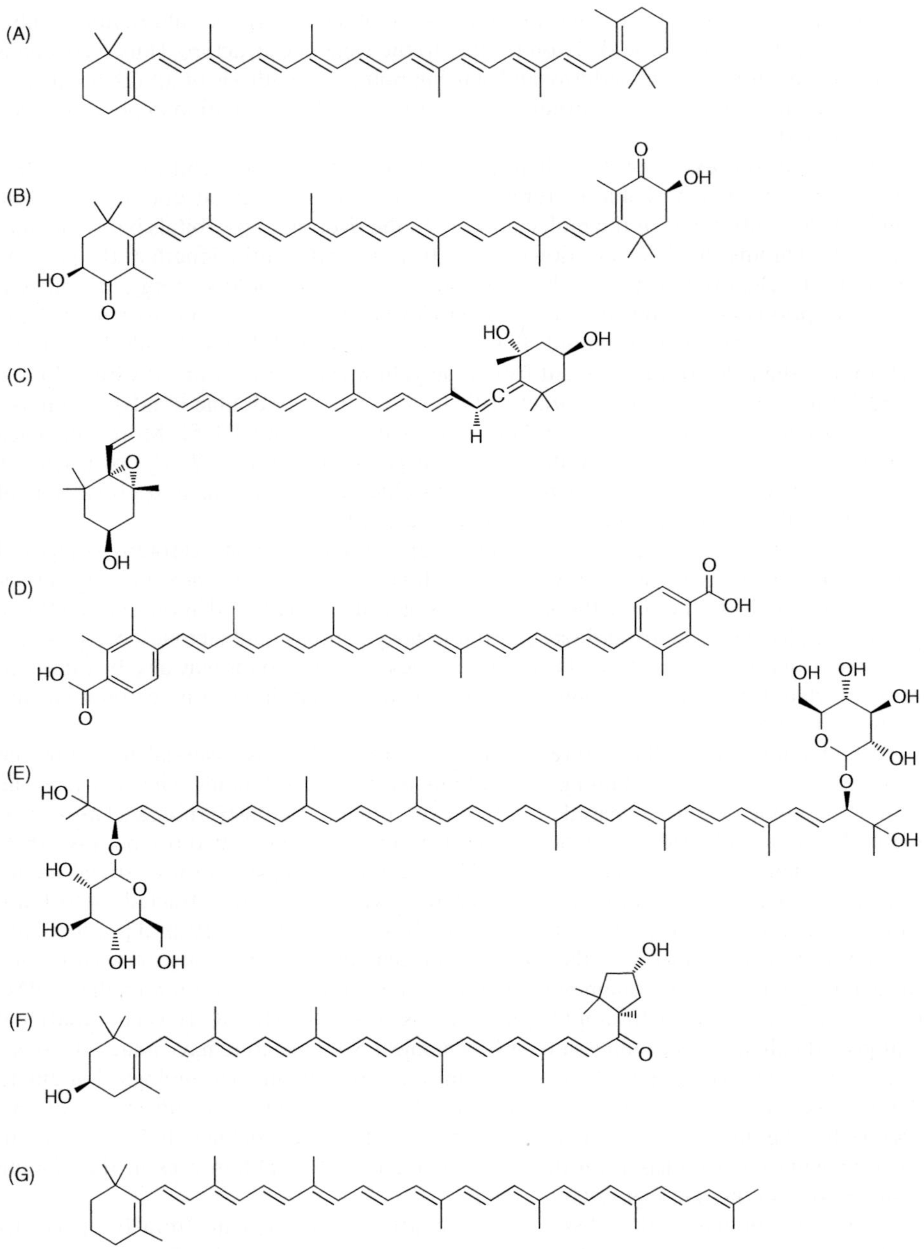

Figure 1.2 Examples of structures of carotenes and xanthophylls; a common natural source of the pigment is given in parentheses. (A) β-carotene (carrot *Daucus carota*); (B) astaxanthin (alga *Haematococcus pluvialis*); (C) neoxanthin (green leafy vegetables, i.e., spinach *Spinacia*); (D) synechoxanthin (cyanobacterium *Synechococcus*); (E) oscillaxanthin (cyanobacterium *Oscillatoria*); (F) capsanthin (paprika *Capsicum annuum*); and (G) torulene (yeast *Rhodotorula* spp.).

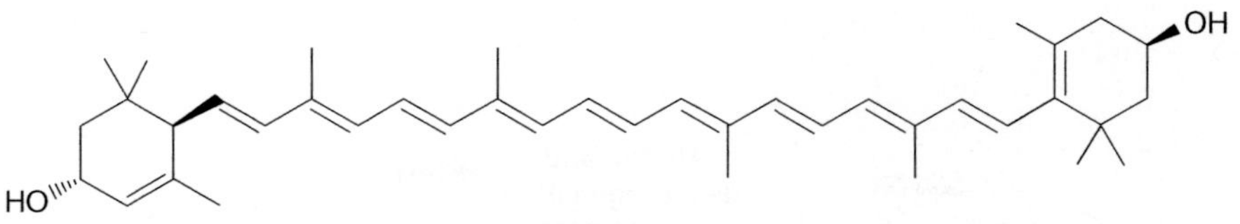

Systematic name: (1R,4R)-4-[(1*E*,3*E*,5*E*,7*E*,9*E*,11*E*,13*E*,15*E*,17*E*)-18-[(4R)-4-hydroxy-2,6,6-trimethylcyclohexen-1-yl]-3,7,12,16-tetramethyloctadeca-1,3,5,7,9,11,13,15,17-nonaenyl]-3,5,5-trimethylcyclohex-2-en-1-ol

Trivial name: lutein (from Latin *luteus*–yellow)

Semi-systematic name: (3R,3′R,6′R)-β,ε-carotene-3,3′-diol

Figure 1.3 The structure of lutein and its names in three naming systems: systematic, trivial, and semisystematic.

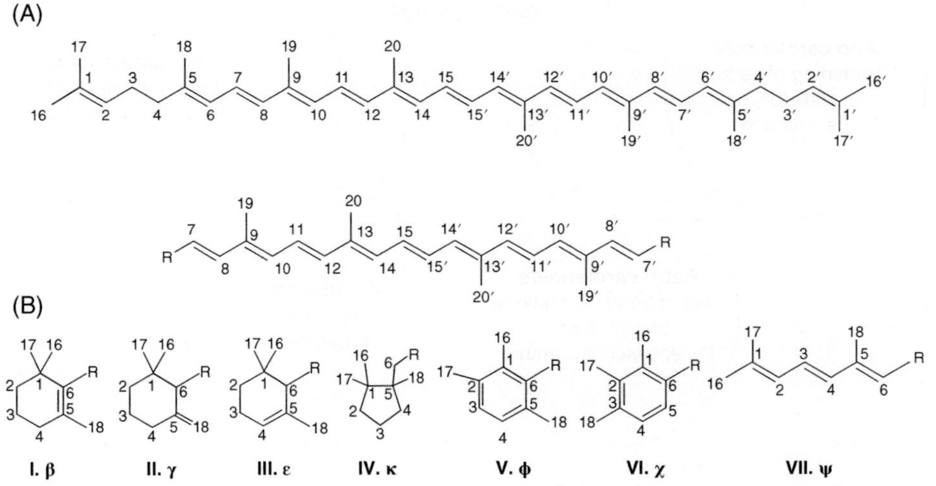

Figure 1.4 (A) The structure of lycopene compared with the structure of the carotenoid polyene chain; and (B) possible end groups found in nature (with prefixes). The numbering scheme for all structures is included.

from the C1 carbon atom, they are marked as below and above the ring plane, respectively. However, when the R group in on the left, that numbering is reversed.

Carotenoid molecules are composed of a hydrocarbon chain core (Fig. 1.4A) and two end groups attached to its opposite edges (Fig. 1.4B). Each terminal group has nine carbon atoms arranged in different structures (e.g., cyclohexene, cyclohexane, and cyclopentane) and is described by Greek-letter prefixes. All names are based on the stem name "carotene" preceded by the prefixes related to both groups occurring in the molecule. The letters should be cited in alphabetical order and doubled if they are identical. Thus, β-carotene is correctly written as β,β-carotene, α-carotene as β,ε-carotene, and so on. If the end groups are dissimilar, the unprimed numbers of carbon atoms are given from the end of the molecule associated with the first Greek letter appearing in the name.

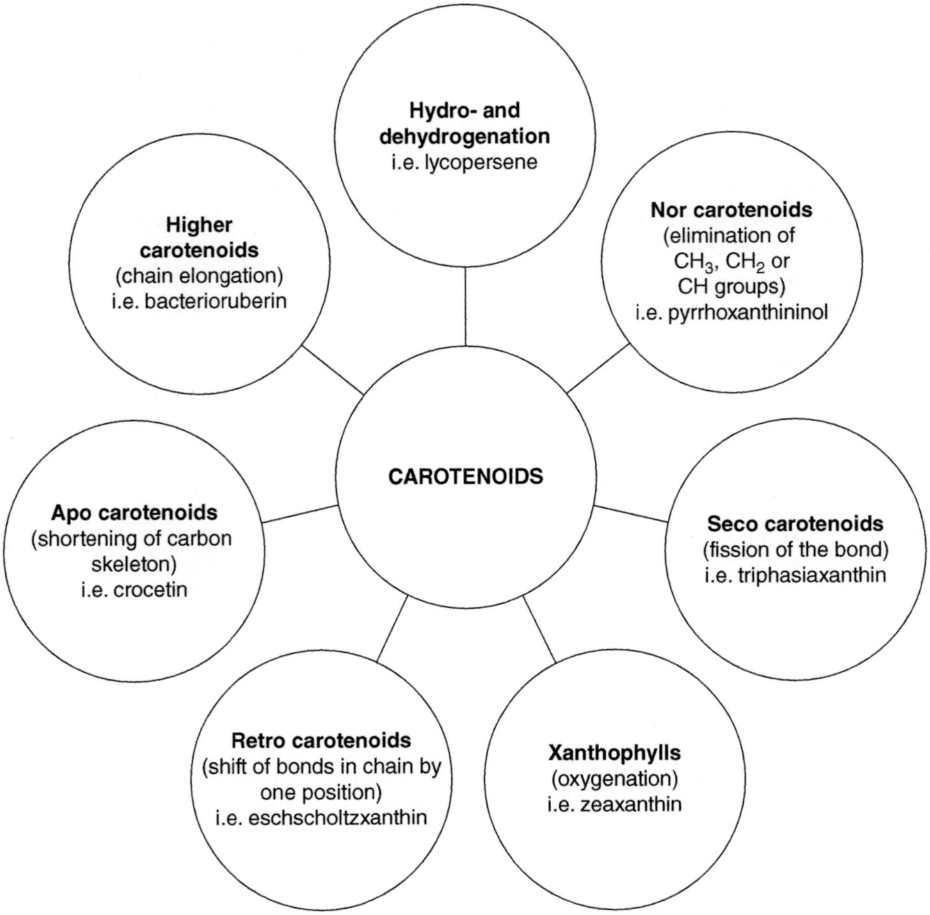

Figure 1.5 Various groups of carotenoid derivatives.

Modifications to both the chain and end groups introduce further rules in the nomenclature of carotenoids. Possible derivatives of carotenoids are presented in Figure 1.5, and the names are explained below:

- For hydrogenated and dehydrogenated derivatives, it is necessary to attach the prefixes "dehydro" and "hydro" when hydrogen atoms are removed or added, respectively, with the locants of the carbon atoms where they occurred. Additional prefixes denoting the number of modifications are used according to the standard organic chemistry principles.
- If one or more CH_3, CH_2, or CH groups has been eliminated from a carotenoid, the prefix "nor" with the locants of removed carbon atoms must be incorporated. In nor carotenoids, the numbering of the remaining carbon atoms is preserved as in the original molecules.
- Seco carotenoids are a subgroup wherein at least one band in the terminal rings has been ruptured. Thus, the name is supplemented by the prefix "seco" and numbers of carbon atoms where a gap occurs.

- Xanthophylls nomenclature follows the rules of the general organic chemistry nomenclature. For alcohols, carboxylic acids, esters of carotenoid alcohols and acids, aldehydes, and ketones, the oxygen-containing group serves as a principal group and is introduced by the use of a proper suffix. Xanthophylls classified as ethers are named in two manners depending on the type of oxygen binding. The non-bridging ethers bring to the name the appropriate "alkoxy" or "aryloxy" prefix, whereas oxygen bridges are introduced by the prefix "epoxy." In both cases, the point of attachment of the oxygen atoms in the molecule must be specified. The numbering in xanthophylls is the same as in other carotenoids only if the two end groups are dissimilar. Otherwise, the unprimed locants are assigned to carbon atoms according to the order of importance: firstly to principal groups, cited as the suffix, then in such a manner to obtain the lowest locants' numbers.
- If all conjugated double bonds are shifted by one position, the prefix "retro" should be included in the name with appropriate locants. The first and second numbers indicate carbon atoms from which protons were removed and added, respectively.
- Apo carotenoids are derivatives in which a carbon skeleton has been shortened by removal of a part of the molecule from one or both ends. The prefix "apo" is introduced with locants indicating that the fragment beyond this carbon atom has been replaced by hydrogen atoms. However, the side-chain methyl groups are not considered to be "beyond" the carbon atom to which it is attached. Additionally, in the case when the locants preceding the "apo" prefix are greater than 5, there is no need to give the Greek letters in the stem name.
- In contrast to apo carotenoids, there are subgroup of higher carotenoids composed of more than eight isoprenoid units. Their names follow the general principle for organic molecules and retain the numbering of the normal carotenoid.

The last step in the procedure of carotenoid naming involves the stereochemistry. The absolute configuration should be determined for each chiral center in the molecule using the R/S convention. Additionally, if any Z (*cis*)-configuration of double bonds is present in the structure, it should be denoted classically. The stem "carotene" indicates a molecule that possesses all C=C bonds in the E (*trans*) configuration.

1.3 Occurrence and functions

The diversity of functions in which carotenoids partake, in both human beings and other organisms, is enormous. Therefore, it is not particularly surprising that the number of literature reports on this topic is rather substantial and well summarized in several review articles published during the last three years (2012–2014) [16, 26–43].

1.3.1 Functions in plants

About 50 carotenoids are fundamental components of the light-harvesting antenna complexes (LHCs) of photosynthetic organisms. The main roles of pigments in LHCs are capturing light, transferring electronic excitations to the acceptor chlorophyll molecules, as well as photoprotection based on regulating the energy flow [43]. Carotenoids also play a role in stabilization of biomembranes and membrane-bound pigment–protein complexes. The function of carotenoids in pigment–protein complexes in relation to their structure is the topic of Chapter 9 of this book.

1.3.2 Antioxidants in humans

Several carotenoids act as potent antioxidants in humans. The omnipotent free-radical scavenger is astaxanthin, which has about 10-fold higher antioxidant activity compared to zeaxanthin, lutein, cantaxanthin, and β-carotene and 100-fold higher activity than α-tocopherol [44]. The antioxidant properties are the basis of preventive function toward many chronic diseases, including *neurodegenerative diseases*: stroke (lutein and astaxanthin), Alzheimer's disease (astaxanthin and β-carotene), and Parkinson's disease (β-carotene); *cardiovascular diseases*: atherosclerosis (lutein, astaxanthin, α-carotene, and crocin) and hypertension (astaxanthin, α-carotene, crocin, and lycopene); *diabetes* (lutein, zeaxanthin, astaxanthin, α-carotene, and lycopene); *cancer* (fucoxanthin, astaxanthin, α-carotene, crocin, and lycopene); and *osteoporosis* (β-cryptoxanthin and crocin) [28, 34, 35 and references cited therein, 37, 38, 45–46]. Moreover, several carotenoids are suggested to have a beneficial influence on the immunological system, decrease drug-withdrawal syndrome, show neuroprotective effect, and possess anti-inflammatory properties [28, 34, 35, 44].

It has been indicated that carotenoids can be used as biomarkers to distinguish between cancerous/malignant and healthy cells and tissues, with practical potential in medical diagnostics [47–49]. This subject is further developed in Chapter 2. Mechanisms of radiation and photoprotection of dietary carotenoids are characterized in Chapter 3.

1.3.3 Role in visual and cognitive function

One of the most important and well-described functions of carotenoids is the pro–vitamin A activity (i.e., their ability to convert into retinol) [43, 50]. Vitamin A is a compound of the key importance for child health and survival, and its deficiency result in disturbances in vision and a number of diverse other pathologies [51].

Two isomeric xanthophylls, lutein and zeaxanthin, play a key role in vision health [33 and references cited therein, 43 and references cited therein]. These pigments, in the forms of lutein, zeaxanthin, and mezo-zeaxathin, formed metabolically from lutein in the human body, are concentrated in the central region of the retina, called the *macula lutea*. Macular carotenoids prevent damage leading to age-related macular degeneration, visual impairment, and cataracts [33 and references cited therein, 43 and references cited therein]. Lutein was also suggested to influence early visual development [52]. This pigment is also a major carotenoid of the human brain, involved in a number of cognitive processes such as learning, memory, language, and executive functions [32 and references cited therein, 33 and references cited therein]. The influence of macular carotenoids on human health is considered in Chapter 4.

1.3.4 Carotenoids in human skin

Skin coloration appears to play an important role in facial attractiveness, with skin yellowness being a desirable feature. Overall, it was suggested that skin coloration is a part of the carotenoid-linked health-signaling system that is of considerable meaning in mate choice [53].

Human skin contains various carotenoids, mainly α-carotene, γ-carotene, β-carotene, lutein, zeaxanthin, lycopene, and their isomers, that serve the living cells as a protection against oxidation [54]. A diet rich in carotenoids prevents cell damage, premature skin aging, skin cancer, and other skin-related diseases as the increase of carotenoid level increases the radical-scavenging activity of the skin and provides a significant protection against stress-induced radical formation [55]. Moreover, the carotenoid level in the skin, which is quite easy to measure with the help of Raman spectroscopy, reflects the antioxidant status [56]. This topic is further developed in this chapter.

1.3.5 Signaling function

Carotenoids are responsible for the color of fruits, vegetables, and flowers, increasing their attractiveness for pollination, seed dispersal, and sexual attraction. Apo carotenoids contribute to the aroma of flowers, fruits, and vegetables. Carotenoid cleavage products are phytohormones and essential signaling molecules [43].

1.3.6 Industrial applications

Astaxanthin, next to β-carotene, is one of the most important carotenoids for industrial applications. Astaxanthin and (to a much lower extent) cantaxanthin, obtained from *de novo* manufacturers, play a crucial function as food colorants in salmonid and crustacean cultures [44]. Algal and yeast cultures are not only feed but also more and more often exploited sources of dietary carotenoids [16 and references cited therein]. Numerous factors influencing carotenoids' synthesis by microorganisms and various tactics that serve optimizing technological processes of carotenoid production are characterized in Chapters 12 and 13. Such microbial cultures are not only environmentally friendly but also, in the future, can function also as "recycling trash-cans" for agro-industrial wastes. Successful carotenoid production by microbial sources cultivated in industrial residues has been already reported [57–59].

Both microorganism-derived and synthetic carotenoids are used commonly as dietary supplements as well as pigments in food and beverages, for instance in fruit juices, soft drinks, and dairy products [16 and references cited therein]. Additionally, they are applied as animal feed and used in the pharmaceutical and cosmetic industries. There are often differences between synthetic and biomanufactured carotenoids in the sense of structures, and therefore their bioavailability. This point is referred to in Chapter 13. A general review of the recent spectroscopic studies regarding structures of carotenoids in *de novo* manufacturers, plants, and animals, also *in situ*, is discussed in Chapters 6–8. Topics related to carotenoids bioavailability from the food matrix and optimization of extraction procedures are included in Chapter 11. Various functions of carotenoids are summarized in Figure 1.6.

1.3.7 Carotenoids of specified properties

Industry is searching for carotenoids of modified properties both for better functionality and for new applications of carotenoids and their derivatives. Particularly, the pharmaceutical industry is interested in more hydrophilic carotenoids, with Cardax™ being an example of this. This disodium disuccinate derivative of astaxanthin is an efficient cardioprotective drug of increased solubility as compared with the original xanthophyll [60].

Various carotenoid-based compounds are synthetized and tested toward many specific applications, with carotenoid–porphyrin–fullerene derivatives being probably one of the most exotic carotenoid derivatives synthetized up to now [61]. Recent achievements, challenges, and perspectives of syntheses with carotenoids are described in Chapter 14.

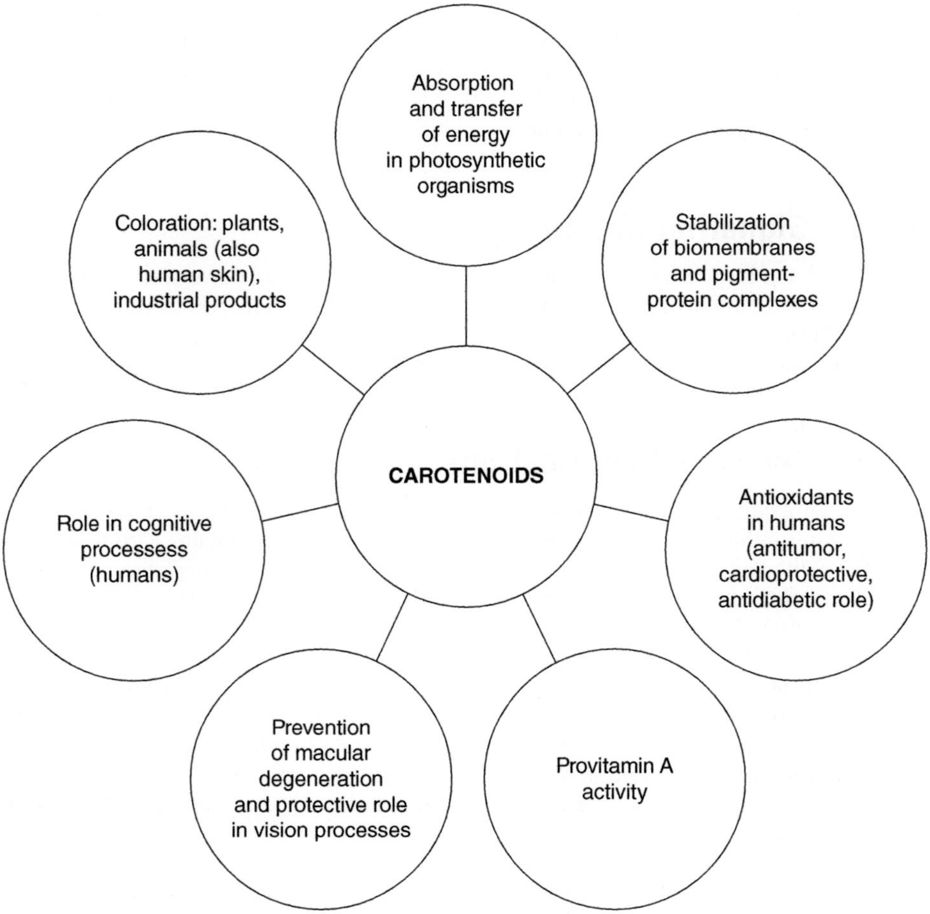

Figure 1.6 Diverse functions of carotenoids.

References

1. G. Britton, "Overview of carotenoid biosynthesis" in "*Carotenoids, vol. 3*" G. Britton, S. Liaaen Jensen and H. Pfander (Eds.), 13–147. Birkhauser, Basel, Switzerland, 1998.
2. M. H. Walter and D. Strack, "Carotenoids and their cleavage products: biosynthesis and functions," *Nat. Prod. Rep.*, **28**, 4, 663–92 (2011).
3. H.-E. Khoo, K. N. Prasad, K.-W. Kong, Y. Jiang, and A. Ismail, "Carotenoids and their isomers: color pigments in fruits and vegetables," *Molecules*, **16**, 2, 1710–38 (2011).
4. C. Zhu, C. Bai, G. Sanahuja, D. Yuan, G. Farré, S. Naqvi, L. Shi, T. Capell, and P. Christou, "The regulation of carotenoid pigmentation in flowers," *Arch. Biochem. Biophys.*, **504**, 1, 132–41 (2010).
5. C. A. Howitt and B. J. Pogson, "Carotenoid accumulation and function in seeds and non-green tissues," *Plant, Cell Environ.*, **29**, 3, 435–45 (2006).

6. D. L. Fox and T. S. Hopkins, "Comparative metabolic fractionation of carotenoids in three flamingo species," *Comp. Biochem. Physiol.*, **17**, 3, 841–56 (1966).
7. A. H. Brush, "Metabolism of carotenoid pigments in birds," *FASEB J.*, **4**, 12, 2969–77 (1990).
8. J. A. Amat, M. A. Rendón, J. Garrido-Fernández, A. Garrido, M. Rendón-Martos, and A. Pérez-Gálvez, "Greater flamingos *Phoenicopterus roseus* use uropygial secretions as make-up," *Behav. Ecol. Sociobiol.*, **65**, 4, 665–73 (2010).
9. N. M. Sachindra, N. Bhaskar, and N. S. Mahendrakar, "Carotenoids in different body components of Indian shrimps," *J. Sci. Food Agric.*, **85**, 1, 167–72 (2005).
10. T. Maoka, "Carotenoids in marine animals," *Mar. Drugs*, **9**, 2, 278–93 (2011).
11. T. Matsuno, "Aquatic animal carotenoids," *Fish. Sci.*, **67**, 5, 771–83 (2001).
12. G. I. Frengova and D. M. Beshkova, "Carotenoids from *Rhodotorula* and *Phaffia*: yeasts of biotechnological importance," *J. Ind. Microbiol. Biotechnol.*, **36**, 163–80 (2009).
13. L. C. Mata-Gómez, J. C. Montañez, A. Méndez-Zavala, and C. N. Aguilar, "Biotechnological production of carotenoids by yeasts: an overview," *Microb. Cell Fact.*, **13**, 1, 12 (2014).
14. C. Echavarri-Erasun and E. A. Johnson, "Fungal carotenoids," *Appl. Mycol. Biotechnol.*, **2**, 45–85 (2002).
15. J. Ávalos, V. Díaz-Sánchez, M. García-Martínez, J. Castrillo, M. Ruger-Herreros, and M. C. Limón, "Carotenoids," in *Biosynthesis and Molecular Genetics of Fungal Secondary Metabolites, Fungal Biology*, J. Martín and C. García-Estrada (Eds.), 149–87, New York: Springer Science+Business Media, 2014.
16. E. Christaki, E. Bonos, I. Giannenas, and P. Florou-Paneri, "Functional properties of carotenoids originating from algae," *J. Sci. Food Agric.*, **93**, 1, 5–11 (2013).
17. A. C. Guedes, H. M. Amaro, and F. X. Malcata, "Microalgae as sources of carotenoids," *Mar. Drugs*, **9**, 4, 625–44 (2011).
18. L. Ma and X.-M. Lin, "Effects of lutein and zeaxanthin on aspects of eye health," *J. Sci. Food Agric.*, **90**, 1, 2–12 (2010).
19. E.-S. M. Abdel-Aal, H. Akhtar, K. Zaheer, and R. Ali, "Dietary sources of lutein and zeaxanthin carotenoids and their role in eye health," *Nutrients*, **5**, 4, 1169–85 (2013).
20. M. Rodriguez-Concepcion and C. Stange, "Biosynthesis of carotenoids in carrot: an underground story comes to light," *Arch. Biochem. Biophys.*, **539**, 2, 110–6 (2013).
21. International Union of Pure and Applied Chemistry and International Union of Biochemistry, *Nomenclature of Carotenoids* (Research Triangle Park, NC: IUPAC, 1974).
22. K. K. Namitha and P. S. Negi, "Chemistry and biotechnology of carotenoids," *Crit. Rev. Food Sci. Nutr.*, **50**, 8, 728–60 (2010).
23. C. I. Cazzonelli, "Goldacre Review: carotenoids in nature: insights from plants and beyond," *Funct. Plant Biol.*, **38**, 11, 833 (2011).
24. G. Britton, "Structure and properties of carotenoids in relation to function," *FASEB J.*, **9**, 15, 1551–8 (1995).
25. A. J. Meléndez-Martínez, G. Britton, I. M. Vicario, and F. J. Heredia, "Relationship between the colour and the chemical structure of carotenoid pigments," *Food Chem.*, **101**, 3, 1145–1150 (2007).
26. P. Giordano, P. Scicchitano, M. Locorotondo, C. Mandurino, G. Ricci, S. Carbonara, M. Gesualdo, A. Zito, A. Dachille, P. Caputo, R. Riccardi, G. Frasso, G. Lassandro, A. Di Mauro, M. M. Ciccone, "Carotenoids and cardiovascular risk," *Curr. Pharm. Des.*, **18**, **34**, 5577–89 (2012).

27. T. Tanaka, M. Shnimizu, and H. Moriwaki, "Cancer chemoprevention by carotenoids," *Molecules*, **17**, 3202–42 (2012).
28. R. G. Fassett and J. S. Coombes, "Astaxanthin in cardiovascular health and disease," *Molecules*, **17**, 2030–48 (2012).
29. R. R. Ambati, P. S. Moi, S. Ravi, and R. G. Aswathanarayana, "Astaxanthin: sources, extraction, stability, biological activities and its commercial applications—a review," *Mar. Drugs*, **12**, 128–52 (2014).
30. J. Avalos and M. C. Limón, "Biological roles of fungal carotenoids," *Curr. Genetics*, DOI:10.1007/s00294-014-0454-x (2014).
31. H. Chang, L. Sheen, and Y. Lei, "The protective role of carotenoids and polyphenols in patients with head and neck cancer," *J. Chinese Med. Assoc.*, **78**, 2, 89–95 (2015).
32. E. J. Johnson, "A possible role for lutein and zeaxanthin in cognitive function in the elderly," *Am. J. Clin. Nutr.*, **96**, 5, 1161S–5S (2012).
33. E. J. Johnson, "Role of lutein and zeaxanthin in visual and cognitive function throughout the lifespan," *Nutr. Rev.*, **72**, 9, 605–12 (2014).
34. S. H. Alavizadeh and H. Hosseinzadeh, "Bioactivity assessment and toxicity of crocin: a comprehensive review," *Food Chem. Toxicol.*, **64**, 65–80 (2014).
35. J. Zhang, Z. Sun, P. Sun, T. Chen, and F. Chen, "Microalgal carotenoids: beneficial effects and potential in human health," *Food Funct.*, **5**, 3, 413–25 (2014).
36. N. D'Orazio, E. Gemello, M. A. Gammone, M. De Girolamo, C. Ficoneri, and G. Riccioni, "Fucoxantin: a treasure from the sea," *Mar. Drugs*, **10**, 3, 604–16 (2012).
37. T. Wolak and E. Paran, "Can carotenoids attenuate vascular aging?" *Vascul. Pharmacol.*, **59**, 3–4, 63–6 (2013).
38. M. Cámara, M. de Cortes Sánchez-Mata, V. Fernández-Ruiz, R. M. Cámara, S. Manzoor, and J. O. Caceres, "Lycopene: a review of chemical and biological activity related to beneficial health effects," *Studies in Natural Products Chemistry*, **40**, 383–426 (2013).
39. S. Takaichi, "Distributions, biosyntheses and functions of carotenoids in algae," *Agro Food Ind. Hi. Tech.*, **24**, 1, 55–8 (2013).
40. K. Jomova and M. Valko, "Health protective effects of carotenoids and their interactions with other biological antioxidants," *Eur. J. Med. Chem.*, **70**, 102–10 (2013).
41. J. J. Heath, D. F. Cipollini, and J. O. Stireman, "The role of carotenoids and their derivatives in mediating interactions between insects and their environment," *Arthropod. Plant. Interact.*, **7**, 1, 1–20 (2013).
42. X. D. Wang, "Lycopene metabolism and its biological significance," *Am. J. Clin. Nutr.*, **96**, 1214–22 (2012).
43. R. Álvarez, B. Vaz, H. Gronemeyer, and Á. R. de Lera, "Functions, therapeutic applications, and synthesis of retinoids and carotenoids," *Chem. Rev.*, **114**, 1, 1–125 (2014).
44. I. Higuera-Ciapara, L. Félix-Valenzuela, and F. M. Goycoolea, "Astaxanthin: a review of its chemistry and applications," *Crit. Rev. Food Sci. Nutr.*, **46**, 185–196 (2006).
45. C. Li, E. S. Ford, G. Zhao, L. S. Balluz, W. H. Giles, and S. Liu, "Serum α-carotene concentrations and risk of death among US adults: the Third National Health and Nutrition Examination Survey Follow-up Study," *Arch. Intern. Med.*, **171**, 6, 507–15 (2011).
46. T. Rokkaku, R. Kimura, C. Ishikawa, and T. Yasumoto, "Anticancer effects of marine carotenoids, fucoxanthin and its deacetylated product, fucoxanthinol, on osteosarcoma," *Int. J. Oncol.*, **43**, 4, 1176–86 (2013).

47. B. Brozek-Pluska, J. Musial, R. Kordek, E. Bailo, T. Dieing, and H. Abramczyk, "Raman spectroscopy and imaging: applications in human breast cancer diagnosis," *Analyst*, **137**, 16, 3773–80 (2012).

48. H. Abramczyk, B. Brozek-Pluska, J. Surmacki, J. Jablonska-Gajewicz, and R. Kordek, "Raman 'optical biopsy' of human breast cancer," *Prog. Biophys. Mol. Biol.*, **108**, 1–2, 74–81 (2012).

49. H. Abramczyk, B. Brozek-Pluska, J. Surmacki, J. Jablonska, and R. Kordek, "The label-free Raman imaging of human breast cancer," *J. Mol. Liq.*, **164**, 1–2, 123–31 (2011).

50. T. Grune, G. Lietz, A. Palou, A. C. Ross, W. Stahl, G. Tang, D. Thurnham, S. Yin, and H. K. Biesalski, "Beta-carotene is an important vitamin A source for humans," *J. Nutr.*, **140**, 2268S–85S (2010).

51. World Health Organization, *Indicators for asssessing vitamin A deficiency and their application in monitoring and evaluating intervention programmes* (Geneva, Switzerland, 1996).

52. B. R. Hammond, "Possible role for dietary lutein and zeaxanthin in visual development," *Nutr. Rev.*, **66**, 12, 695–702 (2008).

53. C. E. Lefevre and D. I. Perrett, "Fruit over sunbed: carotenoid skin colouration is found more attractive than melanin colouration," *Q. J. Exp. Psychol. (Hove)*, **68**, 2, 284–93 (2015).

54. M. E. Darvin, W. Sterry, J. Lademann, and T. Vergou, "The role of carotenoids in human skin," *Molecules*, **16**, 12, 10491–506 (2011).

55. M. C. Meinke, A. Friedrich, K. Tscherch, S. F. Haag, M. E. Darvin, H. Vollert, N. Groth, J. Lademann, and S. Rohn, "Influence of dietary carotenoids on radical scavenging capacity of the skin and skin lipids," *Eur. J. Pharm. Biopharm.*, **84**, 2, 365–73 (2013).

56. M. E. Darvin, A. Patzelt, F. Knorr, U. Blume-Peytavi, W. Sterry, and J. Lademann, "One-year study on the variation of carotenoid antioxidant substances in living human skin: influence of dietary supplementation and stress factors," *J. Biomed. Opt.*, **13**, 4, 044028 (2008).

57. S. Petrik, S. Obruča, P. Benešová, and I. Márová, "Bioconversion of spent coffee grounds into carotenoids and other valuable metabolites by selected red yeast strains," *Biochem. Eng. J.*, **90**, 307–15 (2014).

58. D. B. Rodrigues, É. M. M. Flores, J. S. Barin, A. Z. Mercadante, E. Jacob-Lopes, and L. Q. Zepka, "Production of carotenoids from microalgae cultivated using agroindustrial wastes," *Food Res. Int.*, **65**, 144–8 (2014).

59. E. Valduga, A. Valério, H. Treichel, M. Di Luccio, and A. Furigo Júnior, "Study of the bio-production of carotenoids by *Sporidiobolus salmonicolor* (CBS 2636) using pre-treated agro-industrial substrates," *J. Chem. Technol. Biotechnol.*, **83**, 9, 1267–74 (2008).

60. G. J. Gross and S. F. Lockwood, "Cardioprotection and myocardial salvage by a disodium disuccinate astaxanthin derivative (Cardax)," *Life Sci.*, **75**, 2, 215–24 (2004).

61. T. A. Moore, A. L. Moore, and D. Gust, "The design and synthesis of artificial photosynthetic antennas, reaction centres and membranes," *Philos. Trans. R. Soc. Lond. B. Biol. Sci.*, **357**, 1426, 1481–98 (2002).

Part I

Therapy

2

The Role of Antioxidants in Prevention of Premature Skin Aging

Jürgen Lademann, Maxim Evgen'evich Darvin, Fanny Knorr, Sascha Jung, Leonhard Zastrow, and Martina Claudia Meinke

Charité Universitätsmedizin Berlin, Department of Dermatology, Venerology and Allergology, Center of Experimental and Applied Cutaneous Physiology (CCP), Berlin, Germany

2.1 Introduction

Since ancient times, humans have been trying to keep their skin looking youthful. In our time, the desire for a lasting youthful appearance has become even stronger, as youthfulness and beauty are often considered to be prerequisites for professional and personal success. Plastic surgery is on the rise globally. Cosmetic skin care products are constantly gaining in importance to both female and male consumers. Besides the application of cosmetic products, there are simple behavioral patterns such as eating healthy and reducing stressors that may influence the skin's aging process decisively. The role of the antioxidative status in this process, determined by the carotenoid level as indicator substance, is described in the present chapter.

2.2 State of the art

2.2.1 Solar radiation and skin aging

Solar radiation is a basic requirement for the metabolism of the human species [1, 2]. It induces the synthesis of vitamin D [1] in the skin and stimulates the well-being [3]. If skin is exposed to excessive doses of solar radiation, however, the results may be sunburn, photo-aging, immunosuppression, and even skin cancer [4, 5]. Such damage is predominantly due to the formation of free radicals [6–8]. These highly reactive molecules are

Carotenoids: Nutrition, Analysis and Technology, First Edition. Edited by Agnieszka Kaczor and Malgorzata Baranska.

capable of destroying cells and cell compartments as well as elastin and collagen fibers, and preventing their regeneration [9, 10]. Through antioxidants, nature has evolved a defense system against the destructive effects of excess free radicals. Antioxidants are capable of neutralizing the free radicals before they can begin damaging the body [11, 12]. Although solar radiation is a major cause of premature skin aging, genetic determinants also influence the aging process [13].

2.2.2 Carotenoids and the antioxidants of the human skin

Several of the antioxidants in the multilevel defense system cannot be generated by the human body but must be ingested with a diet rich in antioxidant-containing foods, for instance fruit and vegetables [14]. The antioxidants in the human body comprise carotenoids, vitamins, and specific enzymes [15]. Most of the lipophilic antioxidants are excreted with the sweat and the sebum onto the skin surface, where they disperse homogeneously [16, 17]. Subsequently, they penetrate from the skin surface back into the uppermost layer of the stratum corneum, as if they had been applied topically.

As the antioxidants form protective chains, which allow them to regenerate after neutralizing free radicals, the analysis of one main antioxidant substance is sufficient to yield information regarding the antioxidant status as a whole [18–20]. Using electron paramagnetic resonance (EPR) spectroscopy, it could be demonstrated that, for example, carotenoids represent indicator marker substances for the overall antioxidant status of the epidermis [21].

Formerly, carotenoids were detected using high-pressure liquid chromatography (HPLC) or mass spectroscopy (MS) [22]. These invasive techniques required the use of tissue or blood samples. In addition, excised tissue samples could not be analyzed twice. Thus, kinetic investigations had to be severely restricted in the past.

Through resonance Raman spectroscopy and reflectance spectroscopy, the noninvasive detection of dermal carotenoids has become possible [23–25]. Figure 2.1 (Color Supplement) shows a resonance Raman spectrometer and a reflectance spectroscopy-based skin scanner (biozoom®, Agoura Hills, CA, USA). Both systems are suitable for analyzing the kinetics of the carotenoids in human skin [8].

When the newly developed resonance Raman spectrometer was used for the first time at the CCP in order to detect carotenoids selectively and sensitively, it had not been clear which information could be derived from these measurements. Therefore, the staff of the CCP participated in a one-year study, during which their carotenoids were measured before lunch every workday [26]. The respective measurements took only a few minutes. In addition, the volunteers were surveyed for their nutritional behavior and stressors. As a result, it turned out that the antioxidant status can be considered to be a fingerprint of the specific volunteer. Those volunteers who smoked and lived on relatively unhealthy diets exhibited lower carotenoid concentrations, whereas volunteers who had eaten healthy food containing large amounts of fruit and vegetables displayed higher carotenoid values. A typical example of a volunteer's one-year kinetics is depicted in Figure 2.2 [26]. In the summer and autumn, the measured carotenoid concentrations were distinctly higher than in the spring and winter. The measured values were grouped around a mean value. Distinct enhancements as those visible in Figure 2.2 indicate an increased intake of fruit and vegetables. However, in two cases, the antioxidant status dropped during the measurements. Both cases were due to infections of the upper respiratory tract. Although the affected volunteers did not report in sick because of these infections, they involved considerable stress for them. Moreover, another strong decline was noticed on day 120, which had not been related to a disease, but to a summer night party involving much alcohol and lack of sleep.

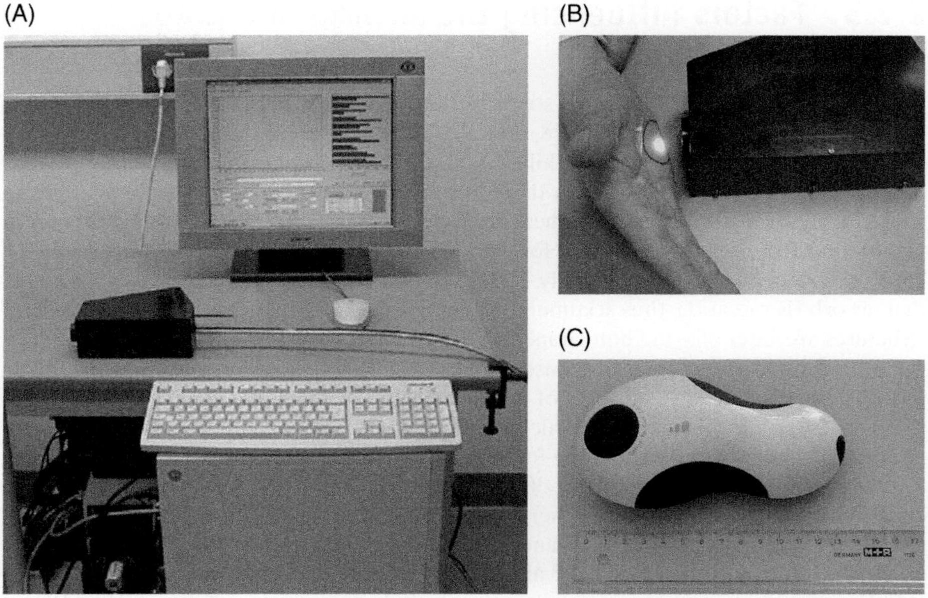

Figure 2.1 (A, B) Raman resonance spectrometer developed at the CCP; and (C) a biozoom® skin scanner based on reflectance spectroscopy for the detection of carotenoids in human skin. (*See insert for color representation of the figure.*)

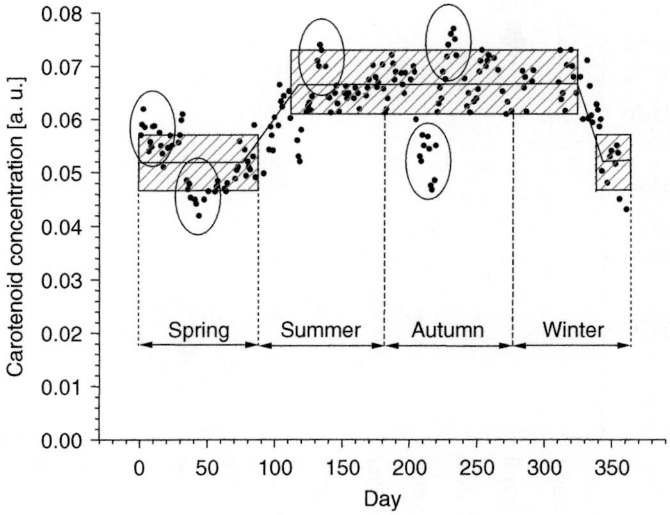

Figure 2.2 Kinetics of carotenoids measured in volunteers over a one-year period on every workday [26]. The encircled values above the mean values correlate with an increased intake of fruit and vegetables as disclosed by the volunteers in the surveys; whereas the lower values encircled around days 40 and 220 correlated with an infection of the upper respiratory tract, and on day 120 with a summer night party involving much alcohol consumption and lack of sleep.

2.2.3 Factors influencing the antioxidant status of the skin

Based on the results of the one-year study, further studies addressed the influence of ultraviolet (UV) [27] and infrared (IR) [18, 19] radiation as well as alcohol consumption [28] on the antioxidant status of the skin. While a depletion of carotenoids due to UV exposure is plausible and has been described in the literature [29–31], the decay of antioxidants as a consequence of IR radiation was rather surprising, as the energy of the IR photons is insufficient for direct radical formation. However, this decay could subsequently be verified by EPR spectroscopy [32]. Consequently, it is assumed that there are structures in human skin that absorb IR radiation, thus accumulating energy and finally inducing free radicals. Such structures are, inter alia, the mitochondria [8, 33].

But the consumption of alcohol also induced free radicals, as shown in Figure 2.3 [28]. In this study, the antioxidant status of the volunteers was measured prior to and at different times after the consumption of alcohol. The volunteers were requested to drink 1 mL of ethanol per kg body weight in the form of vodka or rum containing 40% alcohol within a time period of approximately 15–30 minutes. In Figure 2.3, a strong depletion of the carotenoid concentration can be observed immediately subsequent to the consumption of alcohol [28]. It took up to four days and the intake of a healthy diet for the previous carotenoid level to be restored. Figure 2.3 also shows the points when minimum erythema dose (MED) measurements prior to and after the alcohol intake were performed. The MED is a measure for the UV dose necessary to induce sunburn in the skin. It is clearly shown that volunteers with a disturbed antioxidant protective system are affected by sunburn much more quickly than volunteers whose antioxidant system is intact.

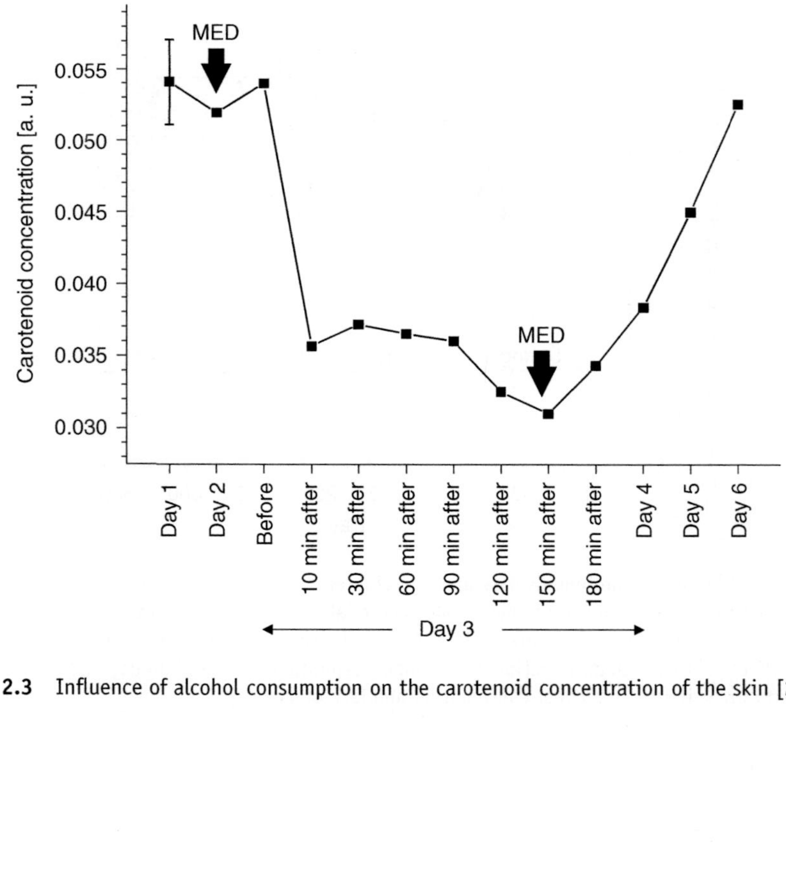

Figure 2.3 Influence of alcohol consumption on the carotenoid concentration of the skin [28].

2.2.4 Antioxidants and sun protection

In the previous paragraph, it was explained that free radicals in the skin can be induced by solar radiation not only in the UV but also in the IR spectral range. In addition, free radicals can also be induced by visible (VIS) light [34]. Sunscreens are designed to protect the human skin against sunburn and damage in the UVB/UVA spectral range, and products with light protection factors beyond 50 are commercially widely available. By using sunscreens, however, people tend to expose themselves to the sun for much longer periods of time than if they did not use sunscreen. Although the sunscreen provides efficient protection in the UV range of the solar spectrum, radical formation in the VIS and IR ranges is enhanced.

Zastrow *et al.* [34] could demonstrate that 50% of the free radicals induced by solar radiation are generated in the UV range, whereas the remaining 50% are formed in the VIS and IR spectral ranges. In the absence of filter substances whose bandwidth would cover the VIS–IR spectra completely, the protective strategy used against UV radiation in sunscreens cannot be transferred to protective measures in the VIS–IR spectral ranges. Therefore, the intrinsic protective mechanisms of the skin must be utilized for these ranges. The first of these mechanisms is hyperkeratosis [35] (i.e., a thickening of the horny layer upon exposure to sunlight radiation). Due to hyperkeratosis, fewer solar photons are able to penetrate into the viable skin layers and can be reflected and scattered more efficiently in the stratum corneum. The second mechanism is tanning [36], which results from an increased melanin production. Melanin is a highly efficient absorber not only in the UV but also in the VIS and IR ranges of the solar spectrum [37]. This means that the solar radiation is reflected and scattered, and fewer photons reach the viable skin. The antioxidants contained in the human skin are the third protective strategy. These antioxidants are capable of neutralizing the free radicals before they become destructive in human tissue. These three protective mechanisms are also contained in some of the modern sunscreens [38]. Pigments, specifically "physical filter" TiO_2, added to the sunscreen formulations ensure that the solar photons are reflected and scattered not only in the UV but also in the VIS and IR spectral ranges for the skin. At the same time, antioxidants that are added to the formulations to stabilize the UV filters have a protective effect in the VIS and IR ranges. In order to investigate this effect, skin areas not treated with sunscreen as well as sunscreens according to COLIPA standard P3 and four commercial sunscreens were tested for their protective efficacy in the IR by EPR spectroscopy. Using this method, spin markers are applied to the skin that are influenced by radical formation in the human skin. This influence can be measured by the EPR system [30]. This study revealed that the untreated skin was affected by the highest radical production subsequent to IR irradiation. The COLIPA standard that contained neither TiO_2 pigments nor antioxidants yielded a result very similar to that of the untreated skin. The sunscreens, however, reduced the radical formation considerably. Although the concentration of antioxidants was not very high in the sunscreen that ranked most effective, it reflected and scattered a high amount of solar photons because it contained a relatively high concentration of TiO_2. Regarding the second-best sunscreen product that differed only slightly from the best one, this sunscreen contained a high concentration of antioxidants, compensating the comparably lower amount of the physical filter TiO_2.

Consequently, there are two mechanisms through which protection in the VIS and IR spectral ranges can be provided. The first mechanism is based on micropigments reflecting and scattering the solar radiation, whereas the second mechanism is based on antioxidants preventing an excess of free radicals before becoming harmful [11]. Meanwhile, the first commercial sunscreens are available that provide protection not only in the UV but also in the VIS and IR spectral ranges, and are declared accordingly.

2.2.5 Antioxidants and skin aging

To date, many volunteers have been investigated with the resonance Raman spectrometer developed at the CCP. As a result, it was found that subjects who exhibited high carotenoid concentrations generally appeared younger looking for their age. This was not observed for the volunteers with low carotenoid concentrations. To objectify this observation, a further study was performed with volunteers aged between 40 and 50 years [39]. These volunteers were measured for their antioxidant status and for photo-aging on the forehead. In this case, photo-aging was determined by the skin roughness index that is based on the density and depth of the furrows and wrinkles. As all volunteers were of a similar age, it can be assumed that their different dermal profiles were due to their individual nutritional and stress behaviorisms. The study involved only volunteers who had not changed their dietary and behavioral manners. A clear correlation was found between the antioxidant status in the skin in the form of lycopene concentration and the skin roughness (Figure 2.4). Volunteers with high lycopene concentrations exhibited considerably less wrinkles than volunteers with lower carotenoid values.

The results of the studies clearly showed that a diet rich in fruit and vegetables is an effective prevention strategy against premature skin aging. Based on these findings, a further study was conducted, this time involving high school students.

2.2.6 Investigations into the antioxidant status of high school students

These investigations were aimed at positively influencing the lifestyles of adolescents, who are still developing their nutritional and behavioral manners, using biofeedback measurements of their antioxidant status. Instead of the resonance Raman system, the easy-to-handle and portable reflectance spectroscopy–based biozoom skin scanner was

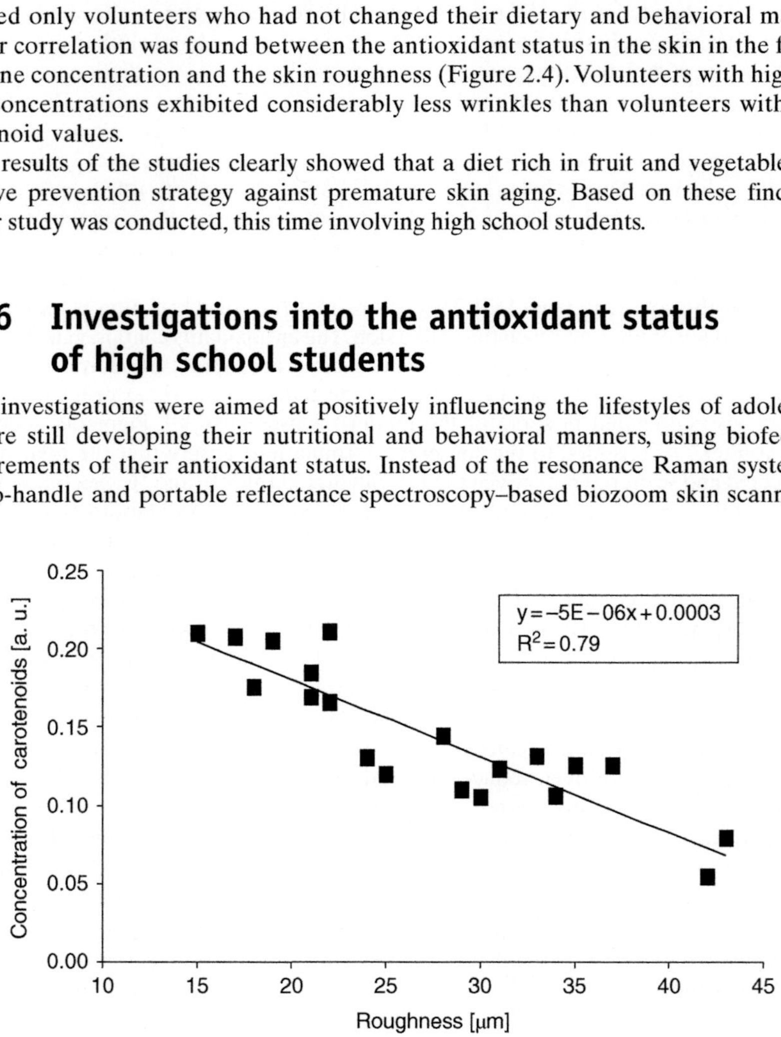

Figure 2.4 Correlation between the antioxidant status of the volunteers in light-exposed skin to skin roughness [39].

used for measuring carotenoids in this study. The measurements were taken over a period of two months. Fifty volunteers were recruited for the study [40].

In month 1, the students were asked not to change their usual lifestyles in terms of nutrition, alcohol consumption, and smoking. They were also requested to keep visiting discotheques and staying up as long as usual. In addition, the students were surveyed regarding their nutritional habits and their stressors. In this phase of the study, the students were not informed of their measuring results.

In month 2, the students were served healthy lunches. In addition, informative courses and lectures were held regarding the positive effects of a healthy nutrition and lifestyle on the antioxidant status and overall health. The students were asked to consume a healthy diet and to avoid stressors to the largest possible extent.

The results of the study showed that the students exhibited relatively high antioxidant values already in month 1. As they were aware of being investigated, they were eager to present themselves in the best light. In phase 2 of the investigations, the initial values were exceeded as the students competed for the highest values. They not only reduced smoking and drinking alcoholic beverages, but also returned home earlier from discotheques. By modifying their lifestyles, the students improved, inter alia, their scholastic performance.

When the students were stressed by preparing for or undergoing exams, their antioxidant status declined [40]. Also, infections of the upper respiratory tract coincided with a reduction of the antioxidant status. On the other hand, the students' high antioxidant values could always be restored by healthy food rich in fruit and vegetables. These results were indeed surprising and gave rise to the question whether the students had changed their habits only for the time of the study or whether they had changed their lifestyles sustainably. Six months after the end of the study, the antioxidant status of the volunteers was therefore determined once more [40], this time without prior notice. It turned out that the students had not only maintained but even slightly improved their measuring values. At the end of the study, the students were asked to briefly summarize their experience from the investigations in writing. Nearly all of the students agreed that they had been reluctant to listen to any advice of their parents or teachers, but would be willing to drastically change their nutritional and behavioral habits now that they have experienced the biofeedback from their own bodies.

2.2.7 Accumulation of antioxidants in human skin by systemic and topical application

In Chapter 1, the importance of antioxidants in the prevention of skin aging was shown, stating that the human body, specifically the skin, can be supplied with antioxidants by healthy food rich in fruit and vegetables. In this context, studies addressing the topical and systemic application of antioxidants were undertaken in which the effects of the verum products were compared to placebo products [41]. Although none of the placebo products induced an increase in the antioxidant status of the volunteer groups, the verum products—both tablets and creams—resulted in a significant enhancement of the carotenoid concentration by almost 100% after eight weeks of application, provided these antioxidants were topically applied as a film or administrated in the form of tablets.

In addition, the combined application of tablets and cream was investigated in this study [41]. The result showed that the simultaneous application of the verum tablets and the verum cream did not result in an antioxidant status that was twice as high as that achieved by the individually applied verum products. The values only slightly exceeded those of the separately applied verum tablets. This was due to the fact that the systemically applied antioxidants are excreted with the sweat and the serum onto the skin surface, where they spread and penetrate back into the skin as when applied topically [41]. If a cream is applied in a nutritious or fatty formulation, the stratum corneum will be saturated by this cream so that the antioxidants being excreted with the sweat and the sebum cannot efficiently penetrate back into the stratum corneum anymore. They remain on the skin surface and will be washed off or removed by textiles such as clothing and desquamation within 24 hours. From these findings, it is evident that the galenics of a verum cream for topical application must be adapted to the specific situation, permitting the cream to penetrate the stratum corneum without saturating it completely. The stratum corneum must still be accessible for antioxidants that are excreted onto the skin surface.

In this context, it must be emphasized that systemically applied food supplements yielded enhanced antioxidant values in the skin for up to six weeks after discontinuance of their ingestion, as the antioxidants taken in systemically are stored in the organism.

When topically applied, the cream was not detectable on the skin surface as early as 24 hours later [41]. Consequently, the combined topical and systemic application of antioxidants was identified as the optimal dosage form. The topical application provides an immediate effect on the skin, although only for approximately 24 hours, and in most cases not on the entire skin surface. By applying antioxidants systemically, the complete skin surface is treated, and long-term protection is thereby induced [41].

Nevertheless, when a cream rich in hyperforin is applied twice daily, after four weeks the radical-scavenging activity was highly enhanced at least 24 hours after the last application. This could be shown using IR irradiation as a stressor [42]. Lower effect could be reached by oral application of curly kale extracts containing carotenoids [22].

When administering antioxidants systemically, it must be considered however that their composition must correlate with the physiological concentrations in the skin. A separate intake of single antioxidants at high concentrations could turn these antioxidants deleterious so that they generate free radicals instead of neutralizing them [14, 20]. This fact will have to be duly considered in future regulatory measures for the production and sale of food supplements.

2.2.8 Ethnic influences on the antioxidant status

The previously described studies revealed that the antioxidant status of the organism, including the skin, is influenced not only by nutritional habits but also by stressors. These findings could be confirmed by another study involving ethnic groups [43]. In this study, the antioxidant statuses of Germans, native Koreans living in South Korea, and volunteers recruited from the Korean community in Berlin were investigated.

The Korean cuisine is deemed to be among the healthiest in the world as it contains a higher amount of vegetables and lower amounts of total fat in comparison to Western or even Japanese and Chinese cuisine [8, 20]. Furthermore, it is based on fermenting (including pickling) or sautéing fruit and vegetables instead of boiling or frying them, thereby preserving larger amounts of antioxidants [8, 20, 27]. It had been hypothesized that the native Korean volunteers would exhibit an antioxidant status that is superior to that of the German volunteers. In this context, it was interesting to elucidate the antioxidant status of the volunteers from the Korean community in Berlin. The aim of the study was to reveal whether their antioxidant status would correlate better with the status of the Korean citizens or with that of the German volunteers.

Contrary to expectations, however, the results obtained from more than 700 volunteers showed only slight differences between the antioxidant values of the German and the native Korean volunteers despite the differences in dietary patterns. Evaluating the surveys, it could be concluded that stress occupies another paradigm in Germany than in Korea [43]. While in Germany the term "stress" is negatively connoted, it linked to high social appreciation in Korea (e.g., in terms of a good family man or diligent employee). Above all, working conditions as well as social and educational environments differ notably from those in Germany. In this study, it could be clearly shown that the positive aspects of the very healthy nutrition on the antioxidant status are compensated by specific stressors.

Interestingly, it turned out from the investigations of the Korean volunteers living in Berlin that immigrant native Koreans exhibited an antioxidant status similar to that of the Korean residents, whereas the antioxidant status of the immigrants' descendants born and raised in Berlin correlated with that of the German volunteers. This can be explained by the mainly Korean dietary pattern of the immigrant Koreans, whereas the younger German-born generations stated to consume more Western food or a mixture of both Korean and Western food.

2.2.9 The antioxidant status in pregnant women and neonates

The investigations regarding the antioxidant status of the skin are interesting not only for cosmetology but also for clinical applications. A further study focused on the antioxidant status of expectant mothers and their newborns [44]. The aim of this study was to find out whether pregnant women with a high antioxidant status would give birth to infants with high antioxidant values and whether the antioxidant status of newborns delivered by women with low antioxidant values would also be low. The pregnant women were investigated in gestational week 39 and at the time they went into labor. In addition, the mothers were measured again for their antioxidant status at days 1 and 5 subsequent to delivery. The results are presented in Figure 2.5. The neonates were measured with the reflectance-based

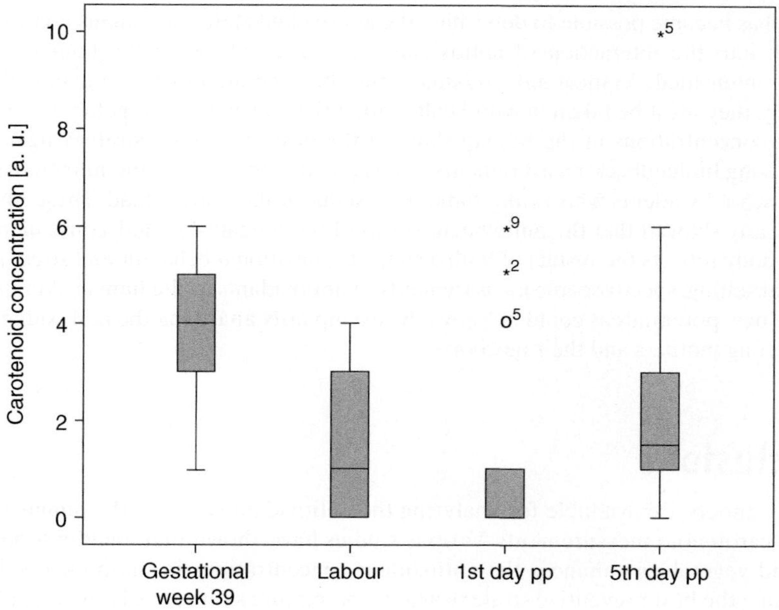

Figure 2.5 Development of the mother's antioxidant potential compared to the value measured in pregnancy week 39 [44].

biozoom hand scanner at the day of birth and at day 5 after birth. As the expectant mothers had ingested antioxidant-containing food supplements during pregnancy, their values were in a normal range.

However, the investigations revealed a distinct decay of the antioxidant status of the expectant mothers from gestational week 39 to the onset of labor [44]. Another slight decline was recorded on day 1 subsequent to delivery, whereas the antioxidant status recovered until day 5 after childbirth. The trend observed for the neonates was vice versa. On the day of birth, their antioxidant status was approximately five times higher than that of their mothers. However, their antioxidant values decayed relatively quickly until day 5 after birth. The results of the study disclosed that the fetuses accumulated as many maternal antioxidants as possible in their bodies in order to be optimally protected against the altered environment in the first hours after birth. As the birth process was highly stressful for the infants, their antioxidant status declined quickly and was compensated only by the intake of breast milk.

Interestingly, it was found that the antioxidant status of mothers who had a normal childbirth declined more strongly than that of mothers who had delivered by caesarean section. Contrary to that, the normally delivered infants exhibited a higher antioxidant status than those delivered by caesarean. It is assumed that a caesarean is in general not performed unless the mother or her infant are directly in danger. Therefore, the stress during birth is higher for infants delivered by a caesarean than for those born naturally.

The study results indicate that in the future, the date of birth could be exactly predictable by measuring the antioxidant status. However, this will require more detailed investigations. A follow-up study to this effect is in the state of preparation.

2.3 Summary

Since it has become possible to determine the antioxidant status in humans noninvasively, research into the interaction of antioxidants and free radicals in the human skin has strongly intensified. As most antioxidants cannot be generated by the human body automatically, they must be taken in with healthy food rich in fruits and vegetables. High antioxidant concentrations in the human skin are the best prevention strategy against skin aging. Using biofeedback measurements, it was possible to improve the nutritional habits of high school students who, at the same time, reduced their stress load. These investigations clearly showed that the antioxidant status of the human skin and, consequently, the human body reflects the results of both a subject's nutritional behavior and stress load. In a clinical setting, spectroscopic measurements of antioxidants in the human skin may also provide new potentials as could be shown by exemplarily analyzing the antioxidant status of expecting mothers and their newborns.

Conclusions

Today, scanners are available for analyzing the antioxidant status of the human skin via dermal carotenoid measurements. Various studies have shown that healthy food rich in fruit and vegetables enhances the antioxidant concentrations in the human skin, thus presenting the best preventive strategy against premature skin aging. However, a healthy lifestyle must be adopted already in adolescence, as it is impossible to regain one's youth by eating a healthy diet in later years. The scanner provides a valuable tool for documenting the consequences of stress for the human body, particularly the skin. Similar to their applicability in nutritional sciences, the scanner measurements will advance the development of new concepts on how to reduce and cope with stress in the human body.

References

1. P. Lips, N. M. van Schoor, and R. T. de Jongh, "Diet, sun, and lifestyle as determinants of vitamin D status," *Ann. NY Acad. Sci.*, **1317**, 92–8 (2014).
2. Y. Gilaberte and J. M. Carrascosa, "Sun protection in children: realities and challenges," *Actas dermo-sifiliograf.*, **105**, 3, 253–62 (2014).
3. S. E. Mancebo, J. Y. Hu, and S. Q. Wang, "Sunscreens: a review of health benefits, regulations, and controversies, *Dermatologic Clin.*, **32**, 3, 427–38, x (2014).
4. A. Perez-Sanchez, E. Barrajon-Catalan, N. Caturla, J. Castillo, O. Benavente-Garcia, M. Alcaraz, *et al.*, "Protective effects of citrus and rosemary extracts on UV-induced damage in skin cell model and human volunteers," *J. Photochem. Photobiol. B, Biol.*, **136**, 12–18 (2014).
5. C. Cole, Y. Appa, and O. Y. Hao, "A broad spectrum high-SPF photostable sunscreen with a high UVA-PF can protect against cellular damage at high UV exposure doses," *Photodermatol. Photo.*, **30**, 4, 212–9 (2014).
6. A. Dhumrongvaraporn and P. Chanvorachote, "Kinetics of ultraviolet B irradiation-mediated reactive oxygen species generation in human keratinocytes," *J. Cosm. Sci.*, **64**, 3, 207–17 (2013).
7. N. Suwannateep, S. Wanichwecharungruang, S. F. Haag, S. Devahastin, N. Groth, J. W. Fluhr, *et al.*, "Encapsulated curcumin results in prolonged curcumin activity in vitro and radical scavenging activity ex vivo on skin after UVB-irradiation," *Euro. J. Pharmaceut. Biopharm.*, **82**, 3, 485–90 (2012).
8. M. J. Lee, B. M. Popkin, and S. Kim, "The unique aspects of the nutrition transition in South Korea: the retention of healthful elements in their traditional diet," *Public Health Nutr.*, **5**, 1A, 197–203 (2002).
9. M. Dalle Carbonare and M. A. Pathak, "Skin photosensitizing agents and the role of reactive oxygen species in photoaging," *J. Photochem. Photobiol. B, Biol.*, **14**, 1–2, 105–24 (1992).
10. H. A. Park, J. S. Lee, S. H. Lee, O. H. Kim, S. W. Oh, and S. K. Lee, "Current status of nutrition transition in South Korea based on the 2005 Korean National Health and Nutrition Survey," *FASEB J.*, **23** (2009).
11. M. C. Meinke, F. Syring, S. Schanzer, S. F. Haag, R. Graf, M. Loch, *et al.*, "Radical protection by differently composed creams in the UV/VIS and IR spectral ranges," *Photochem. Photobiol.*, **89**, 5, 1079–84 (2013).
12. M. C. Meinke, S. Schanzer, S. F. Haag, F. Casetti, M. L. Muller, U. Wolfle, *et al.*, "In vivo photoprotective and anti-inflammatory effect of hyperforin is associated with high antioxidant activity in vitro and ex vivo," *Euro. J. Pharmaceut. Biopharm.*, **81**, 2, 346–50 (2012).
13. P. Elsner, J. W. Fluhr, W. Gehring, M. J. Kerscher, J. Krutmann, J. Lademann, *et al.*, "Anti-aging data and support claims: consensus statement," *J. Deutschen Dermatologischen Gesellschaft*, **9**, S1–S32 (2011).
14. J. Lademann, A. Patzelt, S. Schanzer, H. Richter, M. C. Meinke, W. Sterry, *et al.*, "Uptake of antioxidants by natural nutrition and supplementation: pros and cons from the dermatological point of view," *Skin Pharmacol. Physiol.*, **24**, 5, 269–73 (2011).

15. J. Klein, M. E. Darvin, M. C. Meinke, F. J. Schweigert, K. E. Muller, and J. Lademann, "Analyses of the correlation between dermal and blood carotenoids in female cattle by optical methods," *J. Biomed. Opt.*, **18**, 6 (2013).
16. J. W. Fluhr, P. Caspers, J. A. van der Pol, H. Richter, W. Sterry, J. Lademann, *et al.*, "Kinetics of carotenoid distribution in human skin in vivo after exogenous stress: disinfectant and wIRA-induced carotenoid depletion recovers from outside to inside," *J Biomed Opt.*, **16**, 3, 035002 (2011).
17. S. Ekanayake-Mudiyanselage, A. Tavakkol, T. G. Polefka, Z. Nabi, P. Elsner, and J. J. Thiele, "Vitamin E delivery to human skin by a rinse-off product: penetration of alpha-tocopherol versus wash-out effects of skin surface lipids," *Skin Pharmacol. Physiol.*, **18**, 1, 20–6 (2005).
18. M. E. Darvin, S. Haag, M. Meinke, L. Zastrow, W. Sterry, and J. Lademann, "Radical production by infrared A irradiation in human tissue," *Skin Pharmacol. Physiol.*, **23**, 1, 40–6 (2010).
19. S. Kim and B. M. Popkin, "Salt consumption during the nutrition transition in South Korea: reply to H Kesteloot and J Zhang," *Am. J. Clin. Nutr.*, **72**, 1, 200–1 (2000).
20. S. Kim, S. Moon, and B. M. Popkin, "The nutrition transition in South Korea," *Am. J. Clin. Nutr.*, **71**, 1, 44–53 (2000).
21. S. F. Haag, B. Taskoparan, M. E. Darvin, N. Groth, J. Lademann, W. Sterry, *et al.*, "Determination of the antioxidative capacity of the skin in vivo using resonance Raman and electron paramagnetic resonance spectroscopy," *Exp Dermatol.*, **20**, 6, 483–7 (2011).
22. D. Talwar, T. K. Ha, J. Cooney, C. Brownlee, and D. S. O'Reilly, "A routine method for the simultaneous measurement of retinol, alpha-tocopherol and five carotenoids in human plasma by reverse phase HPLC," *Clinica Chimica Acta*, **270**, 2, 85–100 (1998).
23. M. E. Darvin, W. Sterry, and J. Lademann, "Resonance Raman spectroscopy as an effective tool for the determination of antioxidative stability of cosmetic formulations," *J. Biophotonics*, **3**, 1–2, 82–8 (2010).
24. I. V. Ermakov, M. R. Ermakova, W. Gellermann, and J. Lademann, "Noninvasive selective detection of lycopene and beta-carotene in human skin using Raman spectroscopy," *J. Biomed. Opt.*, **9**, 2, 332–8 (2004).
25. M. Darwin, S. Schanzer, A. Teichmann, U. Blume-Peytavi, W. Sterry, and J. Lademann, "Functional food and bioavailability in the target organ skin," *Hautarzt*, **57**, 4, 286 (2006).
26. M. E. Darvin, A. Patzelt, F. Knorr, U. Blume-Peytavi, W. Sterry, and J. Lademann, "One-year study on the variation of carotenoid antioxidant substances in living human skin: influence of dietary supplementation and stress factors," *J. Biomed. Opt.*, **13**, 4, 044028 (2008).
27. H. Kesteloot and J. J. Zhang, "Salt consumption during the nutrition transition in South Korea," *Am. J. Clin. Nutr.*, **72**, 1, 199–200 (2000).
28. M. E. Darvin, W. Sterry, J. Lademann, and A. Patzelt, "Alcohol consumption decreases the protection efficiency of the antioxidant network and increases the risk of sunburn in human skin," *Skin Pharmacol. Physiol.*, **26**, 1, 45–51 (2013).
29. C. Kohlhardt-Floehr, F. Boehm, S. Troppens, and J. Lademann, and T. G. Truscott, "Prooxidant and antioxidant behaviour of usnic acid from lichens under UVB-light irradiation: studies on human cells," *J. Photochem. Photobiol. B, Biol.*, **101**, 1, 97–102 (2010).
30. M. C. Meinke, S. F. Haag, S. Schanzer, N. Groth, I. Gersonde, and J. Lademann, "Radical protection by sunscreens in the infrared spectral range," *Photochem. Photobiol.*, **87**, 2, 452–6 (2011).
31. V. T. Natarajan, P. Ganju, A. Ramkumar, R. Grover, and R. S. Gokhale, "Multifaceted pathways protect human skin from UV radiation," *Nature Chem. Biol.*, **10**, 7, 542–51 (2014).
32. M. E. Darvin, S. F. Haag, M. C. Meinke, W. Sterry, and J. Lademann, "Determination of the influence of IR radiation on the antioxidative network of the human skin," *J. Biophoton.*, **4**, 1–2, 21–9 (2011).

33. P. Schroeder, J. Lademann, M. E. Darvin, H. Stege, C. Marks, S. Bruhnke, *et al.*, "Infrared radiation-induced matrix metalloproteinase in human skin: implications for protection," *J. Invest. Dermatol.*, **128**, 10, 2491–7 (2008).

34. L. Zastrow, N. Groth, F. Klein, D. Kockott, J. Lademann, R. Renneberg, *et al.*, "The missing link: light-induced (280–1,600 nm) free radical formation in human skin," *Skin Pharmacol. Physiol.*, **22**, 1, 31–44 (2009).

35. H. S. Cho, M. H. Lee, J. W. Lee, K. O. No, S. K. Park, H. S. Lee, *et al.*, "Anti-wrinkling effects of the mixture of vitamin C, vitamin E, pycnogenol and evening primrose oil, and molecular mechanisms on hairless mouse skin caused by chronic ultraviolet B irradiation," *Photodermatol. Photo.*, **23**, 5, 155–62 (2007).

36. K. Jung, M. Seifert, T. Herrling, and J. Fuchs, "UV-generated free radicals (FR) in skin: their prevention by sunscreens and their induction by self-tanning agents," *Spectrochim Acta A*, **69**, 5, 1423–8 (2008).

37. Y. G. Hu, Y. H. Shen, Z. Zhang, and G. Q. Shi, "Melanin and urate act to prevent ultraviolet damage in the integument of the silkworm," *Bombyx Mori. Arch Insect Biochem.*, **83**, 1, 41–55 (2013).

38. M. C. Meinke, S. F. Haag, S. Schanzer, N. Groth, I. Gersonde, J. Lademann, "Radical protection by sunscreens in the infrared spectral range," *Photochem. Photobiol.*, **87**, 2, 452–6 (2011).

39. M. Darvin, A. Patzelt, S. Gehse, S. Schanzer, C. Benderoth, W. Sterry, *et al.*, "Cutaneous concentration of lycopene correlates significantly with the roughness of the skin," *Euro. J. Pharmaceut. Biopharm.*, **69**, 3, 943–7 (2008).

40. R.-X. Yu, W. Köcher, M. E. Darvin, M. Büttner, S. Jung, B. N. Lee, *et al.*, "Spectroscopic biofeedback on cutaneous carotenoids as part of a prevention program could be effective to raise health awareness in adolescents," *J. Biophotonics*, **7**, 11–12, 926–37 (2013).

41. M. E. Darvin, J. W. Fluhr, S. Schanzer, H. Richter, A. Patzelt, M. C. Meinke, *et al.*, "Dermal carotenoid level and kinetics after topical and systemic administration of antioxidants: enrichment strategies in a controlled in vivo study," *J Dermatol Sci.*, **64**, 1, 53–8 (2011).

42. M. S. Lee, M. K. Woo, C. S. Kwak, S. I. Oh, and S. C. Park, "Analysis of traditional Korean food patterns according to the healthy longevity diet based on the database of favorite Korean foods," *Healthy Aging Funct. Longevity*, **928**, 348 (2001).

43. S. Jung, M. E. Darvin, H. S. Chung, B. Jung, S. H. Lee, K. Lenz, *et al.,* "Antioxidants in Asian-Korean and Caucasian skin: the influence of nutrition and stress," *Skin Pharmacol. Physiol.*, **27**, 6, 293–302 (2014).

44. H. G. B. Lademann, D. M. Olbertz, M. E. Darvin, L. Stauf, K. Ueberholz, V. Heinrich, J. Lademann, and V. Briese, "Non-invasive spectroscopic determination of the antioxidative status of gravidae and neonates," *Skin Pharmacol. Physiol.*, **28**, 189–95 (2015).

3

Antitumor Activity of Dietary Carotenoids, and Prospects for Applications in Therapy: Carotenoids and Cancer by Raman Imaging

Halina Abramczyk and Jakub Surmacki

Lodz University of Technology, Institute of Applied Radiation Chemistry, Laboratory of Laser Molecular Spectroscopy, Lodz, Poland

Carotenoids are the pigments that are contained in fruits and vegetables such as mango, pumpkin, apricots, watermelon, carrots, tomatoes, sweet potato, and broccoli. Their vibrant orange, yellow, and green colors are related to unusually high extinction coefficients in the visible (VIS) spectral region. Chemically, carotenoids are classified as belonging to a class of tetraterpenes, and more than 600 natural structures of various size, shape, and polarity have been identified [1].

β-carotene, lycopene, and lutein are all different varieties of carotenoids. Although the full range of biological effects of carotenoids is still unknown, there is more and more evidence that carotenoids play important roles in many biological processes such as anti-oxidative defense, cell-to-cell communication, providing a source of vitamin A, harvesting light for photosynthesis, affecting human health, and preventing disease [1–9].

In contrast to plants, fungi, bacteria, and algae, carotenoids are not synthesized in animals and humans and must be incorporated from their diet. There have been many attempts to uncover the relationships among a carotenoid-rich diet and cancer [2, 5, 10–18].

Carotenoids: Nutrition, Analysis and Technology, First Edition. Edited by Agnieszka Kaczor and Malgorzata Baranska.

Many articles give overviews of the current state of knowledge regarding the cancer-preventing potential of carotenoids [3, 19, 20]. Numerous retrospective and prospective epidemiological studies have shown that a high intake of carotenoids-rich fruits and vegetables is associated with a decreased risk of cancer for a number of pathologies, such as lung, breast, and prostate cancers [8, 21–27].

Mechanisms by which certain carotenoids suppress carcinogenesis are being pieced together bit by bit [1–5, 28]: antioxidative effects, anti-inflammation, immune modulation, induction of cell differentiation, apoptosis induction, antiproliferation, modulation of the nuclear receptor superfamily, enhancement of gap junction communication, and modulation of growth factor and Wnt/β-catenin signaling (Figure 3.1).

Controversial data are reported about the location and distribution of carotenoids in human cells and tissues [1]. Because carotenoids are highly hydrophobic, they are expected to be distributed in lipophilic environments. Analytical obstacles and improvements of analytical instruments to perform the structural elucidation and determine concentrations of carotenoids in cells and tissues are discussed in Ref. [29].

With the exploitation of new technologies such as Raman imaging, the promise of label-free, minimally invasive molecular detection and characterization has driven the field to results unimaginable just a few years ago, and the pace of progress should increase significantly.

Although the difficulty lies in the number and complexity of the biological components in cells and tissues, Raman spectroscopy is a feasible and valid method for noninvasively assessing carotenoids as a biomarker for studies of nutrition, health, disease development, and therapy response.

One of the main advantages of Raman imaging is that it can give spatial information about various chemical constituents in defined cellular compartments, in contrast to other

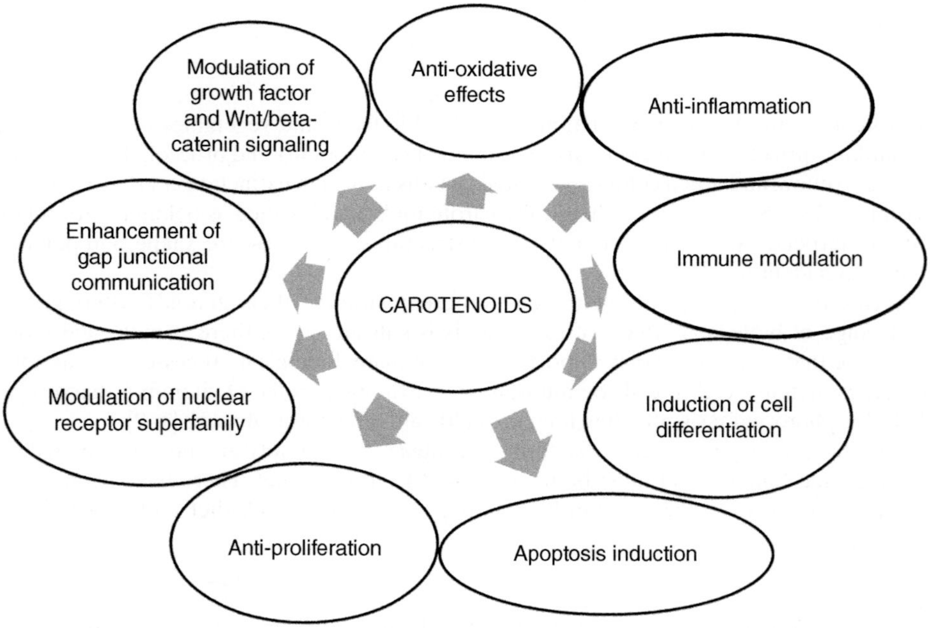

Figure 3.1 Proposed mechanisms by which certain carotenoids suppress carcinogenesis [1–7].

methods (e.g., liquid chromatography–mass spectrometry [LC/MS], nuclear magnetic resonance [NMR], and high-performance LC [HPLC]) that must rely on bulk or fractionated analyses of extracted components.

We will demonstrate how strategies proposed in our laboratory can help in providing a complete and accurate picture of the important biological effects of carotenoids and to uncover the relationships among carotenoids and cancer.

3.1 Results

At the tissue level, a major goal has been the identification and quantification of chemical differences between cancerous and normal tissue. Several groups have successfully demonstrated their ability to analyze human breast cancerous tissues by Raman spectroscopy [30–41].

The results demonstrated negligible contributions of carotenoids in both normal and cancerous breast tissues [30]. The conclusions have been verified by Abramczyk's group [33–41], who showed that carotenoids are the main Raman biomarkers discriminating between normal, benign, and malignant breast tissues.

In this section, we will show the distribution of carotenoids in human breast tissue *ex vivo* [33–42]. We will compare the distribution of carotenoids in the tissue from the safety margin and cancerous human breast tissue from the tumor mass. The assessment of the safety margin of breast cancer is very important in clinical practice during partial mastectomy as a surgical guidance tool. When a tumor is removed, some surrounding tissue is also removed. The safety margin, also known as "margins of resection," is an area within the distance between a tumor and the edge of the surrounding tissue that is removed along with it in the surgery. A pathologist checks the tissue under a microscope to see if the margins are free of cancer cells. Depending upon what the pathologist sees, the margins of a tumor can be classified as:

- *Positive margins*: Cancer cells extend out to the edge of the tissue.
- *Negative margins*: No cancer cells are found.
- *Close margins*: Any situation that falls between positive and negative is considered "close."

Figure 3.2 (Color Supplement) shows the typical Raman and infrared (IR) spectra of the breast tissue surrounding the tumor from the safety margin and the cancerous breast tissue (infiltrating ductal cancer) from the tumor mass of the same patient.

The results presented in Figure 3.2 provide evidence that the Raman spectra and images are very sensitive indicators that allow one to specify the pathology in the human breast tissue.

The most sensitive indicators of cancer can be seen in the following regions:

- The O–H stretching modes of water at around 3200–3500 cm^{-1}
- The C–C coupled with C–CH_3 and C=C stretching mode of carotenoids at 1004 cm^{-1}, 1158 cm^{-1}, and 1518 cm^{-1}
- The vibrational modes of the alkyl chains of lipids (triglycerides and fatty acids): CH_2 symmetric stretching mode at 2854 cm^{-1}, CH_2 asymmetric stretching modes at 2888 cm^{-1} and 2926 cm^{-1}, and (C=C)-C-H asymmetric stretching mode at 3009 cm^{-1}
- The vibrational stretching mode of proteins at around 2940 cm^{-1} [36–38].

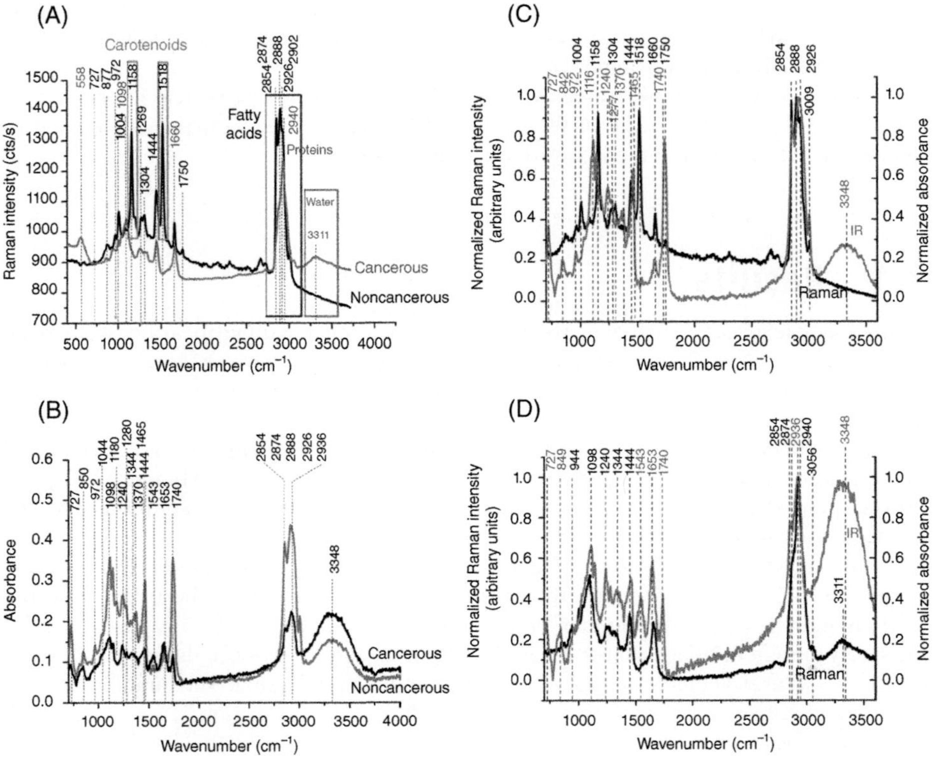

Figure 3.2 The average Raman and infrared (IR) spectra for the noncancerous and cancerous breast tissues (infiltrating ductal carcinoma). (A) Raman spectra of patient P81; (B) IR spectra of patient P83; (C) Raman spectrum for the noncancerous normal breast tissues of patient P81, and IR spectrum for the noncancerous normal breast tissues of patient P83; and (D) Raman spectrum for the cancerous breast tissues of patient P81, and IR spectrum for the cancerous breast tissues of patient P83. Figure reprinted upon Creative Commons Attribution License (http://creativecommons.org/licenses/by/2.0) from Ref. [37]. (*See insert for color representation of the figure.*)

Comparison in Figure 3.2A shows that the normal breast tissue from the safety margin surrounding the tumor contains a markedly higher concentration of carotenoids and monounsaturated triglycerides and fatty acids as compared to the cancerous tissue from the tumor mass.

We have demonstrated (Figure 3.2B) that the Raman method has a markedly higher specificity than IR that allow one to distinguishing between the normal and cancerous breast tissues, thus having the potential to be a better diagnostic tool in breast cancer pathology. Indeed, a detailed inspection into Figure 3.2C demonstrates that the vibrations originating from carotenoids at 1158 cm^{-1} and 1518 cm^{-1}, which are the strongest signals in the Raman spectrum, are not visible in the IR spectrum. The reason is quite obvious, and that is because the excitation with 514 nm (or 532 nm) leads to the resonance Raman enhancement of carotenoids, which is not present in IR measurements.

Raman spectroscopy coupled with various multivariate data analysis techniques allow researchers to quantify chemical differences between normal and diseased tissues. Although identifying human breast cancerous tissue with greater than 90% sensitivity and specificity, our work also quantitatively revealed that normal breast tissue showed higher carotenoids and monounsaturated triglycerides and fatty acids content, whereas tumor tissue had higher protein and nucleic acid content.

Raman and IR imaging has brought a revolution in cancer detection and treatment. These methods are ideally suited to explore the cancer phenotype by monitoring the biochemistry of molecules that are necessary for survival, proliferation, differentiation, cell death, and expression of many cell-type-specific functions [36–39, 43–45].

One step further, Raman imaging could also be used to quantitatively discriminate between distribution of the biochemical components in the epithelial cells of ducts and the extracellular matrix of breast tissue.

Figure 3.3 (Color Supplement) shows the microscopy images, Raman images, and typical Raman spectra of the breast tissue surrounding the tumor from the safety margin and the cancerous breast tissue (infiltrating ductal cancer) from the tumor mass of the same patient.

One can see that the Raman images in Figure 3.3 reveal an inhomogeneous distribution of different compounds in the samples and resemble the microscopy images as well as conventional histological images (not shown here) obtained from thin sections stained with specific dyes (e.g., hematoxylin and eosin [H&E]). Quantitative Raman identification of tissue will surely improve clinical diagnosis of cancer and reduce the number of false-positive diagnoses of patients.

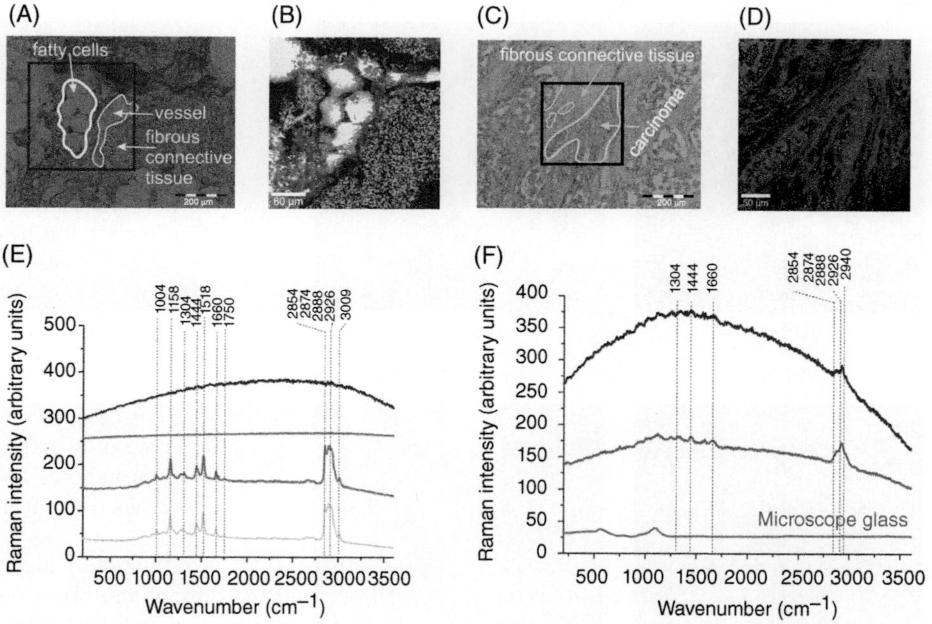

Figure 3.3 Raman image and spectra of the noncancerous and cancerous breast tissue of patient P81. Noncancerous breast tissue: (A) Microscope image (B) Raman image (400 × 400 μm) from the region marked in (A); and (C) Raman spectra (integration time: 0.05 s). Cancerous breast tissue: (D) Microscope image, (E) Raman image (300 × 300 μm) from the region marked in (D), and (F) Raman spectra (integration time: 0.036 s). The colors of the spectra correspond to the colors in the image. Mixed areas are displayed as mixed colors. Figure reprinted upon Creative Commons Attribution License (http://creativecommons.org/licenses/by/2.0) from Ref. [37]. (*See insert for color representation of the figure.*)

Figure 3.4 (Color Supplement) shows the Raman images for the noncancerous (Figure 3.4A) and cancerous (Figure 3.4B) breast tissue for the filters at 1518 cm^{-1}, 2854 cm^{-1}, 2930 cm^{-1}, and 1800 cm^{-1}, corresponding to the vibrational frequency of carotenoids, monounsaturated fatty acids, proteins, and autofluorescence, respectively. A detailed inspection into Figure 3.4 demonstrates that the noncancerous areas in the breast tissue safety margin surrounding the tumor (Figure 3.4A) contain a markedly higher concentration of carotenoids than the cancerous tissue from the tumor mass (Figure 3.4B). One can see that, for the noncancerous tissue, the Raman image at the 1518 cm^{-1} filter (Figure 3.4A) illustrating the distributions of carotenoids is almost identical as that for the 2854 cm^{-1} filter for monounsaturated fatty acids and triglycerides. It clearly indicates that the monounsaturated fatty acids and triglycerides of the adipose tissue act as a dynamic reservoir that supplies carotenoids to the human organs. In contrast, the cancerous breast tissue does not contain any carotenoids, as demonstrated by Figure 3.4B at the 1518 cm^{-1} filter [38].

Of particular interest is the recent demonstration that lipid composition of cytoplasmic lipid droplets in the human breast epithelial cells and in large adipocytes of the breast tissue is different. We have shown that the adipocytes in the cancerous breast tissue are dominated by triglycerides of oleic and linoleic acid [36, 37]. By contrast, nonadipocyte lipid droplets in the cancerous epithelial cells contain triglycerides and fatty acids

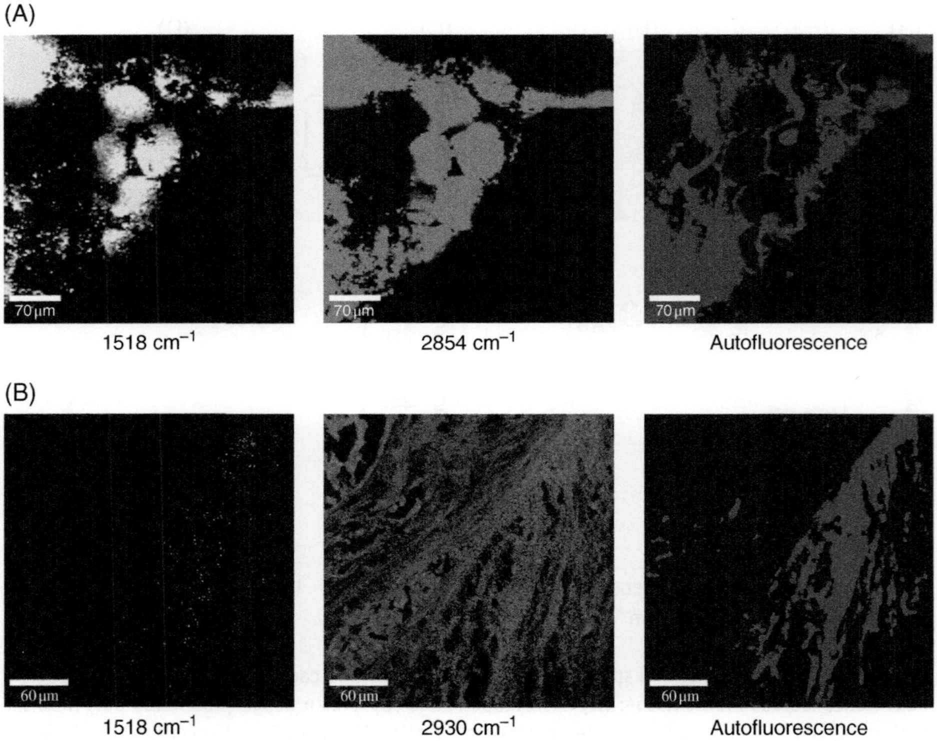

Figure 3.4 Raman images: (A) noncancerous and (B) cancerous breast tissue of patient P81. Filters: carotenoids (1518 cm^{-1}), monounsaturated fatty acids (2854 cm^{-1}), proteins (2930 cm^{-1}), and autofluorescence (1800 cm^{-1}). Figure reprinted upon Creative Commons Attribution License (http://creativecommons.org/licenses/by/2.0) from Ref. [37]. (*See insert for color representation of the figure.*)

dominated by saturated and polyunsaturated fatty acids with a profile typical for arachidonic acid derivatives [38]. It suggests that the lipid droplet synthesis and growth are stimulated by different pathways compared to the adipocytes, thereby affecting the functions of these cells. For example, carotenoids are selectively absorbed by large adipocytes consisting of monounsaturated triglycerides in contrast to the epithelial lipid droplets dominated by saturated and polyunsaturated derivatives. Both profiles represent a lipophilic environment, and highly hydrophobic carotenoids should be expected to be similarly distributed in both environments in contrast to the experimental results that we have obtained recently by Raman imaging [36–38].

Different chemical composition of lipids and distinct distribution of carotenoids suggest that the large adipocytes in the breast tissue play different roles than the lipid droplets in the epithelial breast cells. To answer this fundamental question, let us concentrate on the possible mechanisms. The major role of white adipocytes in the breast tissue is related to storing energy supply. However, our recent results showed that they also serve as a reservoir of anti–reactive oxygen species (ROS) (particularly carotenoids), which may play a protective role against cancer by increasing the resistance of cells to oxidative stress [36, 38, 39]. By contrast, nonadipocyte lipid droplets in the cancerous epithelial cells contain saturated/polyunsaturated triglycerides and fatty acids dominated by an arachidonic acid profile and a lack of carotenoids.

Our results show evidence that lipid droplets in the breast epithelial cells and breast adipocytes differ not only in size but also in biochemical composition. It indicates these lipid bodies must play different roles in cancer pathology. The mechanisms leading to the differences in adipose and lipid droplet composition are unclear, but they are likely to be important for understanding the role of lipid droplets in cancer development.

Recent reviews [46] emphasize the role of lipid synthesis in cancer metabolism and tumor development. Although fatty acid (FA) and cholesterol biosynthesis occurs mainly in liver, adipose, and lactating breast tissues, enhanced *de novo* lipid biosynthesis is also observed in cancerous tissue because it is required for the rapid proliferation of cancer cells. It has been reported that the shift from lipid uptake to *de novo* synthesis in cancer cells leads to increased membrane lipid saturation, resulting in higher levels of saturated and monounsaturated phospholipids, potentially protecting cancer cells from oxidative damage by reducing lipid peroxidation [47].

Increased levels of saturated FAs are found in aggressive breast cancers, suggesting that reduced membrane fluidity is a feature of the advanced disease [48]. Furthermore, depletion of sterol regulatory element-binding transcription factor 1 (SREBP1) and 2 (SREBP2) diminishes levels of monounsaturated FAs, resulting in mitochondrial dysfunction, the accumulation of ROS, and endoplasmic reticulum (ER) stress in immortalized human epithelial cells [49].

The lipid-anti-ROS phenotype was ignored for many years by the Raman scientific community, which has focused almost exclusively on the proteome profile in Raman and IR spectra [50–53]. Substantial progress in understanding the molecular events that may contribute to cancer development made clear that the exclusive proteome approach is not fully justified as there are many signaling pathways and metabolic alterations that are responsible for tumorigenesis. Recent papers suggest that phenotypic heterogeneity in the majority of human cancers represents both genetic and nongenetic inputs [54].

The complexity of cancer cell genotypes provokes a question of whether searching for individual signaling molecules is useful, because thousands of mutations, translocations, and amplifications have been monitored, even among histopathologically identical tumors. However, some of these channels are absolutely required for tumorigenic transformation: (1) rapid adenosine triphosphate (ATP) generation to maintain energy status, (2) increased biosynthesis of macromolecules, and (3) maintenance of appropriate cellular redox status [55]. The link between cancer and the altered metabolism is usually described through the first channel via glycolysis (glycolytic phenotype), known as the Warburg effect, which replaces ATP generation through oxidative phosphorylation by ATP generation through glycolysis, even under normal oxygen concentrations [56]. There is more and more evidence [36, 38, 39, 43, 44, 55, 57] that metabolic alterations in tumors extend beyond the Warburg effect, and pathways (2) and (3) are equally important, particularly those that are crucial for macromolecular building blocks such as reduced nicotinamide adenine dinucleotide phosphate (NADPH), which is also an antioxidant forming the defense against ROS. These paths are also associated with the production of fatty acids and are activated via multiple lipogenic enzymes affected at all levels of regulation, including transcription, translation, protein stabilization, and protein phosphorylation [48, 58].

Our study of human breast cancer showed that noncancerous tissues have increased β-carotene concentration compared to cancerous tissues. The beneficial effects of carotenoids are thought to be due to their role as antioxidants. The chain-breaking antioxidant activity of carotenoids (e.g., β-carotene) is very important in cancer etiology. The interaction of carotenoids with free radicals and singlet oxygen can inhibit the lipid peroxidation processes by quenching or inactivation of the oxidants. The efficacy of carotenoids for physical quenching is related to the number of conjugated double bonds presented in the molecule.

3.2 Conclusions

We have shown that Raman medical diagnostics demonstrate fascinating properties, providing applications that may overturn conventional boundaries in medical imaging in the near future. Thus, it is only a matter of time until the first *in vivo* imaging of live breast tissue will be demonstrated in clinical practice. One of the most important challenges of Raman medical diagnostics is identification and characterization of cancerous and noncancerous human tissues and distribution of the essential constituents of cells.

In this chapter, we present results on the endogenous Raman label-free reporters in human breast tissue that can be useful in clinical practice. The results provide evidence that distribution and composition of carotenoids and lipids in cancerous breast tissue from the tumor mass differ significantly from that of the noncancerous breast tissue and may represent key factors responsible for the mechanisms of carcinogenesis. We have found that fatty acid derivatives composition in the cancerous breast tissue from the tumor mass is markedly different from that of the surrounding breast tissue from the safety margin. The results are of potential importance in clinical assessments, because knowing the removed tissue's type of margin helps in making the right treatment decisions. This is especially important in deciding whether additional surgery is needed. If the margins are negative, one probably does not need more surgery. If the margins are positive, more surgery is needed.

3.3 Perspectives

Cancer diagnosis requires better screening of early stages of pathology and monitoring patient responses to treatment. Current technologies in the clinical sector based on polymerase chain reaction (PCR) amplification or immunofluorescence staining are expensive, sophisticated, and time-consuming. In this chapter, we propose a powerful alternative, double-modality Raman–IR spectroscopy and imaging, which may bring a revolution in cancer detection and treatment. The approach is ideally suited to explore cancer phenotypes by monitoring the biochemistry and morphology of cells necessary for survival, proliferation, differentiation, cell death, and expression of many specific functions. Raman–IR imaging will provide unique insight into vibrational features of cell tissue and intracellular processes in normal and cancerous human tissues as well as localization of chemotherapy drugs and photosensitizers. This goal will be achieved by unsurpassed spatial resolution (nanometers), sensitivity (10^{-15} M), and specificity offered by the double-modality approach. Vibrational signatures will be broadly used to identify and discriminate structures in normal and cancerous tissues. Carotenoids are examples of compounds that have a significant contribution to the observed differences in the spectral profile of cancerous and noncancerous tissues, and the lack of carotenoids can be considered as one of the features confirming the malignant status of the tissue.

It has been demonstrated that our approach has reached a clinically relevant level in regard to cancer diagnosis. Raman–IR imaging will provide an innovative biodiagnostic platform for ultrasensitive, fast, noninvasive, objective cancer diagnosis, therapy monitoring, and imaging based on Raman biomarkers that allows for guidance of intraoperative tumor resection in real surgery time, and is capable of accurately delineating tumor margins (optical biopsy). At the moment, no systems can monitor *in vivo* the biochemical status of the cell in real time with high spatial resolution.

The proposed approach has interdisciplinary character and combines the fields that have already been preserved for physical scientists and, on the other side, for molecular biologists and clinicians. The major limitation in such an interdisciplinary profile of the project is that the physical background is needed to evaluate the technical part of the project and, on the other side, the life science and clinical communities are capable of evaluating its impact on cancer biodiagnostics.

References

1. H. Tapiero, D. M. Townsend, and K. D. Tew, "The role of carotenoids in the prevention of human pathologies," *Biomed. Pharmacother.*, **58**, 2, 100–10 (2004).
2. J. S. Bertram and A. L. Vine, "Cancer prevention by retinoids and carotenoids: independent action on a common target," *Biochimica Biophysica Acta*, **1740**, 2, 170–8 (2005).
3. T. Tanaka, M. Shnimizu, and H. Moriwaki, "Cancer chemoprevention by carotenoids," *Molecules*, **17**, 3, 3202–42 (2012).
4. R. Elliott, "Mechanisms of genomic and non-genomic actions of carotenoids," *Biochimica Biophysica Acta*, **1740**, 2, 147–54 (2005).
5. N. I. Krinsky and E. J. Johnson, "Carotenoid actions and their relation to health and disease," *Mol. Aspects Med.*, **26**, 6, 459–516 (2005).
6. H. Nishino, "Cancer prevention by carotenoids," *Mutation Res.*, **402**, 1, 159–63 (1998).
7. S. Veronica and M. Jisaka, "Lipoxygenase and carotenoids: a co-oxidation story," *African J. Biotechnol.*, **12**, 20, 2786–91 (2013).
8. E. Giovannucci, "Lycopene and prostate cancer risk: methodological considerations in the epidemiologic literature," *Pure Appl. Chem.*, **74**, 8, 1427–34 (2002).
9. T. D. Shultz, B. P. Chew, W. R. Seaman, *et al.*, "Inhibitory effect of conjugated dienoic derivatives of linoleic acid and β-carotene on the in vitro growth of human cancer cells," *Cancer Lett.*, **63**, 2, 125–33 (1992).

10. S. T. Mayne, B. Cartmel, S. Scarmo, *et al.*, "Noninvasive assessment of dermal carotenoids as a biomarker of fruit and vegetable intake," *Amer. J. Clin. Nutr.*, **92**, 4, 794–800 (2010).
11. E. R. Monsen, "Dietary reference intakes for the antioxidant nutrients: vitamin C, vitamin E, selenium, and carotenoids," *J. Amer. Dietetic Assoc.*, **100**, 6, 637–40 (2000).
12. Y. M. Peng, Y. S. Peng, Y. Lin, *et al.*, "Concentrations and plasma-tissue-diet relationships of carotenoids, retinoids, and tocopherols in humans," *Nutrition Cancer*, **23**, 3, 233–46 (1995).
13. A. J. McEligot, C. L. Rock, S. W. Flatt, *et al.*, "Plasma carotenoids are biomarkers of long-term high vegetable intake in women with breast cancer," *J. Nutrition*, **129**, 12, 2258–63 (1999).
14. E. Lanza, A. Schatzkin, C. Daston, *et al.*, "Implementation of a 4-y, high-fiber, high-fruit-and-vegetable, low-fat dietary intervention: results of dietary changes in the Polyp Prevention Trial," *Amer. J. Clin. Nutr.*, **74**, 3, 387–401 (2001).
15. M. Marmot, T. Atinmo, T. Byers, *et al.*, *Food, nutrition, physical activity, and the prevention of cancer: a global perspective*, Washington, DC: World Cancer Research Fund, American Institution for Cancer Research, 2007.
16. S. Liu, J. E. Manson, I. M. Lee, *et al.*, "Fruit and vegetable intake and risk of cardiovascular disease: the Women's Health Study," *Amer. J. Clin. Nutr.*, **72**, 4, 922–8 (2000).
17. A. R. Kristal, A. R. Peters, and J. D. Potter, "Is it time to abandon the food frequency questionnaire?" *Cancer Epidemiol. Biomarkers Prevent.*, **14**, 12, 2826–8 (2005).
18. A. L. Ray, R. D. Semba, J. Walston, *et al.*, "Low serum selenium and total carotenoids predict mortality among older women living in the community: the women's health and aging studies," *J. Nutr.*, **136**, 1, 172–6 (2006).
19. G. van Poppel and H. van den Berg, "Vitamins and cancer," *Cancer Lett.*, **114**, 1, 195–202.
20. G. van Poppel, "Carotenoids and cancer: an update with emphasis on human intervention studies," *Euro. J. Cancer*, **29**, 9, 1335–44 (1993).
21. A. Ruano-Ravina, A. Figueiras, and J. M. Barros-Dios, "Diet and lung cancer: a new approach," *Euro. J. Cancer Prevent.*, **9**, 6, 395–400 (2000).
22. J. J. DiGiovanna, "Retinoid chemoprevention in patients at high risk for skin cancer," *Med. Pediat. Oncol.*, **36**, 5, 564–7 (2001).
23. S. Zhang, D. J. Hunger, M. R. Forman, *et al.*, "Dietary carotenoids and vitamins A, C, and E and risk of breast cancer," *J. Natl. Cancer Inst.*, **91**, 6, 547–56 (1999).
24. N. Cook, M. J. Stampfer, J. Ma, *et al.*, "Beta-carotene supplementation for patients with low baseline levels and decreased risks of total and prostate carcinoma," *Cancer*, **86**, 9, 1783–92 (1999).
25. C. Ritenbaugh, "Carotenoids and cancer," *Nutrition Today*, **21**, 1, 14–19 (1987).
26. R. G. Ziegler, "Vegetables, fruits, and carotenoids and the risk of cancer," *Amer. J. Clin. Nutr.*, **53**, 1, 251S–9S (1991).
27. L. Gallicchio, K. Boyd, G. Matanoski, *et al.*, "Carotenoids and the risk of developing lung cancer: a systematic review," *Amer. J. Clin. Nutr.*, **88**, 2, 372–83 (2008).
28. Y. Sharoni, M. Danilenko, N. Dubi, *et al.*, "Carotenoids and transcription," *Arch. Biochem. Biophys.*, **430**, 1, 89–96 (2004).
29. T. Maoka, "Recent progress in structural studies of carotenoids in animals and plants," *Arch. Biochem. Biophys.*, **483**, 2, 191–5 (2009).
30. A. S. Haka, K. E. Shafer-Peltier, M. Fitzmaurice, *et al.*, "Diagnosing breast cancer by using Raman spectroscopy," *PNAS*, **102**, 12371–6 (2005).
31. A. S. Haka, Z. Volynskaya, J. A. Gardecki, *et al.*, "In vivo margin assessment during partial mastectomy breast surgery using Raman spectroscopy," *Cancer Res.*, **66**, 6, 3317–22 (2006).

32. M. V. Chowdary, K. K. Kumar, J. Kurien, *et al.*, "Discrimination of normal, benign, and malignant breast tissues by Raman spectroscopy," *Biopolymers*, **83**, 5, 556–9 (2006).

33. B. Brożek-Płuska, I. Placek, Z. Kurczewski *et al.*, "Breast cancer diagnostics by Raman spectroscopy," *J. Mol. Liquids*, **141**, 3, 145–8 (2008).

34. H. Abramczyk, J. Surmacki, B. Brożek-Płuska, *et al.*, "The hallmarks of breast cancer by Raman spectroscopy," *J. Mol. Structure*, **924**, 175–82 (2009).

35. H. Abramczyk, B. Brozek-Pluska, J. Surmacki, *et al.*, "The label-free Raman imaging of human breast cancer," *J. Mol. Liquids*, **164**, 1, 123–31 (2011).

36. H. Abramczyk, B. Brozek-Pluska, J. Surmacki, *et al.*, "Raman 'optical biopsy' of human breast cancer," *Prog. Biophys. Mol. Biol.*, **108**, 1, 74–81 (2012).

37. B. Brozek-Pluska, J. Musial, R. Kordek, *et al.*, "Raman spectroscopy and imaging: Applications in human breast cancer diagnosis," *Analyst*, **137**, 16, 3773–80 (2012).

38. J. Surmacki, J. Musiał, R. Kordek, *et al.*, "Raman imaging at biological interfaces: applications in breast cancer diagnosis," *Mol. Cancer*, **12**, 48, 1–12 (2013).

39. H. Abramczyk and B. Brozek-Pluska, "Raman imaging in biochemical and biomedical applications: diagnosis and treatment of breast cancer," *Chem. Rev.*, **113**, 8, 5766–81 (2013).

40. B. Brozek-Pluska, J. Jablonska-Gajewicz, R. Kordek, *et al.*, "Phase transitions in oleic acid and in human breast tissue as studied by Raman spectroscopy and Raman imaging," *J. Med. Chem.*, **54**, 9, 3386–92 (2011).

41. H. Abramczyk, B. Brozek-Pluska, J. Surmacki, *et al.*, "Hydrogen bonds of interfacial water in human breast cancer tissue compared to lipid and DNA interfaces," *J. Biophys. Chem.*, **2**, 2, 159–70 (2011).

42. H. Abramczyk, B. Brozek-Pluska, M. Krzesniak, *et al.*, "The cellular environment of cancerous human tissue. Interfacial and dangling water as a 'hydration fingerprint,'" *Spectrochimica Acta A*, **129**, 609–23 (2014).

43. X. Bi, B. Rexer, C. L. Arteaga, *et al.*, "Evaluating HER2 amplification status and acquired drug resistance in breast cancer cells using Raman spectroscopy," *J. Biomed. Optics*, **19**, 2, 025001 (2014).

44. M. Hedegaard, C. Krafft, H. J. Ditzel, *et al.*, "Discriminating isogenic cancer cells and identifying altered unsaturated fatty acid content as associated with metastasis status, using k-means clustering and partial least squares-discriminant analysis of Raman maps," *Anal. Chem.*, **82**, 7, 2797–802 (2010).

45. I. Notingher and L. L. Hench, "Raman microspectroscopy: a noninvasive tool for studies of individual living cells in vitro," *Expert Rev. Med. Devices*, **3**, 2, 215–34 (2006).

46. F. Baenke, B. Peck, H. Miess, *et al.*, "Hooked on fat: the role of lipid synthesis in cancer metabolism and tumour development," *Dis. Models Mechan.*, **6**, 6, 1353–63 (2013).

47. E. Rysman, K. Brusselmans, K. Scheys, *et al.*, "De novo lipogenesis protects cancer cells from free radicals and chemotherapeutics by promoting membrane lipid saturation," *Cancer Res.*, **70**, 20, 8117–26 (2010).

48. M. Hilvo, C. Denkert, L. Lehtinen, *et al.*, "Novel theranostic opportunities offered by characterization of altered membrane lipid metabolism in breast cancer progression," *Cancer Res.*, **71**, 9, 3236–45 (2011).

49. B. Griffiths, C. A. Lewis, K. Bensaad, *et al.*, "Sterol regulatory element binding protein-dependent regulation of lipid synthesis supports cell survival and tumor growth," *Cancer Metab.*, **1**, 3, 1–21 (2013).

50. A. Mahadevan-Jansen and R. R. Richards-Kortum, "Raman spectroscopy for the detection of cancers and precancers," *J. Biomed. Optics*, **1**, 1, 31–70 (1996).

51. N. J. Kline and P. J.Treado, "Raman chemical imaging of breast tissue," *J. Raman Spectroscopy*, **28**, 2–3, 119–24 (1997).

52. M. Diem, M. Miljkovic, B. Bird, *et al.*, "Applications of infrared and Raman microspectroscopy of cells and tissue in medical diagnostics: present status and future promises," *Spectroscopy*, **27**, 5–6, 463–96 (2012).

53. A. Mahadevan-Jansen, M. F. Mitchell, N. Ramanujamf, *et al.*, "Near-infrared Raman spectroscopy for in vitrodetection of cervical precancers," *Photochem. Photobiol.*, **68**, 1, 123–32 (1998).

54. P. J. Marusyk and K. Polyak, "Cancer cell phenotypes, in fifty shades of grey," *Science*, **339**, 6119, 528–9 (2013).

55. R. A. Cairns, I. S. Harris, and T. W. Mak, "Regulation of cancer cell metabolism," *Nature Rev. Cancer*, **11**, 2, 85–95 (2011).

56. O. Warburg, "On the origin of cancer cells," *Science*, **123**, 3191, 309–14 (1956).

57. C. Nieva, M. Marro, N. Santana-Codina, *et al.*, "The lipid phenotype of breast cancer cells characterized by Raman microspectroscopy: towards a stratification of malignancy," *PLOS One*, **7**, 10, e46456 (2012).

58. K. Bhalla, B. J. Hwang, R. E. Dewi, *et al.*, "PGC1α promotes tumor growth by inducing gene expression programs supporting lipogenesis," *Cancer Res.*, **71**, 21, 6888–98 (2011).

4

Photoprotection and Radiation Protection by Dietary Carotenoids

Fritz Boehm[a], Ruth Edge[b], Terence George Truscott[c], and Christian Witt[d]

[a]*Department of Dermatology, Photobiology Laboratory, Charité Universitätsmedizin Berlin, Berlin, Germany*
[b]*Dalton Cumbrian Facility, The University of Manchester, Westlakes Science & Technology Park, Cumbria, UK*
[c]*School of Physical and Geographical Sciences (Chemistry Section), Keele University, Staffordshire, UK*
[d]*Department of Pneumonology, Charité Universitätsmedizin Berlin, Berlin, Germany*

4.1 Introduction

The dietary carotenoids give photoprotection to photosynthetic systems, the eye, and the skin from reactive oxygen species (aka reactive oxy-species, or ROS). Such ROS are either a range of oxidizing (free) radicals or singlet oxygen (SO), and these arise via two pathways that are often called the Type 1 and Type 2 mechanisms. In both cases, the photosensitizer responsible for the biodamage absorbs light to give the excited singlet state, and these are converted, within a few nanoseconds or less, to the lowest excited triplet state (^{3}sens*). Generally, the excited singlet states are too short-lived to be of significance in photosensitized reactions. Once formed, the ^{3}sens* can (1) undergo electron or hydrogen atom transfer with a substrate (RH) producing free radicals that can then add molecular oxygen to give an oxy-radical ($RO_2^{\bullet}$), or (2) undergo energy transfer to ground state oxygen to produce a damaging oxidizing species, SO. These processes are shown in Figure 4.1 together with possible subsequent reactions of the $RO_2^{\bullet}$ to initiate a chain reaction and of SO to produce oxy-adducts (ROOH).

Additionally, many radicals are produced in the body during normal metabolic processes [1, 2] and, of course, via environmental hazards (e.g., smoking, air pollution, and ionizing radiation). Radicals are usually very reactive species, having one unpaired electron, and

Carotenoids: Nutrition, Analysis and Technology, First Edition. Edited by Agnieszka Kaczor and Malgorzata Baranska.

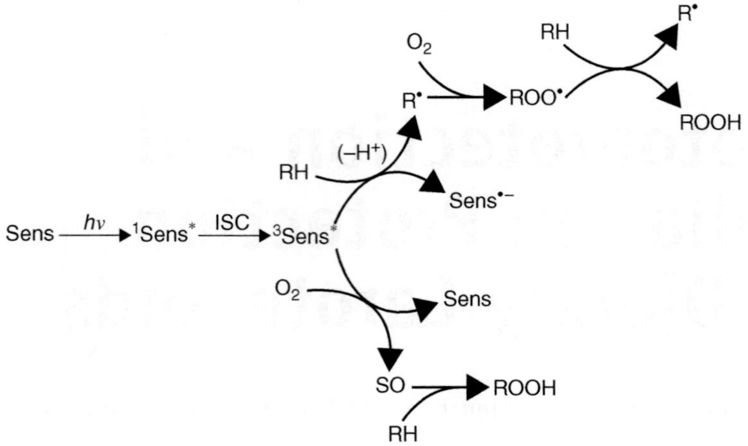

Figure 4.1 Photosensitized schemes for Type 1 and Type 2 reactions.

can be neutral or positively or negatively charged. They are either oxidizing or reducing species, depending on their reduction potentials and those of the substrates they react with, and they can also simply add to substrates [3].

Lipids, proteins, and DNA are all susceptible to attack by both SO and free radicals [4]. Cellular damage is dependent on the location of the sensitizer and permeation of the sensitizer to the target site. It has been suggested that many diseases, including cancer, age-related macular degeneration (AMD), and neurological disorders such as Alzheimer's disease [4, 5], as well as the aging process in general [6], are all associated with SO and/or free radical production.

Many carotenoids (CARs) and oxy-carotenoids (xanthophylls [XANs]) occur naturally in our foodstuffs, and, indeed, several are often added as food colorants, such as β-carotene (β-CAR, yellow-orange), lycopene (LYC, red-orange), lutein (LUT, yellow), canthaxanthin (CAN, orange-red), β-apo-8'-carotenal (APO, orange-red), and astaxanthin (ASTA, red). Some, for example β-CAR, LYC, LUT, and zeaxanthin (ZEA), are used, often in higher concentrations, as dietary supplements.

The C_{40} CARs and XANs comprise one of nature's major antioxidant groups: They are extremely efficient quenchers of SO, simply converting the excess energy of SO to heat, and they often react with oxy-radicals, but here the processes can be much more complex and in a few cases actually lead to deleterious pro-oxidative effects. With the increasing use of CARs (which are even being suggested as "nutraceuticals" and "cosmeceuticals") [7], it is important to establish evidence on the benefit–risk ratio of CARs and XANs in our diet.

4.2 Carotenoids and singlet oxygen

4.2.1 Organic solvents

The extremely efficient quenching of SO by all C_{40} CARs and XANs with 11 conjugated double bonds in "simple" organic solvents such as benzene is well established and reviewed [8, 9], and Figure 4.2 compares these for β-CAR and LYC with CARs with more and less conjugated double bonds.

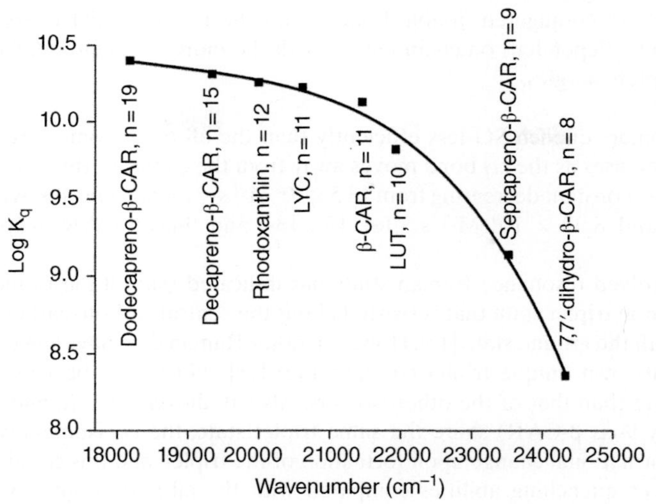

Figure 4.2 Graph showing the relationship between the singlet oxygen (SO) quenching rate constant (k_q) and the wavenumber of the ground state absorption maximum for a range of carotenoids in benzene; adapted from Ref. [8].

Two points are worthy of further discussion:

1. The literature shows lycopene to be a more efficient quencher than β-CAR (and all other C_{40} CARs), but there is disagreement as to the extent of this effect. For example, our own work suggests LYC is only about 20% more efficient than β-CAR [8], whereas Sies and coworkers claimed a much greater efficiency [10]. The reason for the increased efficiency, however big the factor, is probably structural. β-CAR, and all other "common" dietary CARs, have terminal six-membered rings whereas LYC does not. Due to steric hindrance, it has been suggested that a twisting and loss of planarity in all CARs with terminal rings lead to an effective reduction in the length of the conjugated chain [11]. Because, for LYC, this does not arise, it has a somewhat lower triplet energy level than CARs such as β-CAR. For this to be highly important, the CAR triplets must be close in energy to that of SO (94.6 kJ mol^{-1}). This is briefly discussed in point 2.
2. There have been several estimates of the lowest triplet energy level of β-CAR, using a range of techniques such as simple extrapolation of data from shorter chain CARs, weak phosphorescence via Fourier transform luminescence detection techniques, optoacoustic calorimetry, and a temperature study of the SO quenching [12–15]. However, in summary, there is no fully established value except to say the triplet level of β-CAR is below but near that of SO. In agreement with this statement, we note LUT has just one fewer conjugated double bond than β-CAR, so its triplet level will be expected to be a little higher than that of β-CAR and the quenching of SO is reduced from that of β-CAR (13.5×10^9 M^{-1} s^{-1}) to 6.64×10^9 M^{-1} s^{-1} for LUT [9]. With only nine conjugated double bonds, the quenching rate constant for septapreno-β-CAR drops to 1.38×10^9 M^{-1} s^{-1}. It is of interest to note that Rondonuwu [16] used sub-picosecond laser flash photolysis to estimate excited singlet and triplet state lifetimes that led to a measurement of the triplet energy level of lycopene as 82 kJmol^{-1}—which is close to, but probably below, that of β-CAR. They also studied other CARs of differing chain

lengths (9–13 conjugated double bonds), and the lowest triplet energy levels were shown to be dependent on chain length, with the more conjugated CARs having the lower triplet energies.

The *cis* isomers quench SO less efficiently than the all-*trans* isomer. Additionally, the efficiency decreases as the *cis* bond moves away from the center of the molecule, with the quenching rate constant decreasing from $13.5 \times 10^9\ M^{-1}\ s^{-1}$ for all-*trans*-β-CAR to 12.0×10^9, 10.4×10^9, and $8.99 \times 10^9\ M^{-1}\ s^{-1}$ for 15-, 13-, and 9-*cis*-β-CAR, respectively (see Figure 4.3).

A time-resolved resonance Raman study has indicated that all the isomers of β-CAR share a common triplet state that is twisted about the central carbon–carbon double bond compared with the ground state [17]. However, other Raman data have suggested that 9-*cis* β-CAR has its own unique triplet configuration [18], which may be why its quenching ability is lower than that of the other isomers. Also, if all-*trans*, 15-*cis*, and 13-*cis* β-CAR (and possibly 9-*cis* β-CAR) share the same triplet state, the *cis* isomers will undergo a double conformational change upon formation of the triplet, and this could be the reason for their lower quenching abilities compared with the all-*trans* isomer, with the 15-*cis* isomer having the better quenching ability of the three *cis* isomers studied due to the conformational changes being about the same bond. It is interesting to note that, again, the order of the quenching rate constants increases with increasing λ_{max}.

4.2.2 Cell models

Much of this work has concerned micellar and liposomal environments and has been thoroughly reviewed quite recently [9]. For the hydrocarbon CARs, the SO quenching is reduced by, typically, a factor of about 7 in both micelles and unilamellar liposomes

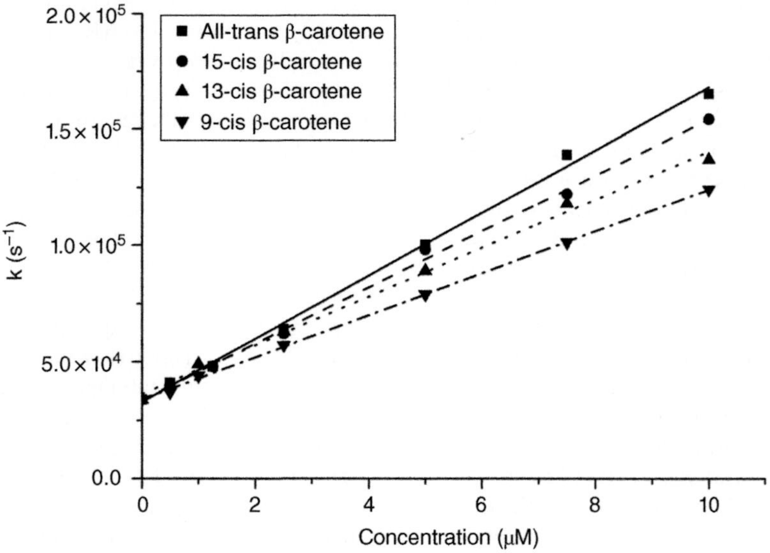

Figure 4.3 Plot of first-order rate constant (k) for the decay of singlet oxygen (SO) against carotenoid concentration in benzene for all-*trans* β-carotene and some *cis* isomers.

compared to organic solvents. For the XANs, there is a much greater loss of efficiency of SO quenching in the liposomes compared to the micelles. Typically, SO quenching by XANs solubilized in unilamellar liposomes is a factor of 70 lower than that observed in organic solvents, whereas for XANs in aqueous micellar solutions the factor stays around 7, as it does for the hydrocarbon CARs. Additionally, there can be a significant effect of concentration of XANs in the liposomes (especially for ZEA) on the measured rate constant, suggesting "stacking" of such XANs in the liposomes [19]. Adamkiewicz *et al.* [20] have recently shown that water molecules can be bound to the aggregated structures formed by ZEA in the form of molecular bridges between the terminal hydroxyl groups of adjacent molecules, whereas for β-CAR, which has no hydroxyl groups, the water molecules are weakly bound via π-type weak hydrogen bonds. An interesting postulate is a molecular ladder mechanism of transferring a proton across the lipid membrane via hopping between the water molecules along the ZEA dimeric structure. It is noteworthy that in these cell model environments, unlike organic solvents, the quenching of SO by LYC and β-CAR is identical to within the experimental error.

4.2.3 Cells

Attempts to measure the SO quenching by CARs, especially β-CAR in cellular environments, are plagued by experimental difficulties. For example, despite washing cells after incubation with a CAR, there is still the possibility that the CAR is attached to the outer surface of a cell rather than being embedded in the lipid membrane [21, 22]. However, a slight decrease in the SO lifetime was detected with lymphoid cells extracted from the blood of individuals who had been treated orally with 25 mg β-CAR three times daily over 4 weeks [22]. In somewhat corresponding work with lycopene, where the volunteers had consumed 500 ml/day tomato juice (pre-boiled) or 400 g/day tomato soup [23], very little SO quenching could be detected via time-resolved luminescence at 1270 nm. However, the cells were protected from damage by SO as measured via standard cell-staining techniques. This possibly illustrates the experimental problems that can arise (due, e.g., to light scattering) when measuring SO directly via its 1270 nm luminescence. Interestingly, these workers observed a much more efficient protection of lycopene-loaded cells from $NO_2^{\bullet}$.

Important new results have been reported by the group of Ogilvy. These workers carefully assessed the concentration of β-CAR in mammalian cells and used a microscope-based SO luminescence technique on single HeLa cells to study the effect of the β-CAR on SO [24]. They report little or no β-CAR-mediated change in the lifetime of intracellular SO (even in D_2O). They conclude that the protective effects of β-CAR in the cellular conditions they used must be via trapping of radicals rather than SO. The results are rationalized in terms of the low rate of diffusion of the SO in the high viscosity of the intracellular environment. In agreement with these findings, we have reported (as discussed in this chapter) only very little quenching of SO luminescence by LYC, which has been introduced into human lymphocytes via a dietary route [23]. It is interesting to note that in the macula, where really efficient antioxidant behavior is critical, the only CARs accumulated are LUT and ZEA. It would be of interest if the single-cell luminescence study could be extended to these XANs in a suitable cellular environment.

It is also of interest to compare these results with the quenching of SO by β-CAR and other CARs in plants that has been established, for many years, as the first line of defense of the plants against the damage due to SO [25]. Here, the CARs are located extremely close to the singlet oxygen generator (triplet chlorophyll), and hence slow diffusion does not arise. Effectively, we have "static" quenching of the SO by the CARs in the photosynthetic reaction center. This, of course, is consistent with the failure to observe SO quenching in cells where diffusion would be required for collisional energy transfer.

A further recent development has shown that chemical (as well as physical) quenching of SO by several CARs in plants can lead to a buildup of oxidation products of the CARs [26, 27]. This work shows that carotene endoperoxides are the major oxidation products and that they provide a useful internal probe of SO production. Additionally, they also show that one of the breakdown products from chemical quenching by CARs (β-cyclocitral) can provoke genetic responses to induce defense mechanisms and increase tolerance to oxidative stress.

4.3 Radicals

One of the earliest studies of electron-donor and electron-acceptor properties of CARs comes from the electrochemical studies of Mairanovsky *et al.* [28]. It is now well established that radicals (from, e.g., environmental pollution, ionizing, or nonionizing radiation) can react with CARs via electron and H-atom transfer and also via addition reactions. Products of such reactions are radical cations and anions of the CARs, neutral radicals, and radical adducts. The best studied reactions are electron transfer reactions, which produce positively charged CAR radical cations, and the subsequent reactions of these radical cations with other bio-substrates. It is these subsequent reactions that can lead to a switch from a CAR acting as an antioxidant to acting as a pro-oxidant. This has been reviewed [9], and only a brief summary of these reactions together with a mention of some speculations on their role in human disease are given below. Unfortunately, it is more difficult to study CAR–radical adducts and neutral CAR radicals partly because of spectral overlap with the parent CAR. Radical anions can be studied more easily, but they have not been observed *in vivo* and are not as biologically relevant as the cations—so rather little work has been reported on these species.

4.3.1 Radical cations

One of the most convenient ways to study radical cations is via pulse radiolysis using fast electrons to generate the primary solvent radicals, although they can also be generated by other means such as pulsed laser methods. These techniques are well established [29] and have allowed the one-electron oxidation potentials of several CARs to be measured in aqueous micellar solution—they are typically near 1000 mV, so that CARs, once converted to their radical cations, become rather strong oxidizing agents [30, 31] themselves. Indeed, unless quenched by some reductant, the CAR radical cations can oxidize important bio-substrates such as cysteine and tyrosine [31]. Pulse radiolysis has also allowed electron transfer to be measured between pairs of CARs so that relative one-electron oxidation potentials have been established [32], and this work has shown that LYC has the lowest potential, that is, it is the most easily oxidized CAR. Thus, in a mixture of CARs (possibly in the *in vivo* environment), it is LYC that is lost preferentially. Indeed, this "sacrificial" behavior of LYC may well mean that it is the most effective free radical quencher (and, as noted, it is also the most efficient SO quencher). Such behavior has been suggested as an explanation of LYC effectiveness against AMD, even though it does not accumulate in the eye [33–35]. The speculation is that LYC protects the LUT and ZEA *en route* to the macula (i.e., if the ZEA or LUT is oxidized in the body, the LYC can reconvert ZEA and LUT radical cations back to ZEA and LUT). Indeed, after solar-simulated UV light exposure, skin LYC is preferentially destroyed over β-CAR [36], suggesting, that in this situation, it is also the sacrificial CAR.

Another interesting speculation from the pulse radiolysis studies arises because it is easy to show that CAR radical cations are converted back to the parent CAR by water-soluble antioxidants such as ascorbic acid [9, 37]. Therefore, any pro-oxidant effect based on the rather high redox potential of CAR radical cations will be mitigated by ascorbic acid. Smokers have low levels of ascorbic acid [38], and free radicals from cigarette smoke can reach the lungs. It has been shown that, for heavy smokers, a high concentration of β-CAR can have a damaging effect [39], and the speculation is that this may be due to these smoke-based free radicals (e.g., $NO_2^{\bullet}$) reacting with β-CAR to generate the CAR radical cation, which can then damage biomolecules (the CAR radical cations can be quite long-lived; indeed, when isolated in sugar-based complexes, they can last for days [40], which increases the possibility of damage to other bio-substrates). As noted above, smokers have low concentrations of ascorbic acid, so they may well exhibit additional lung damage due to a β-CAR supplement.

There has been some interest in the properties of CAR radical cations in the presence of metal ions, with a particular interest in manganese because of its biological relevance in photosynthesis and enzyme activity. Using laser flash photolysis, El-Agamey and Fukuzumi [41] have shown an increase in the lifetime of ASTA radical cations in the presence of a wide range of metal ions in air-saturated solutions, with Mn^{2+} showing the most dramatic increase: The half-life increased by more than three orders of magnitude. The ground state of ASTA has previously been shown to complex metal ions via its oxygen hetero atoms [42, 43], and this was also seen by El-Agamey and Fukuzumi [41]. However, El-Agamey and Fukuzumi [41] also observed increases in radical cation half-life for both CAN and β-CAR, which do not show any ground state spectral changes in the presence of metal ions, suggesting there is no complexation. Although the stabilization of CAN radical cation was (like ASTA) stronger than that for β-CAR, which may indicate that the oxygen in the carbonyl group of CAN can, in fact, interact with the metal ions. The huge effect on the $XAN^{\bullet+}$ lifetime is attributed to a reduction in the back electron transfer involving the positively charged $XAN^{\bullet+}$ and the negatively charged superoxide radical, $O_2^{\bullet-}$.

A slight increase in the half-life in the presence of metal ions was also found in the absence of oxygen (with the half-life further increasing with oxygen concentration up to 5%, then staying stable), although the studies by Polyakov *et al.* [42] that used cyclic voltammetry indicated the opposite effect, with the radical cations having shorter lifetimes in the presence of Ca^{2+}, Zn^{2+}, or Fe^{2+} in deaerated anhydrous acetonitrile.

4.3.2 Carotenoid–radical adducts

It is well established that peroxyl radicals add to CARs. Burton and Ingold [44] suggested that β-CAR scavenges peroxyl radicals via an addition process yielding a resonance-stabilized carbon-centered radical. Others have shown that such adducts can fall apart to generate the CAR radical cation [45–47]. However, this process does depend on the environment and the specific peroxyl radicals being studied [48]. These workers showed that in hexane and benzene the radical cation is not formed from the adducts studied, whereas in polar solvents the radical cation is formed but is not the only product. The overall situation is not fully understood.

Probably the best example of CAR radical addition processes involves sulfur-based radicals [49–52]. These workers used pulse radiolysis and/or laser flash photolysis to observe the reaction of $RS^{\bullet}$ radicals (including the radical generated from glutathione) with β-CAR. No absorption in the region of the radical cations was detected, and the adducts were found to absorb in the same spectral region as the parent CAR. A detailed kinetic analysis allowed the presence of the adduct to be shown.

4.3.3 Neutral radicals

Studies linked to the understanding of the role of CARs in photosynthesis have involved the study of β-CAR, for example, adsorbed onto a silica–alumina solid support and, more recently, a copper-based molecular sieve [53]. These Photosystem II model systems have led to the detection of a neutral radical of β-CAR via deprotonation of the radical cation, and the authors suggest this species explains the previously unassigned near-infrared absorption at 750 nm associated with Photosystem II and may suggest that the extensive secondary electron-transfer pathway in Photosystem II may also be involved in proton transfer. Kispert and coworkers [54] have also shown that, in such microenvironments, the deprotonation "position" depends on the length of the CAR conjugation. The loss of a proton from a methylene group at the end of the conjugation of the radical cation, forming neutral radicals that extend the conjugation, is preferred.

Neutral radicals of the XANs CAN and ASTA have also been observed (in water-based detergents) via protonation of the corresponding radical anions with λ_{max} near 570 nm [55]. Of course, these are different neutral radicals ($XAN(+H)^{\bullet}$), with an extra H atom compared to those studied by Gao *et al.* ($CAR(-H)^{\bullet}$) [53], and they are discussed in more detail in the "Radical anions" section (Section 4.3.4).

In fluid solutions more than one neutral radical of a CAR is possible, and the underlying chemistry is complex and not totally understood. In a recent study, Chen *et al.* [56] claim to have used laser flash photolysis to generate both the hydroxyl radical ($OH^{\bullet}$) and a thiyl radical via 355 nm irradiation of N-hydroxypyridine-2 (1H)-thione. This is a complex system, and several transients arise such as the triplet–triplet absorption of β-CAR, a thiyl radical adduct and a transient with a weak absorption near 750 nm, which the authors assign to a neutral radical of β-CAR via $H^{\bullet}$ abstraction from β-CAR by $OH^{\bullet}$:

$$OH^{\bullet} + \beta\text{-CAR} \rightarrow \beta\text{-CAR}(-H)^{\bullet} + H_2O$$

This assignment was partially based on the disappearance of the transient in the presence of $OH^{\bullet}$ scavengers. This process may be important under extremely oxidizing conditions and appears to only be observed with hydrocarbon CARs and not with the more oxidizing XAN. However, there is now some doubt concerning this assignment of the 750 nm transient absorption. El-Agamey *et al.* [57], also using laser flash photolysis, have studied the effects of pH increase on the reactivity of the β-CAR radical cation to further understand the claims of Chen *et al.* In this recent work the neutral radical was generated by the following reaction:

$$\beta\text{-CAR} - H^{\bullet +} + OH^{-} \rightarrow \beta\text{-CAR} - H^{\bullet} + H_2O$$

El-Agamey showed that oxygen had no effect on the 750 nm transient so generated and therefore, they propose that it is not due to the β-CAR neutral radical, $\beta\text{-CAR}(-H)^{\bullet}$. As a result they suggest that this weak transient species observed by Chen *et al.* is another absorption band due to the CAR radical cation and not a neutral CAR radical.

4.3.4 Radical anions

There has been little development of this topic since that reported in 2006 and 2007 [55, 58]. This has also been reviewed quite recently [9], so only a summary is given here. However, there has been recent interest in the interactions of CARs with superoxide radical anions, and these are discussed here.

As with the radical cations, the relative ordering of the one-electron reduction potentials has been obtained [58]. These increase in the following order:

$$\text{ZEA} < \beta\text{-CAR} = \text{LUT} < \text{LYC} < \text{APO} = \text{CAN} < \text{ASTA}$$

This sequence shows that, unlike the oxidation potentials where LYC is the most easily oxidized CAR (and therefore acts as the sacrificial CAR in mixtures), LYC is not the most easily reduced and XANs with carbonyl substituents are more easily reduced. The reduction potentials for β-CAR and ZEA have been shown to be −2075 ± 75 mV against NHE (normal hydrogen electrode) [55], showing such radicals to be very strong reducing species. Thus, there are virtually no biological or *in vivo* situations where we can expect a "natural" radical anion to be quenched by a CAR via a direct electron transfer to generate the radical anion of the CAR—in contrast to the situation of the radical cations discussed in this chapter. Also, of course, CAR radical anions, unlike the radical cations, do react with oxygen—the product of this reaction is not reported, but the generation of the superoxide radical anion would seem to be a possibility. In unpublished work we have shown that, in hexane, the radical anion of β-CAR reacts with oxygen about twice as fast as that of LYC.

4.3.5 The interaction of CARs with the superoxide radical and its protonated conjugated acid

The superoxide radical anion ($O_2^{\bullet-}$) is generally regarded as unreactive, unlike its conjugate acid, $HO_2^{\bullet}$ (the pK_a of $O_2^{\bullet-}/HO_2^{\bullet}$ is 4.7). Indeed, it is possible that any reactions claimed to involve $O_2^{\bullet-}$, even at pH near neutrality, could be due to the small amounts of $HO_2^{\bullet}$ present at such pH values. However, because of the importance of $O_2^{\bullet-}$ in biochemical processes, there have been studies of the possible reaction(s) between $O_2^{\bullet-}$ and CARs over the last 20 years or so, and more recent work suggests that CARs do react with $O_2^{\bullet-}$. An early experimental study [59] showed a reaction between $O_2^{\bullet-}$ and β-CAR in aqueous Triton X detergent, which they interpreted as formation of an adduct—however, reanalysis suggests this was the formation of the β-CAR radical cation. These workers also studied the interaction between LYC and $O_2^{\bullet-}$ but could make no measurements in detergent systems due to the low solubility of the lycopene. Using hexane as solvent, they suggested a reversible electron transfer—however, the transients observed are so weak that these results are not unambiguous.

In unpublished work, we have investigated the possible interaction between three CARs (ASTA, ZEA, and crocetin) and $O_2^{\bullet-}/HO_2^{\bullet}$. In pulse radiolysis studies using aqueous 2% Triton X in water with 0.1 M sodium formate, we generate virtually only $O_2^{\bullet-}/HO_2^{\bullet}$—the formate, in the presence of air, converts the primary radicals, e_{aq} and $OH^{\bullet}$, to $O_2^{\bullet-}$. Monitoring the formation of the ZEA radical cation (λ_{max} 940 nm) as a function of pH from 0.96 to 5.80, our results show very little detectable reaction at pH 5.80 but significant reaction below pH 3 (see Figure 4.4), consistent with a reaction between $HO_2^{\bullet}$ and ZEA and no measureable reaction between $O_2^{\bullet-}$ and ZEA:

$$\text{ZEA} + HO_2^{\bullet} \xrightarrow{H^+} \text{ZEA}^{\bullet+} + H_2O_2$$

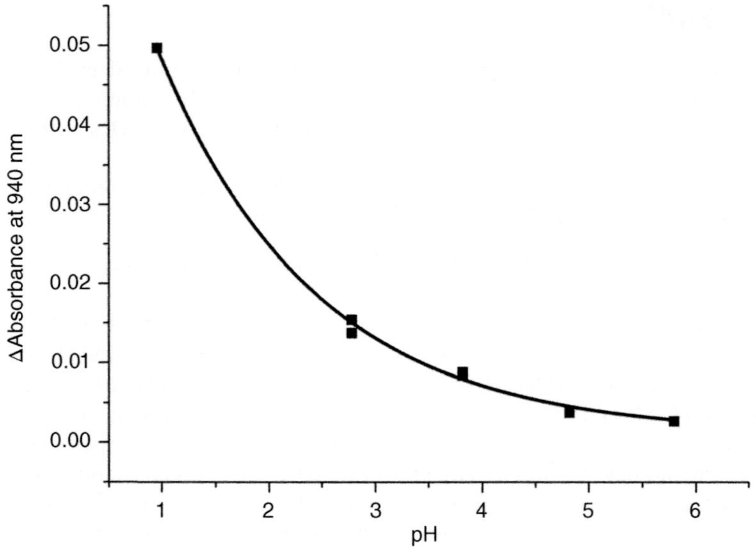

Figure 4.4 Plot of absorbance change at 940 nm against pH, showing the increase in the zeaxanthin (ZEA) radical cation at low pH after pulse radiolysis of an aqueous 2% Triton X solution containing 0.1 M sodium formate and 10 μM ZEA.

Further increases in the yield of $CAR^{\bullet+}$ at lower pH values are due to other processes, possibly direct reaction of the CAR with the hydroxyl radical—the efficiency of the formate to convert the hydroxyl radical to the superoxide radical anion being reduced in acid conditions.

In an attempt to further understand the role of $O_2^{\bullet-}$, we have studied the effect of γ-radiation on CARs in "simple" solutions—ASTA solubilized in Triton X detergents, and crocetin in water. We choose crocetin, a water-soluble CAR, to eliminate any effects due to the detergents themselves. Our results show there is virtually no absorbance change of ASTA or crocetin in air-saturated water γ-irradiated to 25 Gy in the presence of 0.1 M sodium formate compared to an un-irradiated sample, suggesting no detectable reaction between both ASTA and crocetin with $O_2^{\bullet-}$ at this low dose. The result with crocetin is the same as previously reported by Bors *et al.* [60], who also used pulse radiolysis of aqueous solutions containing sodium formate.

However, the situation concerning CAR reactions with $O_2^{\bullet-}$ has become more uncertain with both theoretical studies and experimental work on solubilized CARs, suggesting a reaction involving $O_2^{\bullet-}$ itself. Galano *et al.* [61], using computational studies, show a reaction between many CARs and $O_2^{\bullet-}$ and suggest that such a reaction is extremely efficient with a diffusion-controlled rate constant. Cardounel *et al.* [62] have studied a water-soluble derivative of ASTA (disodium disuccinate astaxanthin) with an activated human neutrophil assay and showed that this ASTA derivative nearly completely eliminated the electron paramagnetic resonance (EPR) signal from $O_2^{\bullet-}$.

Finally, in a recent study, Chetia *et al.* [63] studied the scavenging properties of β-CAR (and a flavonoid, naringenin) against a wide range of free radicals, including $O_2^{\bullet-}$. These workers used a phenazine methosulphate–NADH system to generate $O_2^{\bullet-}$ and a spectrophotometric analysis method based on nitroblue tetrazolium superoxide. They found concentration-dependent quenching of $O_2^{\bullet-}$ for β-CAR, which was comparable to the quenching of superoxide radical by vitamin C.

Clearly where a radiation method (pulse radiolysis or γ-radiation) is used to directly generate $O_2^{\bullet-}$, there seems no evidence of a significant reaction with CARs unless the pH is low enough to convert the radical to $HO_2^{\bullet}$. Other indirect techniques for generating the superoxide radical anion and also computational studies suggest there is a direct and (according to the computational work) efficient reaction between CARs and $O_2^{\bullet-}$. More work is needed to resolve this dilemma, which is discussed further in this chapter.

4.4 Future prospects and challenges

Although the efficient quenching of SO (often diffusion controlled) by dietary CARs in "simple" solvents and some micro-heterogeneous environments (e.g., detergent micelles) is a rather straightforward and well-understood process, the effect of different types of CAR–XAN aggregation is not totally clear, leading in some cases to a much less efficient quenching. Therefore, it would be worthwhile to measure the reactivity of carefully characterized CAR aggregates with SO. Furthermore, as shown by Adamkiewicz *et al.* [20], water molecules can be bound to ZEA aggregated structures as molecular bridges between the terminal hydroxyl groups of adjacent molecules. A molecular ladder mechanism of transferring a proton across the lipid membrane via hopping between the water molecules along the ZEA dimeric structure suggests new challenges to understand all the roles of CARs in cellular environments. Also, it is noteworthy that in cell model environments, unlike organic solvents, the quenching of SO by LYC and β-CAR is identical to within experimental error despite many old (but often repeated) claims in the literature that lycopene is a more efficient quencher of SO than other dietary CARs. Finally, the possibility that SO is not efficiently quenched by CARs in mammalian cells [24] should be a subject of future research.

As noted here, not all free radical–CAR interactions are fully understood. For example, although the radical cations and anions of the CARs are now quite well characterized, the study of the various neutral CAR radicals is much more experimentally difficult, and extensive work, possibly expanding the studies of Chen *et al.* and El-Agamey *et al.* [56, 57], is now required. There is also confusion related to the interactions of CARs with (the biologically important) superoxide radical anion, $O_2^{\bullet-}$. We have studied the possible reaction between $O_2^{\bullet-}$ and crocetin, a water-soluble CAR. This allowed us to study the interactions without any possible contribution(s) for detergents or liposomes, which are usually needed to solubilize the CAR. Our results clearly show that little reaction between crocetin and $O_2^{\bullet-}$ can be detected. This result, with crocetin, is more or less the same as previously reported [60]. We have made the same observation (i.e., no reaction) for other non-water-soluble CARs (in the presence of detergents). However, the situation concerning CAR reactions with $O_2^{\bullet-}$ has become more uncertain with both theoretical studies and experimental work on solubilized CARs, suggesting there is a reaction. Galano *et al.* [61], using computational studies, show an efficient reaction between many CARs and $O_2^{\bullet-}$, and Cardounel *et al.* [62] have studied a water-soluble derivative of ASTA and observed a nearly completely eliminated $O_2^{\bullet-}$ EPR signal. Clearly, future studies are needed to resolve this apparent contradiction, especially as $O_2^{\bullet-}$ is such an important radical for the *in vivo* situation.

4.5 Conclusion

Virtually all dietary CARs are regarded as efficient quenchers of ROS—SO and oxy-radicals. It is straightforward to observe the very efficient quenching of SO by such CARs in organic solvents, micellar solutions, and various cell models with rate constants near the diffusional limit. However, it is not easy to observe such quenching in cells themselves, and this may indicate that the major protective role of dietary CARs *in vivo* is via free radical quenching. Such quenching of free radicals leads to other CAR radical species such as radical adducts, radical cations, neutral radicals, and, in rare cases, radical anions. The reactivity of these "new" radical species, especially the oxidizing ability of the radical cations, can be significant and may well account for the switch in behavior of CARs from anti- to pro-oxidants in some environments. This potential damaging switch may, for example, be associated with the increased risk of lung cancer by smokers who ingest large amounts of β-CAR.

Another significant aspect of CAR radical cations concerns the effect of metal ion, especially manganese (a metal ion of biological importance), on ASTA. The metal ion can link to the ASTA molecule at both ends via the hydroxyl and adjacent carbonyl groups on this CAR (a 2:1 complex) and, in a process involving oxygen, there is a spectral shift in the ASTA radical cation absorption spectrum and, despite complex decay kinetics, a clear and dramatic increase in the lifetime of the $ASTA^{\bullet+}$. This huge effect on the $ASTA^{\bullet+}$ lifetime is probably related to a reduction in the back electron transfer involving the positively charged ASTA cation and the negatively charged superoxide radical, $O_2^{\bullet-}$.

The possible interactions of CARs with the superoxide radical anion have led to recent controversy. Direct generation of the superoxide radical via various high-energy radiation methods appears to lead to little reactivity with the CARs studied but reactivity, at lower pH due to $HO_2^{\bullet}$, whereas computational studies and other methods of generating the superoxide radical anion appear to show efficient reactions between this radical and several CARs. More work is needed to resolve our understanding of the reactivity of CARs with superoxide radical anion.

Acknowledgments

We would like to thank Drs S. Navaratnam and E. J. Land for experimental help with some of the unpublished results discussed.

References

1. H. Nohl, "Is redox-cycling ubiquinone involved in mitochondrial oxygen activation?" *Free Rad. Res. Comms.*, **8**, 307–15 (1990).
2. J. Fiedor and K. Burda, "Potential role of carotenoids as antioxidants in human health and disease," *Nutrients*, **6**, 466–88 (2014).
3. P. Neta, M. Z. Hoffman, and M. Simic, "Electron spin resonance and pulse radiolysis studies of the reactions of OH and O^- radicals with aromatic and olefinic compounds," *J. Phys. Chem.*, **76**, 847–53 (1972).
4. J. P. Kehrer and C. V. Smith, "Free radicals in biology: sources, reactivities, and roles in the etiology of human diseases," in B. Frei (ed.), *Natural antioxidants in human health and disease*, New York: Academic Press, 1994, pp. 25–62.
5. G. E. Marak, Y. de Kozak, and J. P. Faure, "Free radicals and antioxidants in the pathogenesis of eye diseases," in I. Emerit, L. Packer, and C. Auclair (eds.), *Antioxidants in therapy and preventative medicine* (Advances in Experimental Medicine and Biology, vol. 264), New York: Plenum Press, 1990, pp. 513–27.
6. C. L. Greenstock, "The role of free radicals in radiation chemical aging," *Proc. React. Kinet.*, **14**, 249–65 (1986).

7. T. P. Anunciato and P. A. Rocha-Filho, "Carotenoids and polyphenols in nutricosmetics, nutraceuticals and cosmeceuticals," *J. Cos. Dermatol.*, **11**, 51–4 (2012).
8. R. Edge, D. J. McGarvey, and T. G. Truscott, "The carotenoids as antioxidants—a review," *J. Photochem. Photobiol. B: Biol.*, **41**, 189–200 (1997).
9. R. Edge and T. G. Truscott, "Properties of carotenoid radicals and excited states and their potential role in biological systems," in J. T. Landrum (ed.) *Carotenoids: physical, chemical, and biological functions and properties*, Boca Raton, FL: CRC Press, pp. 283–307.
10. P. Di Mascio, S. Kaiser, and H. Sies, "Lycopene as the most efficient biological carotenoid singlet oxygen quencher," *Arch. Biochem. Biophys.*, **274**, 532–8 (1989).
11. B. C. L. Weedon and C. P. Moss, "Structure and nomenclature," in G. Britton (ed.), *Carotenoids: spectroscopy*, vol. **1A**, Basel: Birkhäuser, 1995, pp. 27–70.
12. R. Bensasson, E. J. Land, and B. Maudinas, "Triplet states of carotenoids from photosynthetic bacteria studied by nansecond ultraviolet and electron pulse irradiation," *Photochem. Photobiol.*, **23**, 189–93 (1976).
13. G. Marston, T. G. Truscott, and R. P. Wayne, "Phosphorescence of β-carotene," *J. Chem. Soc. Farad. Trans.*, **91**, 4059–61 (1995).
14. C. Lambert and R. W. Redmond, "Triplet energy level of β-carotene," *Chem. Phys. Lett.*, **228**, 495–8 (1994).
15. A. A. Gorman, I. Hamblett, C. Lambert, B. Spencer, and M. C. Standen, "Identification of both preequilibrium and diffusion limits for reaction of singlet oxygen, O_2 ($^1\Delta_g$), with both physical and chemical quenchers: variable-temperature, time-resolved infrared luminescence studies," *J. Am. Chem. Soc.*, **110**, 8053–9 (1988).
16. F. S. Rondonuwu, Y. Watanabe, R. Fujii, and Y. Koyama, "A first detection of singlet to triplet conversion from the $1^1B_u^-$ to the 1^3A_g state and triplet internal conversion from the 1^3A_g to the 1^3B_u state in carotenoids: dependence on the conjugation length," *Chem. Phys. Lett.*, **376**, 292–301 (2003).
17. J. Teraoka, H. Hashimoto, S. Matsudaira, and Y. Koyama, "Resonance Raman spectra of excited triplet states of β-carotene isomers," *Chem. Lett.*, **14**, 311–14 (1985).
18. H. Hashimoto and Y. Koyama, "Time-resolved resonance Raman spectroscopy of the triplet β-carotene produced from all-trans, 7-cis, 9-cis, 13-cis, and 15-cis isomers and high-pressure liquid chromatography analyses of photoisomerisation via the triplet state," *J. Phys. Chem.*, **92**, 2101–8 (1988).
19. W. Okulski, A. Sujak, and W. I. Gruszecki, "Dipalmatoylphosphatidylcholine membranes modified with zeaxanthin: numeric study of membrane organization," *Biochem. Biophys. Acta*, **1509**, 216–28 (2000).
20. P. Adamkiewicz, A. Sujak, and W. I. Gruszecki, "Spectroscopic study on formation of aggregated structures by carotenoids: role of water," *J. Mol. Struct.*, **1046**, 44–51 (2013).
21. F. Böhm, J. Haley, T. G. Truscott, and W. Schalch, "Cellular bound β-carotene quenches singlet oxygen in man," *J. Photochem. Photobiol. B: Biol.*, **21**, 219–21 (1993).
22. J. H. Tinkler, F. Böhm, W. Schalch, and T. G. Truscott, "Dietary carotenoids protect human cells from damage," *J. Photochem. Photobiol. B: Biol.*, **26**, 283–5 (1994).
23. F. Böhm, R. Edge, M. Burke, and T. G. Truscott, "Dietary uptake of lycopene protects human cells from singlet oxygen and nitrogen dioxide: ROS components of cigarette smoke," *J. Photochem. Photobiol. B: Biol.*, **64**, 176–8 (2001).
24. G. N. Bosio, T. Breitenbach, J. Parisi, *et al.*, "Antioxidant β-carotene does not quench singlet oxygen in mammalian cells," *J. Am. Chem. Soc.*, **135**, 272–9 (2013).
25. R. J. Cogdell and H. A. Frank, "How carotenoids function in photosynthetic bacteria," *Biochim. Biophys. Acta*, **895**, 63–79 (1987).

26. F. Ramel, S. Birtic, C. Ginies, *et al.*, "Carotenoid oxidation products are stress signals that mediate gene responses to singlet oxygen in plants," *PNAS*, **109**, 5535–40 (2012).

27. F. Ramel, S. Birtic, S. Cuiné, *et al.*, "Chemical quenching of singlet oxygen by carotenoids in plants," *Plant Physiol.*, **158**, 1267–78 (2012).

28. V. G. Mairanovsky, A. A. Engovatov, N. T. Ioffe, and G. I. Samokhvalov, "Electron-donor and electron-acceptor properties of carotenoids: electrochemical study of carotenes," *J. Electroanal. Chem.*, **66**, 123–37 (1975).

29. R. Bensasson, E. J. Land, and T. G. Truscott, *Excited states and free radicals in biology and medicine: contributions from flash photolysis and pulse radiolysis*, Oxford: Oxford University Press, 1993.

30. R. Edge, E. J. Land, D. J. McGarvey, M. Burke, and T. G. Truscott, "The reduction potential of the β-carotene$^{•+}$/β-carotene couple in an aqueous micro-heterogeneous environment," *FEBS Lett.*, **271**, 125–7 (2000).

31. M. Burke, R. Edge, E. J. Land, D. J. McGarvey, and T. G. Truscott, "One-electron reduction potentials of dietary carotenoid radical cations in aqueous micellar environments," *FEBS Lett.*, **500**, 132–6 (2001).

32. R. Edge, E. J. Land, D. J. McGarvey, L. Mulroy, and T. G. Truscott, "Relative one-electron reduction potentials of carotenoid radical cations and the interactions of carotenoids with the vitamin E radical cation," *J. Am. Chem. Soc.*, **17**, 4087–90 (1998).

33. J. A. Mares-Perlman, W. E. Bracy, R. Klein, *et al.*, "Serum antioxidants and age-related macular degeneration in a population based control study," *Arch. Opthalmol.*, **113**, 1518–23 (1995).

34. F. Simonelli, F. Zarrilli, S. Mazzeo, *et al.*, "Serum oxidative and antioxidative parameters in a group of Italian patients with age-related maculopathy," *Clin. Chim. Acta*, **320**, 111–15 (2002).

35. N. Cardinault, J.-H. Abalain, B. Sairafi, *et al.*, "Lycopene but not lutein nor zeaxanthin decreases in serum and lipoproteins in age-related macular degeneration patients," *Clin. Chim. Acta*, **357**, 34–42 (2005).

36. J. D. Ribaya-Mercado, M. Garmyn, B. A. Gilchrest, and R. M. Russell, "Skin lycopene is destroyed preferentially over β-carotene during ultraviolet irradiation in humans," *J. Nutr.*, **125**, 1854–9 (1995).

37. M. Burke, R. Edge, E. J. Land, and T. G. Truscott, "Characterisation of carotenoid radical cations in liposomal environments: interaction with vitamin C," *J. Photochem. Photobiol, 'B' (Biol.)*, **60**, 1–6 (2001).

38. L. van Antwepen, A. J. Theron, S. Meyer, *et al.*, "Cigarette smoke-mediated oxidant stress, phagocytes, vitamin C, vitamin E and tissue injury," *Ann. New York Acad. Sci.*, **686**, 53–65 (1993).

39. G. S. Omenn, G. E. Goodman, M. D. Thornquist, *et al.*, "Effects of a combination of beta carotene and vitamin A on lung cancer and cardiovascular disease," *New Eng. J. Med.*, **334**, 1150–5 (1996).

40. N. E. Polyakov, T. V. Leshina, E. S. Meteleva, A. V. Dushkin, T. A. Konovalova, and L. D. Kispert, "Water soluble complexes of carotenoids with arabinogalactan," *J. Phys Chem B*, **113**, 275–82 (2009).

41. A. El-Agamey and S. Fukuzumi, "The remarkable effect of the manganese ion with dioxygen on the stability of π-conjugated radical cations," *Chem. Eur. J.*, **18**, 14660–70 (2012).

42. N. E. Polyakov, A. L. Focsan, M. K. Bowman, and L. D. Kispert, "Free radical formation in novel carotenoid metal ion complexes of astaxanthin," *J. Phys Chem B*, **114**, 16968–77 (2010).

43. E. Hernandez-Marin, A. Barbosa, and A. Martinez, "The metal cation chelating capacity of astaxanthin: does this have any influence on antiradical activity?" *Molecules*, **17**, 1039–54 (2012).

44. G. W. Burton and K. U. Ingold, "β-Carotene: an unusual type of lipid antioxidant," *Science*, **224**, 569–73 (1984).

45. J. E. Packer, J. S. Mahood, V. O. Mora-Arellano, T. F. Slater, R. L. Willson, and B. S. Wolfenden, "Free radicals and singlet oxygen scavengers: reaction of a peroxy-radical with β-carotene, diphenyl furan and 1,4-diazobicyclo (2,2,2)-octane," *Biochem. Biophys. Res. Commun.*, **98**, 901–6 (1981).

46. T. J. Hill, E. J. Land, D. J. McGarvey, W. Schalch, J. H. Tinkler, and T. G. Truscott, "Interactions between carotenoids and the $CCl_3O_2^\bullet$ radical," *J. Am. Chem. Soc.*, **117**, 8322–6 (1995).

47 A. Mortensen and L. H. Skibsted, "Kinetics of photobleaching of β-carotene in chloroform and formation of transient carotenoid species absorbing in the near infrared," *Free Rad. Res.*, **25**, 355–68 (1996).

48. A. El-Agamey and D. J. McGarvey, "Evidence for a lack of reactivity of carotenoid radicals towards oxygen: a laser flash photolysis study of the reactions of carotenoids with acylperoxyl radicals in polar and non-polar solvents," *J. Am. Chem. Soc.*, **125**, 3330–40 (2003).

49. S. A. Everett, S. C. Kundu, S. Maddix, and R. L. Willson, "Mechanisms of free-radical scavenging by the nutritional antioxidant β-carotene," *Biochem. Soc. Trans.*, **23**, 230S (1995).

50. S. A. Everett, M. F. Dennis, K. B. Patel, S. Maddix, S. C. Kundu, and R. L. Willson, "Scavenging of nitrogen dioxide, thiol, and sulphonyl free radicals by the nutritional antioxidant β-carotene," *J. Biol. Chem.*, **271**, 3988–94 (1996).

51. A. Mortensen, "Mechanism and kinetics of scavenging of the phenylthiyl radical by carotenoids: a laser flash photolysis study," *Asian Chem. Lett.*, **4**, 135–43 (2000).

52. A. Mortensen and L. H. Skibsted, "The importance of carotenoid structure in radical scavenging reactions," *J. Agric. Food Chem.*, **45**, 2970–7 (1997).

53. Y. Gao, K. E. Shinopoulos, C. A. Tracewell, A. L. Focsan, G. W. Brudvig, and L. D. Kispert, "Formation of carotenoid neutral radicals in photosystem II," *J. Phys. Chem. B*, **113**, 9901–8 (2009).

54. A. L. Focsan, M. K. Bowman, P. Molnar, J. Deli, and L. D. Kispert, "Carotenoid radical cation formation: dependence on conjugation length," *J. Phys. Chem. B*, **115**, 9495–506 (2011).

55. A. El-Agamey, R. Edge, S. Navaratnam, E. J. Land, and T. G. Truscott, Carotenoid radical anions and their protonated derivatives," *Org. Lett.*, **8**, 4255–8 (2006).

56. C.-H. Chen, R.-M. Han, R. Liang, *et al.*, "Direct observation of the β-carotene reaction with hydroxyl radical," *J. Phys. Chem. B*, **115**, 2082–9 (2011).

57. A. El-Agamey, M. A. El-Hagrasy, T. Suenobu, and S. Fukuzumi, Influence of pH on the decay of β-carotene radical cation in aqueous Triton X-100: A laser flash photolysis study. *J. Photochem. Photobiol. B: Biol.* **146**, 68–73 (2015).

58. R. Edge, A. El-Agamey, E. J. Land, S. Navaratnam, and T. G. Truscott, "Studies of carotenoid one-electon reduction radicals," *Arch. Biochem. Biophys.*, **458**, 104–10 (2007).

59. P. F. Conn, C. Lambert, E. J. Land, W. Schalch, and T. G. Truscott, "Carotene-oxygen radical interactions," *Free Radic. Res. Commun.*, **16**, 401–8 (1992).

60. W. Bors, M. Saran, and C. Michel, "Radical intermediates involved in the bleaching of the carotenoid crocin: hydroxyl radicals, superoxide anions and hydrated electrons," *Int. J. Radiat. Biol.*, **41**, 493–501 (1982).

61. A. Galano, R. Vargas, and A. Martinez, "Carotenoids can act as antioxidants by oxidising the superoxide radical anion," *Phys. Chem. Chem. Phys.*, **12**, 193–200 (2010).

62. A. Cardounel, C. Dumitrescu, J. L. Zweier, and F. Lockwood, "Direct superoxide scavenging by a disodium disuccinate astaxanthin derivative: Relative efficacy of individual stereoisomers versus the statistical mixture of stereoisomers by electron paramagnetic resonance imaging," *Biochem. Biophys. Res. Comm.*, **307**, 704–12 (2003).

63. P. Chetia, A. Bala, B. Khandelwal, and P. K. Haldar, "Comparative *in vitro* free radical scavenging property of β-carotene and nagingenin wirh respect to vitamin C and N-acetyl cysteine," *Pharmacologia*, **3**, 724–8 (2012).

5

Macular Carotenoids: Human Health Aspects

Aruna Gorusupudi and Paul S. Bernstein

Moran Eye Center, University of Utah School of Medicine, Salt Lake City, Utah, USA

5.1 Introduction

The *macula lutea* is the central part of the human retina and is responsible for the high-acuity vision required for reading, driving, and recognizing faces. It is a visibly yellow spot that consists of two dietary carotenoids, lutein and zeaxanthin, along with their metabolite *meso*-zexanthin in the ratio of 1:1:1. They are collectively referred to as the *macular carotenoids* or *macular pigment* (MP). The macular carotenoids are thought to play a major role in filtration of potentially phototoxic blue light and in protection against singlet oxygen radicals and other reactive oxygen species. The presence of the macular carotenoids in areas of the eye highly enriched in polyunsaturated fatty acids is consistent with their antioxidant roles. Most investigations into the relationship between the macular carotenoids and eye disease have focused on age-related macular degeneration (AMD), a disease in which the oxidative damage plays a major role. Epidemiological studies have indicated an inverse relationship between the levels of the macular carotenoids in the diet and eye and the incidence of AMD, and that supplementation of macular carotenoids can reduce the risk of advanced AMD [1–3]. Biological plausibility for the protective functions of macular carotenoids against AMD are supported by (1) the chemical structures and biochemical properties of macular carotenoids; (2) the topographic distribution of the macular carotenoids in the macula; and (3) the specific uptake of macular carotenoids from a much more diverse pool of circulating dietary carotenoids. In this chapter, we review the functional role of macular carotenoids, and their stereochemistry, absorption, and metabolism.

Carotenoids: Nutrition, Analysis and Technology, First Edition. Edited by Agnieszka Kaczor and Malgorzata Baranska.

5.2 Macular pigment distribution

Around 600 carotenoids exist in nature, 30–40 carotenoids are found in the human diet, and about 15 are detectable in human serum, but only lutein, zeaxanthin, and *meso*-zeaxanthin are present in human macula. The ratio of lutein:zeaxanthin:*meso*-zeaxanthin is 3:1:0 in blood and liver, 2:1:0.5 in the peripheral retina and 1:1:1 in the macula [1]. The human fovea has the highest concentration of lutein and zeaxanthin found anywhere in the human body at around 0.1 to 1 mM [1, 2]. The concentration of macular carotenoids declines over 100-fold just a few millimeters from the center of the fovea. Cross-sectionally, macular carotenoids are deposited preferentially in the Henle fiber layer of the fovea and in the inner plexiform layers of the parafovea (Figure 5.1, Color Supplement) [3, 4].

The macular carotenoids are hydroxylated, which makes them xanthophylls with no vitamin A activity, and they are characterized by a conjugated polyene chain and two terminal hydroxyl groups. This unique structure makes them well suited antioxidant components of biological membranes rich in polyunsaturated phospholipids that are susceptible to free radical–induced damage [5]. Lutein and zeaxanthin have been shown to increase the rigidity of lipid bilayers and act as "molecular rivets" because of their orientation within the membrane [6]. Zeaxanthin adopts a roughly perpendicular orientation to the plane of the membrane, while lutein and its isomers follow perpendicular as well as parallel orientations [7]. These direct effects of macular carotenoids on lipid membranes, particularly their effects on the membranes' structural and dynamic properties, seem to decrease lipid susceptibility to oxidative degradation [8].

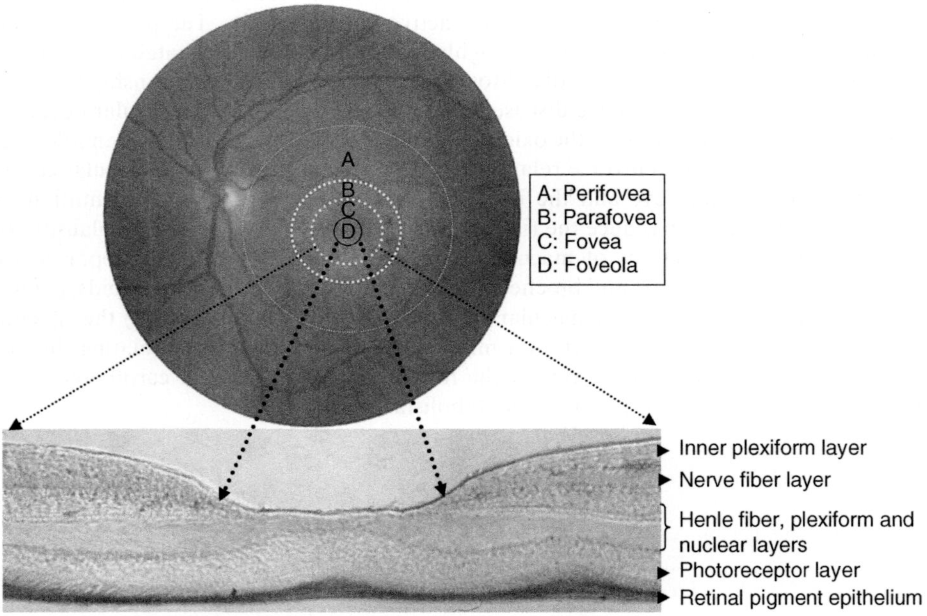

Figure 5.1 Schematic diagram demonstrating the distribution of macular pigment in the retina: fundus (top) and cross-section (bottom). (*See insert for color representation of the figure.*)

Lutein is the most abundant xanthophyll in the photosynthetic apparatus of plants. Lutein and zeaxanthin are mainly bound to major light-harvesting complex proteins of both photosystem I and photosystem II [9], where they reduce non-photochemical quenching and prevent photo-oxidative damage to the photosynthetic apparatus [10, 11]. Lutein specifically quenches harmful excited triplet chlorophyll species, formed by photo-oxidation, thus preventing the formation of reactive oxygen species in plants [12].

5.3 Human health aspects

The human retina is at high risk of oxidative damage due to light exposure, which generates free radicals and reactive oxygen species from the endogenous photosensitizers like retinal, lipofuscin, A2E, and melanin [13]. The high abundance of polyunsaturated fatty acids in retina makes it more vulnerable to oxidative damage [14]. The lipophilic macular carotenoids can effectively absorb the short wavelength portion of the visible light spectrum, which enables them to prevent or reduce free radical formation in the retina. They also directly quench free radicals, lipid peroxy radicals, hydroxyl radicals, and superoxide anions [15, 16].

5.4 Age-related macular degeneration (AMD)

AMD is an eye disease that typically affects older adults >50 years old; its prevalence rises dramatically in the elderly population older than 70 years. There are two common forms of AMD, wet (neovascular) and dry (non-neovascular). Around 80–90% of AMD cases are the dry form, characterized by the presence of drusen under the macular retina. Drusen are formed due to oxidized lipids, protein adducts and inflammatory material that may accumulate as a result of oxidative damage. An autopsy study by Bone *et al.* [2] using human donor eyes (56 AMD and 56 control) revealed that maculae from patients with AMD have lower concentrations of macular carotenoids compared to the maculae from control patients. Epidemiological evidence also suggests an inverse relationship between dietary intake [17, 18] and increased serum levels [19, 20] of lutein and zeaxanthin with incidence of AMD. Acute light damage studies on primate retinas also suggested that lutein and zeaxanthin supplementation can protect the fovea from blue light–induced oxidative damage, which may thereby reduce the risk of AMD [21].

The association between AMD risk and lutein and zeaxanthin supplementation has been explored in several large-scale epidemiological studies. The Eye Disease Case Control Study found that the risk for advanced exudative AMD was reduced by 43% in participants in the highest quintile of dietary carotenoid intake when compared with those in the lowest quintile [18]. In 2006, the Carotenoids in Age-Related Eye Disease Study (CAREDS) concluded that lutein- and zeaxanthin-rich diets may protect against intermediate AMD in female patients younger than 75 years of age [22]. In a case control study using resonance Raman measurement of macular pigment conducted at a time when lutein-containing supplements were just entering the American market, the group of AMD patients regularly consuming high-dose lutein supplements had MP levels significantly higher than those of their cohorts not using lutein supplements ($p=0.038$) and were indistinguishable from those of normal subjects ($p=0.829$) [17]. More recently, the Blue Mountain Eye Study [23] reported that higher dietary lutein and zeaxanthin intake reduced the risk of AMD incidence over 5 and 10 years. Participants in the top tertile of intake (≥942 μg/day) had a decreased risk of incident neovascular AMD, and those with above-median intakes (743 μg) had a reduced risk of indistinct soft or reticular drusen when compared with the remaining population. The original Age-Related Eye Disease Study (AREDS) did not provide the subjects with lutein–zeaxanthin supplementation, but dietary lutein–zeaxanthin intake (as determined by a food frequency questionnaire at enrollment) was inversely associated with prevalent neovascular AMD, geographic atrophy, and large or extensive intermediate drusen when the highest versus lowest quintiles were compared [24]. Although studies have shown that macular pigment optical density (MPOD) is partially related to dietary intake or serum levels of lutein and zeaxanthin [25], the results relating MPOD to AMD have been less consistent across populations and are influenced by many factors that affect uptake and distribution of these carotenoids in the body. Recent reports from the CAREDS group [26] and Hammond *et al.* [27] could not find a consistent cross-sectional association between MPOD and AMD [26], and they suggested that prospective studies were needed to further explore this relationship.

In the Age-Related Eye Disease Study 2 (AREDS2), subjects were given the carotenoids lutein (10 mg per day) and zeaxanthin (2 mg per day), alone or in combination with the omega-3 fatty acids, docosahexaenoic acid (DHA) (350 mg per day) and eicosapentaenoic acid (EPA) (650 mg per day), to assess their influence on progression to advanced AMD in individuals at high risk for the disease with bilateral large, soft drusen and/or advanced AMD in one eye. In June 2008, 80 participating US centers recruited over 4000 AMD patients for the study, with each patient scheduled to receive their assigned treatment in a randomized, placebo-controlled, double-blind manner for five years [28, 29]. This study showed that daily supplementation of lutein–zeaxanthin had no statistically significant effect on cataract surgery or vision loss [30]. DHA–EPA and varying doses of zinc appeared to have no effect, whereas lutein–zeaxanthin had a favorable effect on progression to late AMD. These reports suggest that supplementation of lutein–zeaxanthin along with β-carotene compared to β-carotene alone was beneficial in reducing the risk for late AMD and neovascular AMD. Thus, lutein–zeaxanthin may be important carotenoids to consider for the AREDS supplement [31]. Although primary analysis from the AREDS2 did not reveal any benefit from daily supplementation with lutein–zeaxanthin on AMD progression, secondary exploratory analyses suggested that lutein–zeaxanthin were helpful in reducing this risk, so they are recommended as replacements for β-carotene, which had been associated with increased risk of lung cancer in current and former smokers [32].

Infant retinas are more vulnerable to oxygen insult due to clear lenses and higher metabolic activity. They have incompletely formed and diffuse maculae with lutein predominance over zeaxanthin in the ratio of 1.49:1 [33], which changes to a more adult ratio as age increases. The change in macular carotenoid ratio appears to be closely related to anatomical development [34]. Macular development coincides with progressive shifts in the distribution of lutein, zeaxanthin, and *meso*-zeaxanthin within the developing macula [35], and nutritional status may affect this process [36]. Animal experiments with monkeys suggested that lutein and zeaxanthin are necessary for macular development [37], and deficient diets failed to induce yellow pigmentation of the macular area [38]. Newborn may have low carotenoid levels due to decreased placental nutrient transfer in uterus, similar to the decrease in placental transfer of macronutrients, which has been implicated as a mechanism for intrauterine growth restriction [39, 40]. Recent studies in our laboratory suggest that maternal serum zeaxanthin levels correlated with infant MPOD [41], and supplementation of macular carotenoids to improve visual development and cognition in infants deserves further study.

5.5 Macular carotenoid absorption

The macular carotenoids lutein and zeaxanthin are the most common xanthophylls in green leafy vegetables, whereas *meso*-zeaxanthin is uncommon in nature. Because humans cannot produce lutein and zeaxanthin *de novo*, we depend on natural dietary sources. These xanthophylls are commonly present in green leafy vegetables, fruits, egg yolk, milk, and cream. Recently, microbial sources of carotenoids such as algae are also gaining attention as an alternative for lutein and zeaxanthin supplementation [42]. Reliable data on carotenoids in agricultural produce may provide information on food sources that are crucial for dietary intake of lutein and zeaxanthin, which also offers a basis for studies on their physiologic actions [43].

Bioavailability is defined as the "fraction of nutrient from ingested dose that is absorbed." Lutein and zeaxanthin absorption strongly depends on a number of factors that include mainly the release of carotenoids from the food matrix, their incorporation into mixed micelles, the transfer of carotenoids from micelles to the mucosa for passive or facilitated absorption (via SR-BI proteins) and their sequestration into chylomicrons [44]. Carotenoid absorption in humans is higher from oils containing supplements than from complex food matrixes [45] such as spinach, kale, or yellow carrots [46]. Chung *et al.* [47] studied higher lutein absorption from lutein-enriched eggs when compared to supplements and spinach, indicating lutein absorption is higher and improved in the presence of fat. Dietary fiber has a negative effect on carotenoid absorption by entrapping them and increasing excretion of bile acids and fecal output, inhibiting lipase activity [48, 49]. Lutein and zeaxanthin are dissolved with dietary fat to form an emulsion in the gut with the aid of lipolytic enzymes and bile acids to form mixed micelles. These mixed micelles become accessible for intestinal absorption. Dietary factors play a major role in the absorption of lutein and zeaxanthin by affecting the size and formation of the micelles. A certain amount of fat is necessary for micellarization, chylomicron secretion and carotenoid absorption, but which type of fat or fatty acid goes along with carotenoid is still uncertain.

Intestinal absorption is a complex process, and studies using caco-2 intestinal cell cultures suggest that receptor proteins play a role in the uptake of dietary carotenoids [50, 51]. Cell culture and knockout mouse models have shown that scavenger receptor B1 (SR-B1) [51, 52] and CD36 [53] mediate lutein and zeaxanthin absorption into cells along with other carotenoids and tocopherols [54, 55]. Recently, Lobo *et al.* [56] identified ISX, a gut-specific homeodomain transcription factor that controls SR-B1 and β-carotene 15,15′-monooxygenase (BCO1) messenger RNA (mRNA) expression, suggesting that retinoic acid produced from dietary precursors affects intestinal absorption of carotenoids. The adenosine triphosphate (ATP)-binding cassette G5 (ABCG5) gene, which plays an important role in cholesterol absorption, also helps in lutein absorption along with other lipids [57, 58]. Genetic variation in BCO1 and CD36 can modulate plasma lutein and retinal concentrations [59].

The carotenoids are further transported into the hepatic system by chylomicrons and to the rest of the body tissues by general circulation. In the blood, albumin, low-density lipoprotein (LDL), high-density lipoprotein (HDL), and very low-density lipoprotein (VLDL) play important roles as the carriers of carotenoids to the target tissues [60]. Lutein and zeaxanthin are relatively equally distributed between LDL and HDL [61, 62] with a progressive decrease in the content of lutein and zeaxanthin from light to dense LDL. HDL plays an important role in the transport of macular carotenoids from serum to the retina [63].

Although our understanding of the transport processes of macular carotenoids from the source to sink is still incomplete, the currently available data suggest that the uptake of carotenoids to the retinal pigment epithelium (RPE), a tissue with a moderate concentration of a diverse range of carotenoids [1], probably shares the transport pathway with cholesterol and that HDL and the receptors for HDL such as SR-B1 may be involved in this delivery process (Figure 5.2, Color Supplement). Although not yet proven, we speculate that carotenoids are delivered from the RPE to the retina by the pathway analogous to the one used for retinoid transport that employs inter-photoreceptor retinoid binding protein (IRBP) to facilitate transport of the hydrophobic ligands across the inter-photoreceptor space [64] because retinoids and the macular carotenoids share equal affinities with IRBP [65] as shown in Figure 5.2.

Whenever a tissue exhibits such exquisite selectivity of uptake and long-term stability, specific, high-affinity-binding proteins are almost always involved along with appropriate transport proteins and metabolic enzymes. Our laboratory has been investigating the specific binding proteins for macular carotenoids for a considerable time. Using a classical biochemical approach for protein purification and identification consisting of tissue homogenization and protein solubilization followed by density gradient centrifugation and column chromatography, we identified GSTP1 as the human macular zeaxanthin-binding protein [66, 67]. Pharmacological and spectroscopic studies with human recombinant GSTP1 demonstrated that its interactions with zeaxanthin closely match

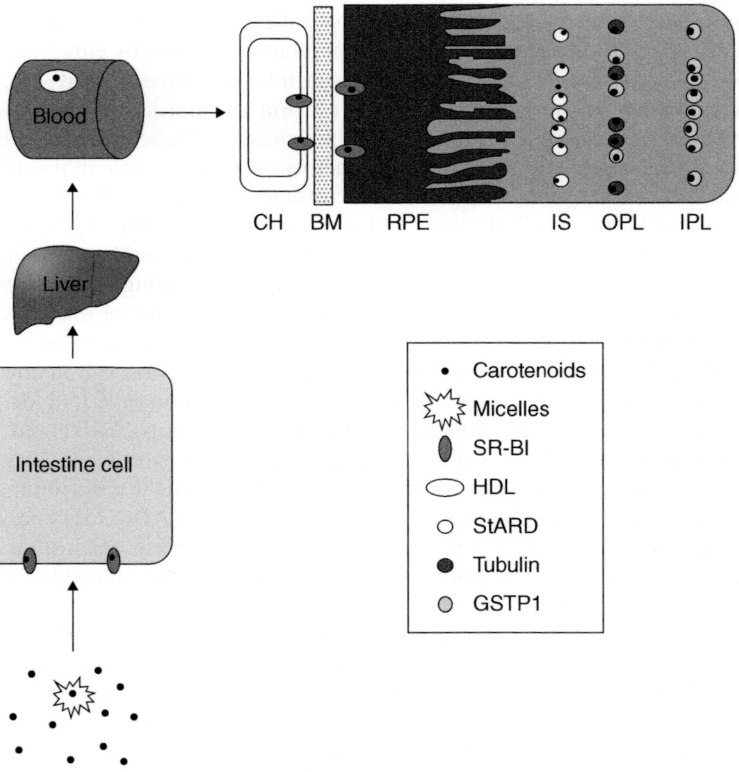

Figure 5.2 Possible pathway for macular carotenoid transport and accumulation in human retina [64] (reproduced by permission of The Royal Society of Chemistry [RSC] on behalf of the European Society for Photobiology, the European Photochemistry Association, and RSC). (*See insert for color representation of the figure.*)

those of the endogenous xanthophyll-binding protein purified from human maculae [66]. Li *et al.* [68] provided evidence to identify StARD3 as the human lutein-binding protein based on database searching, Western blotting and immunohistochemistry. Surface plasma resonance binding assays have confirmed the selective high-affinity binding of GSTP1 with zeaxanthin and *meso*-zeaxanthin and of StARD3 with lutein [69].

5.6 Stereochemistry and metabolism of macular carotenoids

The macular carotenoids lutein and zeaxanthin act as protective antioxidants in the eye, and in certain situations, they undergo oxidation and a series of transformations to protect the macula [1, 70, 71]. Bone *et al.* [72] identified the stereoisomers of lutein and zeaxanthin in human retina using high-performance liquid chromatography–mass spectrometry (HPLC-MS). They are characterized by an internally symmetrical form with a conjugated polyene chain and two terminally hydroxylated ionone rings. Structurally, the macular carotenoids have hydroxyl groups attached at the 3 and 3′ positions of the terminal ionone rings, as shown in Figure 5.3. The position of the double bond in lutein at the 4′, 5′ position is shifted to the 5′, 6′ position in zeaxanthin and *meso*-zeaxanthin, and the double-bond shift in zeaxanthin converts a more chemically reactive allylic hydroxyl end group into a molecule with an extra conjugated double bond. The extra conjugated double bond makes zeaxanthin and *meso*-zeaxanthin more stable and better antioxidants in comparison to lutein.

The lutein component of the macular pigment consists of a single stereoisomer of lutein [(3R, 3′R, 6′R)- β, ε-carotene-3,3′-diol], whereas the zeaxanthin component consists of two

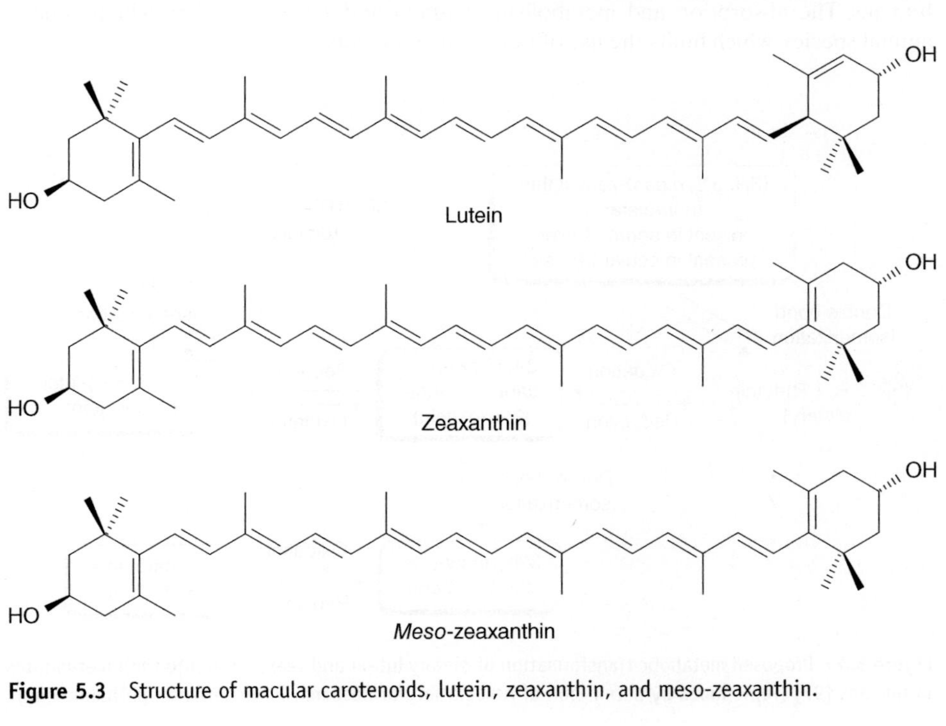

Figure 5.3 Structure of macular carotenoids, lutein, zeaxanthin, and meso-zeaxanthin.

major stereoisomers: dietary zeaxanthin itself [(3R,3′R)-β, β-carotene-3,3′-diol] and nondietary *meso*-zeaxanthin [(3R,3′S)-β, β-carotene-3,3′-diol] [35, 72]. They observed that a base-catalyzed reaction known to isomerize lutein to zeaxanthin yielded only *meso*-zeaxanthin, suggesting that *meso*-zeaxanthin is a conversion product derived from retinal lutein. *meso*-Zeaxanthin was not detected in the human plasma or liver but was present in the human macula, retina, and choroid [1], indicating that there is specific conversion of lutein to *meso*-zeaxanthin in the eye tissue. When xanthophyll-deficient monkeys were supplemented with lutein, both lutein and *meso*-zeaxanthin were incorporated in the retinas, whereas dietary zeaxanthin supplementation resulted solely in the untransformed delivery of zeaxanthin to the retina, further indicating that lutein is the precursor for *meso*-zeaxanthin [73] (Figure 5.4).

Khachik *et al.* [74] first identified oxidation products and isomers of lutein *in vivo*, in human serum. Anhydrolutein and dihydroxy lutein were observed as metabolites of lutein in human breast milk and serum using HPLC-MS [75, 76] and monkey serum [77] formed as a result of dehydration and in acidic conditions similar to those of the stomach using HPLC and LC-MS. 3-Hydroxy β, ε-caroten-3′-one was identified as the direct oxidation product of lutein present in monkey retinas [70], quail ocular tissue [78], chicken [79], rats [80], and human retinas [81], and it was quantified in human retina by Bhosale and Bernstein [82] using HPLC-MS. The presence of the direct oxidation product in the retina confirms *in vivo* metabolic oxidation of retinal lutein [83]. 3-Methoxyzeaxanthin was also identified in the macula of donor eyes using HPLC-MS and was present only in aged donors, indicating that methylation of carotenoids may be an important age-related metabolic pathway [84]. Mein *et al.* [85] identified the formation of apocarotenoids (whose biological functions are unknown) from lutein and zeaxanthin in the presence of β-carotene 9′, 10′ dioxygenase (BCO2). *In vitro* studies using azo compounds and other radicals oxidize lutein to various metabolites [80, 86], but these metabolites are not identified in humans. The absorption and metabolism of lutein and zeaxanthin vary widely among animal species, which limits the use of most animal models.

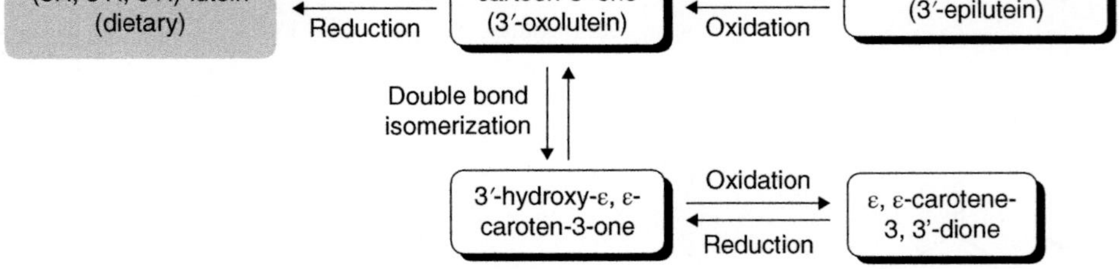

Figure 5.4 Proposed metabolic transformation of dietary lutein and zeaxanthin into their metabolites in humans [97] (reproduced by permission of Association for Research in Vision and Ophthalmology).

Macular pigment remains stable for long periods in humans, but unlike humans, other animal models such as mice do not accumulate macular carotenoids in their eyes even when their serum levels are high. The spatially and chemically specific accumulation of lutein and zeaxanthin in retina is a unique feature of the primate retina relative to other mammals, but the biochemical basis for this high degree of specificity is unclear. Recent studies in our laboratory indicate that human retinal BCO2 is an inactive enzyme, whereas mouse BCO2 is an active carotenoid cleavage enzyme, responsible for eccentric cleavage of carotenes and xanthophylls [87]. Naturally occurring BCO2 mutations in sheep result in yellow flesh due to xanthophyll deposition in various tissues, and bovine BCO2 mutants produce yellow milk [88, 89].

5.7 Measurement of macular carotenoids

Accurate assessment of the amount of macular pigment in eyes is necessary to investigate the role of macular carotenoids and their presumed functions. HPLC is the "gold standard" technique for measurement of carotenoids from extracted samples, but it requires significant amounts of precious biological tissue. Bone *et al.* [4] first used this technique to preliminarily identify the macular carotenoids and they subsequently completed their stereochemical characterization a few years later [72].

In recent years, there has been considerable interest in developing quantitative methods to measure macular pigment optical density (MPOD) noninvasively in humans to facilitate observational and interventional studies of AMD. MPOD can be measured by various reported methods, including heterochromatic flicker photometry (HFP), autofluorescence attenuation imaging (AFI), reflectometry, and resonance Raman spectrometry (RRS). HFP is a psychophysical measure of macular pigment levels that uses advantageously low light levels, but subjects require extensive prior training for reproducible results [90]. The measurement is accomplished by viewing a small circular stimulus that alternates between a test wavelength that is absorbed by the macular pigment and a reference wavelength that is not absorbed [91]. The major downside of heterochromatic flicker photometry is its poor spatial resolution and the fact that its intrasubject variability can be more than 50% [92]. Fundus reflectometry is based on the observation that the spectra of light reflected from central and peripheral retina are different [93]. AFI measures MPOD levels by determining the macular pigment's attenuation of the fluorescence of lipofuscin in the retinal pigment epithelium [94]. More recently, RRS has been developed to measure the MPOD. It is an objective, rapid, sensitive, specific, and highly reproducible method for estimating macular pigment in patients with a wide variety of macular pathological features [92]. It measures the excitation of bond vibrations within molecules, which are directly proportional to the concentration of macular pigment existing in the irradiated area. For measurement, a subject fixes on a 1 mm spot of low-power argon laser light that resonantly excites the macular carotenoids for 0.2 seconds. The intensity of the Raman-scattered light at the carotenoids' conjugated carbon double-bond frequency of 1525 cm^{-1} is quantified after subtraction of the background fluorescence. The use of this technique was first described by Bernstein *et al.* in 1998 in monkey eyes with HPLC confirmation of correlation with tissue levels [95], and the device was soon developed for clinical studies [96]. In our recently published AREDS2 ancillary study, we analyzed MPOD and macular pigment distribution using a dual-wavelength autofluorescence imaging system along with skin carotenoid levels by RRS [28] and found that MPOD did not correlate with skin or serum measurements. This study provided the baseline information regarding lutein and zeaxanthin concentrations in AREDS2 participants.

5.8 Conclusions and perspectives

Evidence suggests that macular carotenoids enhance central vision and are effective in absorption of blue light and filtration of free radical species. Their effective disposition in polyunsaturated phospholipid membranes makes them susceptible to free radical damage; consecutively, they operate as antioxidants. Although studies suggest an inverse relationship between dietary intake of lutein and zeaxanthin and the progression of AMD, correlation studies of MPOD and serum lutein–zeaxanthin levels need further investigation. Supplementation of macular carotenoids to improve visual development and cognition in infants also deserves further study. Recent advancements in the noninvasive quantification of macular pigment density provide a means to gather relevant data, which may strengthen the correlation between carotenoids in tissues and ocular health.

Recent studies in our laboratory indicate that human retinal BCO2 is an inactive enzyme, whereas mouse BCO2 is an active carotenoid cleavage enzyme that is responsible for eccentric cleavage of macular carotenoids, which makes them an unsuitable model for carotenoid studies. Development of suitable animal models for studies on carotenoids could provide valuable information regarding the metabolism of lutein and zeaxanthin in the retina. The discovery of specific binding proteins and genes responsible for concentrating these carotenoids in the macula helps us understand the transport of lutein and zeaxanthin from blood to the retina. Further study into transport proteins and the genes responsible for successful uptake of macular carotenoids into the human body will increase our knowledge regarding healthy aging of the eye.

References

1. F. Khachik, F. F. de Moura, D. Y. Zhao, C. P. Aebischer, and P. S. Bernstein, "Transformations of selected carotenoids in plasma, liver, and ocular tissues of humans and in nonprimate animal models," *Invest. Opthalm. Visual Sci.*, **43**, 11, 3383–92 (2002).
2. R. A. Bone, J. T. Landrum, S. T. Mayne, C. M. Gomez, S. E. Tibor, and E. E. Twaroska, "Macular pigment in donor eyes with and without AMD: a case-control study," *Invest. Opthalm. Visual Sci.*, **42**, 1, 235–40 (2001).
3. D. M. Snodderly, J. D. Auran, and F. C. Delori, "The macular pigment. II. Spatial distribution in primate retinas," *Invest. Opthalm. Visual Sci.*, **25**, 6, 674–85 (1984).
4. R. A. Bone, J. T. Landrum, and S. L. Tarsis, "Preliminary identification of the human macular pigment," *Vision Res.*, **25**, 11, 1531–5 (1985).
5. J. Widomska and W. K. Subczynski, "Why has nature chosen lutein and zeaxanthin to protect the retina?" *J. Clin. Experimental Ophthalm.*, **5**, 1, 326 (2014).
6. J. Gabrielska and W. I. Gruszecki, "Zeaxanthin (dihydroxy-beta-carotene) but not beta-carotene rigidifies lipid membranes: a 1H-NMR study of carotenoid-egg phosphatidylcholine liposomes," *Biochimica Biophys. Acta*, **1285**, 2, 167–74 (1996).
7. A. Sujak, J. Gabrielska, W. Grudzinski, R. Borc, P. Mazurek, and W. I. Gruszecki, "Lutein and zeaxanthin as protectors of lipid membranes against oxidative damage: the structural aspects," *Arch. Biochem. Biophys.*, **371**, 2, 301–7 (1999).
8. W. I. Gruszecki and K. Strzalka, "Carotenoids as modulators of lipid membrane physical properties," *Biochimica Biophys. Acta*, **1740**, 2, 108–15 (2005).
9. R. Croce, S. Weiss, and R. Bassi, "Carotenoid-binding sites of the major light-harvesting complex II of higher plants," *J. Biol. Chem.*, **274**, 42, 29613–23 (1999).

10. Y. Z. Ma, N. E. Holt, X. P. Li, K. K. Niyogi, and G. R. Fleming, "Evidence for direct carotenoid involvement in the regulation of photosynthetic light harvesting," *Proc. Natl. Acad. Sci. USA*, **100**, 8, 4377–82 (2003).

11. Z. Li, T. K. Ahn, T. J. Avenson, M. Ballottari, J. A. Cruz, D. M. Kramer, R. Bassi, G. R. Fleming, J. D. Keasling, and K. K. Niyogi, "Lutein accumulation in the absence of zeaxanthin restores nonphotochemical quenching in the Arabidopsis thaliana npq1 mutant," *Plant Cell*, **21**, 6, 1798–812 (2009).

12. L. Dall'Osto, C. Lico, J. Alric, G. Giuliano, M. Havaux, and R. Bassi, "Lutein is needed for efficient chlorophyll triplet quenching in the major LHCII antenna complex of higher plants and effective photoprotection in vivo under strong light," *BMC Plant Biol.*, **6**, 32 (2006).

13. P. R. Trumbo and K. C. Ellwood, "Lutein and zeaxanthin intakes and risk of age-related macular degeneration and cataracts: an evaluation using the Food and Drug Administration's evidence-based review system for health claims," *Amer. J. Clin. Nutr.*, **84**, 5, 971–4 (2006).

14. S. J. Fliesler and R. E. Anderson, "Chemistry and metabolism of lipids in the vertebrate retina," *Prog. Lipid Res.*, **22**, 2, 79–131 (1983).

15. B. Li, F. Ahmed, and P. S. Bernstein, "Studies on the singlet oxygen scavenging mechanism of human macular pigment," *Arch. Biochem. Biophys.*, **504**, 1, 56–60 (2010).

16. C. C. Trevithick-Sutton, C. S. Foote, M. Collins, and J. R. Trevithick, "The retinal carotenoids zeaxanthin and lutein scavenge superoxide and hydroxyl radicals: a chemiluminescence and ESR study," *Molecular Vis.*, **12**, 1127–35 (2006).

17. P. S. Bernstein, D. Y. Zhao, S. W. Wintch, I. V. Ermakov, R. W. McClane, and W. Gellermann, "Resonance Raman measurement of macular carotenoids in normal subjects and in age-related macular degeneration patients," *Ophthalmology*, **109**, 10, 1780–7 (2002).

18. J. M. Seddon, U. A. Ajani, R. D. Sperduto, R. Hiller, N. Blair, T. C. Burton, M. D. Farber, E. S. Gragoudas, J. Haller, D. T. Miller, *et al.*, "Dietary carotenoids, vitamins A, C, and E, and advanced age-related macular degeneration. Eye Disease Case-Control Study Group," *JAMA*, **272**, 18, 1413–20 (1994).

19. J. Curran-Celentano, B. R. Hammond, Jr., T. A. Ciulla, D. A. Cooper, L. M. Pratt, and R. B. Danis, "Relation between dietary intake, serum concentrations, and retinal concentrations of lutein and zeaxanthin in adults in a Midwest population," *Amer. J. Clin. Nutr.*, **74**, 6, 796–802 (2001).

20. E. E. Connolly, S. Beatty, J. Loughman, A. N. Howard, M. S. Louw, and J. M. Nolan, "Supplementation with all three macular carotenoids: response, stability, and safety," *Invest. Opthalm. Visual Sci.*, **52**, 12, 9207–17 (2011).

21. F. M. Barker, 2nd, D. M. Snodderly, E. J. Johnson, W. Schalch, W. Koepcke, J. Gerss, and M. Neuringer, "Nutritional manipulation of primate retinas, V: effects of lutein, zeaxanthin, and n-3 fatty acids on retinal sensitivity to blue-light-induced damage," *Invest. Opthalm. Visual Sci.*, **52**, 7, 3934–42 (2011).

22. S. M. Moeller, N. Parekh, L. Tinker, C. Ritenbaugh, B. Blodi, R. B. Wallace, J. A. Mares, and Group CRS, "Associations between intermediate age-related macular degeneration and lutein and zeaxanthin in the Carotenoids in Age-related Eye Disease Study (CAREDS): ancillary study of the Women's Health Initiative," *Arch. Ophthalm.*, **124**, 8, 1151–62 (2006).

23. J. S. Tan, J. J. Wang, V. Flood, E. Rochtchina, W. Smith, and P. Mitchell, "Dietary antioxidants and the long-term incidence of age-related macular degeneration: the Blue Mountains Eye Study," *Ophthalmology*, **115**, 2, 334–41 (2008).

24. Age-Related Eye Disease Study Research Group, J. P. SanGiovanni, E. Y Chew, T. E. Clemons, F. L. Ferris 3rd, G. Gensler, A. S. Lindblad, R. C. Milton, J. M. Seddon, and

R. D. Sperduto, "The relationship of dietary carotenoid and vitamin A, E, and C intake with age-related macular degeneration in a case-control study: AREDS Report No. 22," *Arch. Ophthalm.*, **125**, 9, 1225–32 (2007).

25. J. A. Mares, T. L. LaRowe, D. M. Snodderly, S. M. Moeller, M. J. Gruber, M. L. Klein, B. R. Wooten, E. J. Johnson, R. J. Chappell, Group CMPS, *et al.*, "Predictors of optical density of lutein and zeaxanthin in retinas of older women in the Carotenoids in Age-Related Eye Disease Study, an ancillary study of the Women's Health Initiative," *Amer. J. Clin. Nutr.*, **84**, 5, 1107–22 (2006).
26. T. L. LaRowe, J. A. Mares, D. M. Snodderly, M. L. Klein, B. R. Wooten, R. Chappell, and Group CMPS, "Macular pigment density and age-related maculopathy in the Carotenoids in Age-Related Eye Disease Study. An ancillary study of the women's health initiative," *Ophthalmology*, **115**, 5, 876–83, e871 (2008).
27. C. J. Hammond, S. H. Liew, F. J. Van Kuijk, S. Beatty, J. M. Nolan, T. D. Spector, and C. E. Gilbert, "The heritability of macular response to supplemental lutein and zeaxanthin: a classic twin study," *Invest. Opthalm. Visual Sci.*, **53**, 8, 4963–8 (2012).
28. P. S. Bernstein, Ahmed F, Liu A, Allman S, Sheng X, Sharifzadeh M, I. Ermakov, W. Gellermann, "Macular pigment imaging in AREDS2 participants: an ancillary study of AREDS2 subjects enrolled at the Moran Eye Center," *Invest. Opthalm. Visual Sci.*, **53**, 10, 6178–86 (2012).
29. AR Group, E. Y Chew, T. Clemons, J. P. SanGiovanni, R. Danis, A. Domalpally, W. McBee, R. Sperduto, and F. L. Ferris, "The Age-Related Eye Disease Study 2 (AREDS2): study design and baseline characteristics (AREDS2 report number 1)," *Ophthalmology*, **119**, 11, 2282–9 (2012).
30. Age-Related Eye Disease Study 2 Research Group, E. Y Chew, J. P. SanGiovanni, F. L. Ferris, W. T. Wong, E. Agron, T. E. Clemons, R. Sperduto, R. Danis, S. R. Chandra, *et al.*, "Lutein/zeaxanthin for the treatment of age-related cataract: AREDS2 randomized trial report no. 4," *JAMA Opthalm.*, **131**, 7, 843–50 (2013).
31. Age-Related Eye Disease Study 2 Research G, E. Y Chew, T. E. Clemons, J. P. Sangiovanni, R. P. Danis, F. L. Ferris 3rd, M. J. Elman, A. N. Antoszyk, A. J. Ruby, D. Orth, *et al.*, "Secondary analyses of the effects of lutein/zeaxanthin on age-related macular degeneration progression: AREDS2 report No. 3," *JAMA Opthalm.*, **132**, 2, 142–9 (2014).
32. M. E. Aronow and E. Y Chew, "Age-related Eye Disease Study 2: perspectives, recommendations, and unanswered questions," *Curr. Opin. Opthalm.*, **25**, 3, 186–90 (2014).
33. R. A. Bone, J. T. Landrum, L. Fernandez, and S. L. Tarsis, "Analysis of the macular pigment by HPLC: retinal distribution and age study," *Invest. Opthalm. Visual Sci.*, **29**, 6, 843–9 (1988).
34. J. P. Zimmer and B. R. Hammond, Jr., "Possible influences of lutein and zeaxanthin on the developing retina," *Clinical Opthalm.*, **1**, 1, 25–35 (2007).
35. R. A. Bone, J. T. Landrum, L. M. Friedes, C. M. Gomez, M. D. Kilburn, E. Menendez, I. Vidal, and W. Wang, "Distribution of lutein and zeaxanthin stereoisomers in the human retina," *Exper. Eye Res.*, **64**, 2, 211–18 (1997).
36. L. P. Rubin, G. M. Chan, B. M. Barrett-Reis, A. B. Fulton, R. M. Hansen, T. L. Ashmeade, J. S. Oliver, A. D. Mackey, R. A. Dimmit, E. E. Hartmann, *et al.*, "Effect of carotenoid supplementation on plasma carotenoids, inflammation and visual development in preterm infants," *J. Perinatol.*, **32**, 6, 418–24 (2012).
37. I. Y. Leung, M. M. Sandstrom, C. L. Zucker, M. Neuringer, and D. M. Snodderly, "Nutritional manipulation of primate retinas, II: effects of age, n-3 fatty acids, lutein, and zeaxanthin on retinal pigment epithelium," *Invest. Opthalm. Visual Sci.*, **45**, 9, 3244–56 (2004).

38. M. R. Malinow, L. Feeney-Burns, L. H. Peterson, M. L. Klein, and M. Neuringer, "Diet-related macular anomalies in monkeys," *Invest. Opthalm. Visual Sci.*, **19**, 8, 857–63 (1980).

39. B. J. Song, Z. E. Jouni, and M. G. Ferruzzi, "Assessment of phytochemical content in human milk during different stages of lactation," *Nutrition*, **29**, 1, 195–202 (2013).

40. V. C. Jewell, C. B. Mayes, T. R. Tubman, C. A. Northrop-Clewes, and D. I. Thurnham, "A comparison of lutein and zeaxanthin concentrations in formula and human milk samples from Northern Ireland mothers," *Euro. J. Clin. Nutr.*, **58**, 1, 90–7 (2004).

41. B. S. Henriksen, G. Chan, R. O. Hoffman, M. Sharifzadeh, I. V. Ermakov, W. Gellermann, and P. S. Bernstein, "Interrelationships between maternal carotenoid status and newborn infant macular pigment optical density and carotenoid status," *Invest. Opthalm. Visual Sci.*, **54**, 8, 5568–78 (2013).

42. P. Vachali, P. Bhosale, and P. S. Bernstein, "Microbial carotenoids," *Methods Mol. Biol.*, **898**, 41–59 (2012).

43. D. B. Rodriguez-Amaya, "Food carotenoids: analysis, composition and alterations during storage and processing of foods," *Forum Nutr.*, **56**, 35–7 (2003).

44. A. During and E. H. Harrison, "Intestinal absorption and metabolism of carotenoids: insights from cell culture," *Arch. Biochem. Biophys.*, **430**, 1, 77–88 (2004).

45. P. Riso, A. Brusamolino, S. Ciappellano, and M. Porrini, "Comparison of lutein bioavailability from vegetables and supplement," *Intl. J. Vitamin Nutr. Res.*, **73**, 3, 201–5 (2003).

46. K. L. Molldrem, J. Li, P. W. Simon, and S. A. Tanumihardjo, "Lutein and beta-carotene from lutein-containing yellow carrots are bioavailable in humans," *Amer. J. Clin. Nutr.*, **80**, 1, 131–6 (2004).

47. H. Y. Chung, H. M. Rasmussen, and E. J. Johnson, "Lutein bioavailability is higher from lutein-enriched eggs than from supplements and spinach in men," *J. Nutr.*, **134**, 8, 1887–93 (2004).

48. K. J. Yeum and R. M. Russell, "Carotenoid bioavailability and bioconversion," *Ann. Rev. Nutr.*, **22**, 483–504 (2002).

49. B. S. Mamatha and V. Baskaran, "Effect of micellar lipids, dietary fiber and beta-carotene on lutein bioavailability in aged rats with lutein deficiency," *Nutrition*, **27**, 9, 960–6 (2011).

50. P. Borel, "Factors affecting intestinal absorption of highly lipophilic food microconstituents (fat-soluble vitamins, carotenoids and phytosterols)," *Clin. Chem. Lab. Med.*, **41**, 8, 979–94 (2003).

51. E. Reboul, L. Abou, C. Mikail, O. Ghiringhelli, M. Andre, H. Portugal, D. Jourdheuil-Rahmani, M. J. Amiot, D. Lairon, and P. Borel, "Lutein transport by Caco-2 TC-7 cells occurs partly by a facilitated process involving the scavenger receptor class B type I (SR-BI)," *Biochem. J.*, **387**, Pt. 2, 455–61 (2005).

52. A. van Bennekum, M. Werder, S. T. Thuahnai, C. H. Han, P. Duong, D. L. Williams, P. Wettstein, G. Schulthess, M. C. Phillips, and H. Hauser, "Class B scavenger receptor-mediated intestinal absorption of dietary beta-carotene and cholesterol," *Biochemistry*, **44**, 11, 4517–25 (2005).

53. M. Moussa, E. Gouranton, B. Gleize, C. E. Yazidi, I. Niot, P. Besnard, P. Borel, and J. F. Landrier, "CD36 is involved in lycopene and lutein uptake by adipocytes and adipose tissue cultures," *Mol. Nutr. Food Res.*, **55**, 4, 578–84 (2011).

54. P. Borel, Lietz G, Goncalves A, Szabo de Edelenyi F, Lecompte S, Curtis P, Goumidi L, Caslake MJ, Miles EA, Packard C, *et al.*, "CD36 and SR-BI are involved in cellular uptake of provitamin A carotenoids by Caco-2 and HEK cells, and some of their genetic variants are associated with plasma concentrations of these micronutrients in humans," *J. Nutr.*, **143**, 4, 448–56 (2013).

55. E. Reboul, Klein A, Bietrix F, Gleize B, Malezet-Desmoulins C, Schneider M, Margotat A, Lagrost L, Collet X, and P. Borel, "Scavenger receptor class B type I (SR-BI) is involved in vitamin E transport across the enterocyte," *J. Biol. Chem.*, **281**, 8, 4739–45 (2006).

56. G. P. Lobo, S. Hessel, A. Eichinger, N. Noy, A. R. Moise, A. Wyss, K. Palczewski, and J. von Lintig, "ISX is a retinoic acid-sensitive gatekeeper that controls intestinal beta, beta-carotene absorption and vitamin A production," *FASEB J.*, **24**, 6, 1656–66 (2010).

57. E. Kotake-Nara and A. Nagao, "Absorption and metabolism of xanthophylls," *Marine Drugs*, **9**, 6, 1024–37 (2011).

58. K. L. Herron, M. M. McGrane, D. Waters, I. E. Lofgren, R. M. Clark, J. M. Ordovas, and M. L. Fernandez, "The ABCG5 polymorphism contributes to individual responses to dietary cholesterol and carotenoids in eggs," *J. Nutr.*, **136**, 5, 1161–5 (2006).

59. P. Borel, de F. S. Edelenyi, Vincent-Baudry S, Malezet-Desmoulin C, Margotat A, Lyan B, Gorrand JM, Meunier N, Drouault-Holowacz S, and Bieuvelet S, "Genetic variants in BCMO1 and CD36 are associated with plasma lutein concentrations and macular pigment optical density in humans," *Annals Med.*, **43**, 1, 47–59 (2011).

60. E. Loane, J. M. Nolan, O. O'Donovan, P. Bhosale, P. S. Bernstein, and S. Beatty, "Transport and retinal capture of lutein and zeaxanthin with reference to age-related macular degeneration," *Survey Ophthalm.*, **53**, 1, 68–81 (2008).

61. J. W. Erdman, Jr., T. L. Bierer, and E. T. Gugger, "Absorption and transport of carotenoids," *Annals NY Acad. Sci.*, **691**, 76–85 (1993).

62. S. Goulinet and M. J. Chapman, "Plasma LDL and HDL subspecies are heterogenous in particle content of tocopherols and oxygenated and hydrocarbon carotenoids. Relevance to oxidative resistance and atherogenesis," *Arterioscler. Thromb. Vasc. Biol.*, **17**, 4, 786–96 (1997).

63. E. Loane, J. M. Nolan, and S. Beatty, "The respective relationships between lipoprotein profile, macular pigment optical density, and serum concentrations of lutein and zeaxanthin," *Invest. Opthalm. Visual Sci.*, **51**, 11, 5897–905 (2010).

64. B. Li, P. Vachali, and P. S. Bernstein, "Human ocular carotenoid-binding proteins," *Photochem. Photobiol. Sci.*, **9**, 11, 1418–25 (2010).

65. P. Vachali, B. M. Besch, F. Gonzalez-Fernandez, and P. S. Bernstein, "Carotenoids as possible interphotoreceptor retinoid-binding protein (IRBP) ligands: a surface plasmon resonance (SPR) based study," *Arch. Biochem. Biophys.*, **539**, 2, 181–6 (2013).

66. P. Bhosale, A. J. Larson, J. M. Frederick, K. Southwick, C. D. Thulin, and P. S. Bernstein, "Identification and characterization of a Pi isoform of glutathione S-transferase (GSTP1) as a zeaxanthin-binding protein in the macula of the human eye," *J. Biol. Chem.*, **279**, 47, 49447–54 (2004).

67. P. Bhosale and P. S. Bernstein, "Vertebrate and invertebrate carotenoid-binding proteins," *Arch. Biochem. Biophys.*, **458**, 2, 121–7 (2007).

68. B. Li, P. Vachali, J. M. Frederick, and P. S. Bernstein, "Identification of StARD3 as a lutein-binding protein in the macula of the primate retina," *Biochemistry*, **50**, 13, 2541–9 (2011).

69. P. Vachali, B. Li, K. Nelson, and P. S. Bernstein, "Surface plasmon resonance (SPR) studies on the interactions of carotenoids and their binding proteins," *Arch. Biochem. Biophys.*, **519**, 1, 32–7 (2012).

70. F. Khachik, P. S. Bernstein, and D. L. Garland, "Identification of lutein and zeaxanthin oxidation products in human and monkey retinas," *Invest. Opthalm. Visual Sci.*, **38**, 9, 1802–11 (1997).

71. F. Khachik, "An efficient conversion of (3R,3′R,6′R)-lutein to (3R,3′S,6′R)-lutein (3′-epilutein) and (3R,3′R)-zeaxanthin," *J. Natl. Prod.*, **66**, 1, 67–72 (2003).

72. R. A. Bone, J. T. Landrum, G. W. Hime, A. Cains, and J. Zamor, "Stereochemistry of the human macular carotenoids," *Invest. Opthalm. Visual Sci.*, **34**, 6, 2033–40 (1993).

73. E. J. Johnson, M. Neuringer, R. M. Russell, W. Schalch, and D. M. Snodderly, "Nutritional manipulation of primate retinas, III: Effects of lutein or zeaxanthin supplementation on adipose tissue and retina of xanthophyll-free monkeys," *Invest. Opthalm. Visual Sci.*, **46**, 2, 692–702 (2005).

74. F. Khachik, G. R. Beecher, M. B. Goli, W. R. Lusby, and J. C. Smith, Jr., "Separation and identification of carotenoids and their oxidation products in the extracts of human plasma," *Analytical Chem.*, **64**, 18, 2111–22 (1992).

75. F. Khachik, G. Englert, G. R. Beecher, and J. C. Smith, Jr., "Isolation, structural elucidation, and partial synthesis of lutein dehydration products in extracts from human plasma," *J. Chromatog. B, Biomed. Appl.*, **670**, 2, 219–33 (1995).

76. F. Khachik, C. J. Spangler, J. C. Smith, Jr., L. M. Canfield, A. Steck, and H. Pfander, "Identification, quantification, and relative concentrations of carotenoids and their metabolites in human milk and serum," *Anal. Chem.*, **69**, 10, 1873–81 (1997).

77. G. I. Albert, U. Hoeller, J. Schierle, M. Neuringer, E. J. Johnson, and W. Schalch, "Metabolism of lutein and zeaxanthin in rhesus monkeys: identification of (3R,6′R)- and (3R,6′S)-3′-dehydro-lutein as common metabolites and comparison to humans," *Compar. Biochem. Physiol. B*, **151**, 1, 70–8 (2008).

78. P. Bhosale, B. Serban, Y. Zhao da, and P. S. Bernstein, "Identification and metabolic transformations of carotenoids in ocular tissues of the Japanese quail *Coturnix japonica*," *Biochemistry*, **46**, 31, 9050–7 (2007).

79. J. K. Tyczkowski, J. L. Schaeffer, C. Parkhurst, and P. B. Hamilton, "3′-Oxolutein, a metabolite of lutein in chickens," *Poultry Sci.*, **65**, 11, 2135–41 (1986).

80. R. Lakshminarayana, G. Aruna, R. K. Sangeetha, N. Bhaskar, S. Divakar, and V. Baskaran, "Possible degradation/biotransformation of lutein in vitro and in vivo: isolation and structural elucidation of lutein metabolites by HPLC and LC-MS (atmospheric pressure chemical ionization)," *Free Radical Biol. Med.*, **45**, 7, 982–93 (2008).

81. P. S. Bernstein, F. Khachik, L. S. Carvalho, G. J. Muir, D. Y. Zhao, and N. B. Katz, "Identification and quantitation of carotenoids and their metabolites in the tissues of the human eye," *Exper. Eye Res.*, **72**, 3, 215–23 (2001).

82. P. Bhosale and P. S. Bernstein, "Quantitative measurement of 3′-oxolutein from human retina by normal-phase high-performance liquid chromatography coupled to atmospheric pressure chemical ionization mass spectrometry," *Anal. Biochem.*, **345**, 2, 296–301 (2005).

83. S. Beatty, M. Boulton, D. Henson, H. H. Koh, and I. J. Murray, "Macular pigment and age related macular degeneration," *Brit. J. Ophthalm.*, **83**, 7, 867–77 (1999).

84. P. Bhosale, D. Y. Zhao, B. Serban, and P. S. Bernstein, "Identification of 3-methoxyzeaxanthin as a novel age-related carotenoid metabolite in the human macula," *Invest. Opthalm. Visual Sci.*, **48**, 4, 1435–40 (2007).

85. J. R. Mein, G. G. Dolnikowski, H. Ernst, R. M. Russell, and X. D. Wang, "Enzymatic formation of apo-carotenoids from the xanthophyll carotenoids lutein, zeaxanthin and beta-cryptoxanthin by ferret carotene-9′,10'-monooxygenase," *Arch. Biochem. Biophys.*, **506**, 1, 109–21 (2011).

86. A. A. Woodall, S. W. Lee, R. J. Weesie, M. J. Jackson, and G. Britton, "Oxidation of carotenoids by free radicals: relationship between structure and reactivity," *Biochimica Biophys. Acta*, **1336**, 1, 33–42 (1997).

87. B. Li, P. Vachali, A. Gorusupudi, Z. Shen, H. Sharifzadeh, B. M. Besch, K. Nelson, M. M. Horvath, J. M. Frederick, W. Baehr, *et al.*, "Inactivity of human beta, beta-

carotene-9',10'-dioxygenase (BCO2) underlies retinal accumulation of the human macular carotenoid pigment," *Proc. Natl. Acad. Sci. USA*, **111**, 28, 10173–8 (2014).

88. S. D. Berry, S. R. Davis, E. M. Beattie, N. L. Thomas, A. K. Burrett, H. E. Ward, A. M. Stanfield, M. Biswas, A. E. Ankersmit-Udy, P. E. Oxley, *et al.*, "Mutation in bovine beta-carotene oxygenase 2 affects milk color," *Genetics*, **182**, 3, 923–6 (2009).
89. D. I. Vage and I. A. Boman, "A nonsense mutation in the beta-carotene oxygenase 2 (BCO2) gene is tightly associated with accumulation of carotenoids in adipose tissue in sheep (*Ovis aries*)," *BMC Genet.*, **11**, 10 (2010).
90. K. Neelam, N. O'Gorman, J. Nolan, O. O'Donovan, H. B. Wong, K. G. Au Eong, and S. Beatty, "Measurement of macular pigment: Raman spectroscopy versus heterochromatic flicker photometry," *Invest. Opthalm. Visual Sci.*, **46**, 3, 1023–32 (2005).
91. B. R. Wooten, B. R. Hammond, Jr., R. I. Land, and D. M. Snodderly, "A practical method for measuring macular pigment optical density," *Invest. Opthalm. Visual Sci.*, **40**, 11, 2481–9 (1999).
92. P. S. Bernstein and W. Gellermann, "Measurement of carotenoids in the living primate eye using resonance Raman spectroscopy," *Methods Mol. Biol.*, **196**, 321–9 (2002).
93. J. van de Kraats, T. T. Berendschot, S. Valen, and D. van Norren, "Fast assessment of the central macular pigment density with natural pupil using the macular pigment reflectometer," *J. Biomed. Optics*, **11**, 6, 064031 (2006).
94. F. C. Delori, D. G. Goger, B. R. Hammond, D. M. Snodderly, and S. A. Burns, "Macular pigment density measured by autofluorescence spectrometry: comparison with reflectometry and heterochromatic flicker photometry," *J. Optic. Soc. Amer. A*, **18**, 6, 1212–30 (2001).
95. P. S. Bernstein, M. D. Yoshida, N. B. Katz, R. W. McClane, and W. Gellermann, "Raman detection of macular carotenoid pigments in intact human retina," *Invest. Opthalm. Visual Sci.*, **39**, 11, 2003–11 (1998).
96. D. Y. Zhao, S. W. Wintch, I. V. Ermakov, W. Gellermann, and P. S. Bernstein, "Resonance Raman measurement of macular carotenoids in retinal, choroidal, and macular dystrophies," *Arch. Ophthalm.*, **121**, 7, 967–72 (2003).
97. F. Khachik, F. F. de Moura, E. Y Chew, L. W. Douglass, F. L. Ferris 3rd, J. Kim, and D. J. Thompson, "The effect of lutein and zeaxanthin supplementation on metabolites of these carotenoids in the serum of persons aged 60 or older," *Invest. Opthalm. Visual Sci.* 2006, **47**, 12, 5234–42.

Part II

Spectroscopy

6 Vibrational Spectroscopy as a Tool to Investigate Carotenoids

Jan Cz. Dobrowolski

Institute of Chemistry and Nuclear Technology, and National Medicines Institute, Warsaw, Poland

6.1 Introduction

The chapter is composed of two parts: The first one focuses on the principal factors that determine the vibrational spectra of carotenoids, and the second focuses on vibrational spectroscopy studies published after 2008 devoted to natural carotenoids in bacteria, lichens, and algae, as well as in geological deposits, biominerals, and even art and archaeological objects. The chapter ends with a brief comment on possible future applications of new vibrational spectroscopy techniques in the investigation of carotenoids.

6.2 Vibrations of carotenoids

Carotenoids are built from a polyene chain most often terminated with one or two cyclic end groups. The chain is formally derivable from the acyclic lycopene, and the end groups are either oxygenated (in xanthophylls) or not (in carotenes). Usually, methyl groups are attached to every fifth carbon atom of the polyene chain [1]. The exceptional vibrational spectroscopy properties of carotenoids originate primarily from the polyene chain and only secondarily from the methyls and the end groups. Therefore, let us first have a closer look at the properties and optical spectroscopy of polyene chains.

Due to specific carotenoid biosynthesis pathways in plants and carotenogenic bacteria [2], the chain in carotenes usually has an odd number (from 3 to 13) of conjugated C=C double bonds. In addition, the bonds may be conjugated with the other C=C or C=O double bonds of the end groups [3]. The number n of the conjugated C=C double bonds

Carotenoids: Nutrition, Analysis and Technology, First Edition. Edited by Agnieszka Kaczor and Malgorzata Baranska.

has direct consequences on the following carotenoid features: (1) geometry; (2) geometrical *cis-trans* isomerism; (3) syn-periplanar (s-*cis*) or anti-periplanar (s-*trans*) conformation at single bonds; (4) π-electron delocalization; (5) the nature, shape, and energy of the electronic ground and excited states; (6) electron affinity, ionization, reduction, and oxidation potentials; (7) the nature and shape of molecular vibrations and the vibrational coupling pattern; and so on. Finally, the end groups and (8) the methyl groups attached to the polyene chain also play a role. Clearly, all these factors exert a potent influence on optical molecular spectra of polyenes and carotenoids.

6.2.1 Geometry

The alteration of single and double bonds in conjugated all-*trans* polyenes results in the double bond's elongation and the synchronous single bond's shortening by about twice as much as the double bond lengthens. The changes with n are not linear. The path contributions to both the single bonds and the double bonds decay exponentially with n with the same decay constant [4]. The conjugation effects extend out through approximately six neighboring double bonds. Thus, a polyene bond is the most significantly influenced by the neighboring six conjugated double bonds. Importantly, several polyene properties, such as band gaps [5] and characteristic ultraviolet (UV) and vibrational frequencies [6–8], extrapolate smoothly as an inverse of conjugation length unless the number of double bonds exceeds seven. Thus, conjugation through at least six bonds probably determines the properties of polyenes and carotenoids [4]. The decay in the bond length alternation with respect to the length of the polyene chain is also observed for regularly altering *cis-trans* types of configurations; however, the decay is slightly slower and the point of convergence is slightly higher than for all-*trans* isomers [9].

6.2.2 Geometrical *cis-trans* isomerism

The presence of n-conjugated bonds in the polyene chain theoretically enables the formation of 2^n geometrical *cis-trans* isomers. However, desaturases catalyzing the formation of all-*trans* lycopene and further carotenoids from 15-*cis*-phytoene in the carotenoid biosynthetic pathways are additionally mediating in a single *cis*-to-*trans* isomerization [2, 10]. The enzymes favor the formation of only selected geometrical isomers, simultaneously restricting the presence of a possible plethora of *cis-trans* isomers in biosystems [2]. Yet, biotic as well as abiotic stress such as heat, light, acidic environment, enzymatic or nonenzymatic oxidation, or the presence of an active surface may promote *trans*-to-*cis* carotenoid isomerization in both plant and animal tissue. Notice that the presence of a double bond of a *cis* configuration in an "almost-all-*trans*" polyene chain perturbs the single- and double-bond distances, the regularity of bond alteration changes, and the conditions necessary for π-electron delocalization. When considering the idealized all-*cis* and all-*trans* structures in the different forms in which they may be present in polyacetylene polymers, we find that they exhibit varying geometrical, and thus electrical and spectroscopic, features [11]. However, in natural carotenoids, there are at most only a few *cis* moieties in the polyene chain [12–14] and considering the *cis* structures in full generality is not necessary. Since the *cis*- and *trans*-isomers of carotenoids exhibit different bioactivities and bioavailabilities (e.g., [15]), it is important to quantify their geometrical isomers in plants, animals, food, and human tissues [16–18].

6.2.3 Syn-periplanar (s-*cis*) or anti-periplanar (s-*trans*) conformations

Hypothetically, there is also a possibility of carotenoids adopting syn-periplanar (s-*cis*) or anti-periplanar (s-*trans*) arrangements at each of the (n–1) single bonds separating the conjugated double bonds, which would again increase the number of conformers by 2^{n-1}. However, the presence of s-*cis* or s-*trans* conformers in carotenoids is stirred up only scarcely. This is because the s-*trans* conformation of double bonds in a *trans* configuration minimizes the steric hindrance of the neighboring fragments [3]. Nevertheless, the s-*cis* conformation was reported in β-ionone and retinals [19], as well as in spiralene: A *cis* conjugated triene isomer exists in the bis-s-*cis* conformation [20]. It was also demonstrated that the 7-*cis*,8-s-*cis* okenone isomer's nuclear magnetic resonance (NMR) and electronic absorption spectra exhibit regions clearly different than that of the 7-*cis* isomer, whereas the resonance Raman spectra are barely distinguishable [21]. Again, one should consider the s-*cis* and s-*trans* polyenes in general and discuss the consequences of the formation of (s-*trans*)-*trans*, (s-*cis*)-*trans*, (s-*trans*)-*cis*, and (s-*cis*)-*cis* as well as mixed types of polyene conformers [11]. However, although such a discussion is of great importance to conducting polymers chemistry [22, 23], it can be restricted to only one or a few particular bonds in the case of the chemistry of (natural) carotenoids.

6.2.4 π-electron delocalization

The all-*trans* configuration of the polyene chain establishes good conditions for π-electron delocalization. They are manifested in the decrease of the bond length alternation as the length of the chain is increased but also in a significant energetic stabilization, estimated to approach in long chains ca. 8 kcal/mol per double bond [4]. Interestingly, the path contributions to the stabilization energy decay exponentially with respect to n with the same decay constant as the geometric parameters [4]. The slower decay in the bond length alternation in all-*cis* isomers than in all-*trans* ones indicates a decreased electron delocalization in the *cis* chains compared to the *trans* ones [24].

6.2.5 The nature, shape, and energy of the electronic ground and excited states

The increasing π-electron delocalization in the all-*trans* polyenes results in the shift of transition energies to lower energies with increasing conjugations, which can be expressed approximately by $\Delta E = a/n + b$. One of the most important consequences of the conjugation is that the low-energy, symmetry-forbidden $1^1A_g^- \rightarrow 2^1A_g^-$ transition lies below the strongly allowed $1^1A_g^- \rightarrow 1^1B_u^+$ transitions associated with the transfer of an electron from HOMO (highest occupied molecular orbital) to LUMO (lowest unoccupied molecular orbital) [25–27]. As a consequence, in long polyene systems, emissions from the low-lying $2^1A_g^-$ state are often dominated by nonradiative decay processes. Considering energy gaps between several different excited states in polyenes leads to the conclusion that they follow similar trends, linear with $1/n$ [28]. The magnitude of the $S_0 \rightarrow S_2$ ($1^1A_g^- \rightarrow 1^1B_u^+$) energy gap has important consequences for the polyene Raman scattering because there is a linear correlation between the ν_1 Raman band wavenumber and the electronic transition energy [29].

6.2.6 Electron affinity, ionization, reduction, and oxidation potentials

The longer the polyene chain, the higher the electron affinity and the lower the ionization potential. Analogously, the reduction potentials are higher and the oxidation potentials are lower [30]. As before, the trends are nearly linear with $1/n$. For polyene radical cations, the energy of the first two excited configurations decreases and the energy gap between them gets smaller [31]. Thus, the linear polyene-conjugated molecules are effective electron donors and thereby good antiradicals and antioxidants [32]. Yellow and red carotenoids are also good antiradicals because they are effective electron acceptors and simultaneously good antireductants [32]. In polyene radical cations, both spin and charge are delocalized over the entire chain with maxima at the central bonds [31]. The bond length alternation in radicals and radical cations follows the same trends as in neutral closed-shell polyenes [33]. The vertical excitation energies obtained for the five lowest excited states of linear polyenyl radical cations decrease regularly with the chain lengths [33]. The electron paramagnetic resonance (EPR) and electron nuclear double resonance (ENDOR) parameters of carotenoid radicals indicate a polyene π-cation radical structure where the unpaired electron is delocalized throughout the entire carbon backbone [34, 35]. The resonance Raman study of carotenoid cation radicals exhibits the frequencies of the characteristic C=C stretchings as decreased by 30–40 cm^{-1}, whereas those of C–C stretchings increased by 15–30 cm^{-1}, which also suggests the delocalization of unpaired electron density throughout the entire polyene chain [36].

6.2.7 The nature and shape of molecular vibrations and vibrational coupling patterns

Understanding the vibrational spectra of polyenes requires the consideration of three basic facts: the C_{2h} symmetry of the (idealized) all-*trans* isomers, the increase in the number of vibrational modes by 3 with each added C=C bond in the conjugated chain, and the facilitation of the UV-Vis resonance conditions as the electronic states gap is narrowed with increasing n. The C_{2h} symmetry of the all-*trans* structure means that the polyene has a symmetry center, the infrared (IR) active modes are silent in Raman scattering, and conversely the Raman active modes are silent in the IR absorption spectra. For a finite all-*trans* polyene of n double bonds, there are $12n$ normal modes out of which the in-plane vibrations belong to the $A_g(4n+1)$ and $B_u(4n)$ irreducible representations and the remaining $4n+1$ out-of-plane modes belong to the $A_u(2n)$ and $B_g(2n+1)$ irreducible representations [37]. The A_g and B_g modes are active in the Raman scattering, and the A_u and B_u ones are active in the IR spectra. Taking into account the number of nodes formed by the alternations of stretches and contractions [38], the analysis of the band position with increasing n demonstrates an increasingly complex pattern [37]. However, the normal mode analysis for the infinite *trans*- and *cis*-polyacetylene chains [39, 40] juxtaposed with the experimental IR [41] and Raman spectra [42, 43] shows that for the all-*trans* polyacetylene, one can consider only five Raman ($4A_g+B_g$) and three IR (A_u+2B_u) active modes. On the other hand, four bands are usually considered in the vibrational spectra of natural carotenoids [44]: ν_1 located at ca. 1500–1530 cm^{-1}, primarily assigned to the C=C stretching vibrations; ν_2 placed at ca. 1150–1160 cm^{-1}, mainly assigned to the C–C stretching vibrations; ν_3 at ca. 1000 cm^{-1}, assigned to the in-plane rocking vibrations of the CH_3 groups attached to the conjugated chain coupled with the in-plane bending vibrations of the adjacent C–H bonds; and ν_4 at ca. 960 cm^{-1}, assigned to the C–H out-of-plane wagging vibrations coupled with the C=C out-of-plane torsional twists of the carbon backbone [44, 45]. The frequencies of ν_1 and ν_2 decrease nearly linearly with $1/n$ and intercorrelate [6, 44]. The ν_2 region (1100–1300 cm') is very sensitive and unique to the *cis-trans* configuration of the chain [46]. The Raman ν_1 and ν_2 bands shift along with the change of energy gap between the electronic states [6]. Moreover, the intensity ratio of the Raman ν_1 and ν_2 bands in a thick trans-polyacetylene film increases significantly as the incident laser line changes from 647.1 nm through 488.0 nm to 350.7 nm [47]. Even at a single exciting line frequency, the Raman activity of the ν_1 (and some other modes) increases rapidly as the number of double bonds exceeds nine, and the IR intensity of this band also increases rapidly with n (Figure 6.1) [38, 48–50].

6.2.8 The role of methyl groups attached to the polyene chain and the end groups

In contrast to the unsubstituted all-*trans* polyenes, the carotenoids are not strictly linear but have a slightly bowing, S-shaped form of the chain. This is a result of the steric hindrance between the methyl groups distributed along the chain. The curvature of the polyene chain in β-carotene with the methyl groups on the convex side was already stated in the mid-1960s based on X-ray studies [51, 52] and was observed earlier for the shorter chain in retinoic acid [53]. Today, it is well documented that the polyene chain methyl groups of each half of β-carotene and other all-*trans* C_{40} carotenoids are arranged on opposite sides of the chain, and there is a pronounced S-shape of the polyene chain to minimize steric hindrance [54–59]. It was demonstrated that, along with the decreasing number of methyl groups linked to the conjugated carbon chain, the ν_1 mode is practically unaffected, the ν_2 mode shows a downshift when the number of methyl groups decreases, whereas the ν_4 mode is upshifted and its intensity is decreased [59]. Recently, the ν_4 Raman mode in synthetic and natural coral polyenes has been carefully studied [60]. It has been shown that the methyl groups connected to the conjugated chain of carotenoids induce a splitting of the ν_1 Raman band [29].

Although the conformation of the end groups is not a primary factor determining the vibrational spectrum of carotenoids, it affects the carotenoid's ability to selectively bind to proteins [61, 62], the ground and excited states' geometries and electronic spectra [63, 64], and the vibrational spectra [65, 66]. Studies have pointed out that similar rotational-angle dependencies of the ν_1 and ν_2 mode frequencies in the β-carotene prove the contribution of the C=C stretch vibrations to the ν_2 mode and that the β-rings play an important role in ν_2 Raman and IR bands, especially for the all-*trans* isomer [65]. Also, it has been demonstrated that lycopene's greater pressure effect on the ν_1 frequency compared to β-carotene can be ascribed to the β-ring rotation, which relieves the pressure effect on the C=C bond length [67].

6.3 Recent applications of vibrational spectroscopy to study natural carotenoids

The vibrational spectroscopy techniques are mainly used to study natural carotenoids in plant, animal, and human tissues; in food; in geological deposits and biominerals; in art and archaeological objects; and in material chemistry samples. Quite a number of vibrational spectroscopy papers on carotenoids are also devoted to problems related to their physical

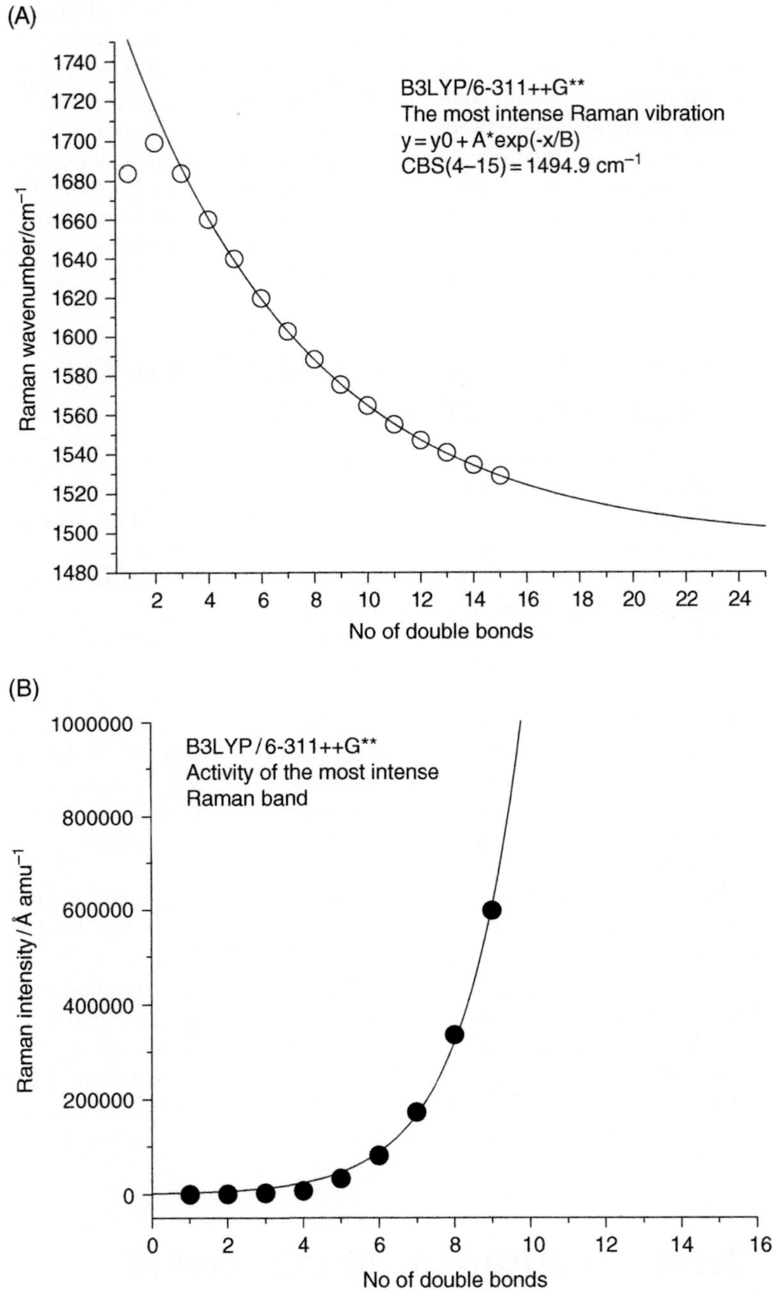

Figure 6.1 Decrease of the wavelength (A) and increase of the intensity (B) of the most intense ν_1 Raman band as function of the number of double bonds in all-*trans*-polyenes calculated at the B3LYP/6-311++G** level. Reproduced from Ref. [50] with kind permission of Wiley-Liss, Inc.

chemistry and the spectroscopy itself. In this review, we will mainly focus on papers published after 2008 on bacteria and algae, including those found in geological deposits, biominerals, art, and archaeological objects. The topics related to carotenoids in plant, animal, and human tissues will be covered in detail in Chapters 2 and 8. Several important reviews have been published recently on Raman spectroscopy analysis of carotenoids in biological samples [14], the use of resonance Raman technique in the field of photosynthesis [68], the possibility for noninvasive online measuring of carotenoids in skin by using resonance Raman spectroscopy [69], measuring macular pigment (lutein, zeaxanthin, and meso-zeaxanthin) and optical density using Raman spectroscopy [70], the use of Raman imaging in diagnostics of human breast cancer [71], the applications of Raman spectroscopy (but also of mass spectrometry and NMR) in diagnosing and healing cancers [72], the application of Raman spectroscopy to determine the role of carotenoids in biological membranes [73], recent progress in enhancing signals in different Raman techniques for the *in vivo* analysis of individual living cells [74], the application of Raman spectroscopy for the analysis of carotenoids in oocytes [75], Raman spectroscopy as one of the analytical tools for the analysis of carotenoids in diverse materials [76], the use of Raman spectroscopy in the analysis of algae [77], and the potential of Raman spectroscopy in the study of selected plant metabolites, including carotenoids, in plants, algae, lichens, and fungi [78].

6.3.1 Bacteria lichens and algae

The effectiveness of Raman spectroscopy for *in situ* analysis in plants, algae, and bacteria is repeatedly emphasized in many papers. Different analytical approaches requiring the time-consuming isolation of unstable carotenoid molecules extracted from horse chestnut, mahaleb cherry, large-leaved linden, and sallow pollen were compared with *in situ* Raman analysis of the $\nu_1 \div \nu_6$ as well as the overtone and combination carotenoid bands [79]. This comparison proves the Raman technique's advantage of including spectral features that arise from the association of carotenoid molecules with the biological matrix. It has also been demonstrated that observing the $\nu_1 \div \nu_4$ Raman bands can serve as an alternative method to high-performance liquid chromatography (HPLC) and UV-Vis for the quantification of carotenoids in *Blakeslea trispora*, a fungal plant pathogen used for the commercial production of β-carotene, and similar organisms [80]. The ν_1 Raman bands of carotenoids present in two algal species, *Chlorella sorokiniana* and *Neochloris oleoabundans*, both considered to be viable candidates for the production of biofuels, allowed for identifying compounds of interest (and triglycerides) within a single cell down to a few microns and drawing up chemical maps of the compounds using confocal Raman microscopy [81]. The *Klebsormidium flaccidum* algal cells, encapsulated within silica gels, were shown to maintain their ability to form an intracellular suspension with gold nanoparticles and to reduce gold salts by *in situ* Raman imaging of entrapped cells, and thus to preserve photosynthetic activity [82]. The carotenoids were detected by observing the $\nu_1 \div \nu_3$ Raman bands and 514 and 633 nm excitation lines. The gold nanoparticles most likely additionally enhanced the signals of carotenoids by the surface-enhanced Raman spectroscopy (SERS) effect. Research suggests that the coupling of sol–gel encapsulation and Raman imaging should allow for the future development of novel photosynthesis-based cellular biosensors.

6.3.1.1 Bacteria Dynamic processes caused by the high-temperature treatment of single spores of *Bacillus cereus*, *Bacillus megaterium*, and *Bacillus subtilis* were monitored by observing the carotenoids' ν_1 and ν_2 Raman bands, present in the inner membranes of spores, by using dual-trap laser tweezers Raman spectroscopy (LTRS) and elastic light scattering

(ELS) [83]. Changes in the intensity of the ν_1 and ν_2 bands possibly reflect changes in the environment and structure of the spore's inner membrane during thermal treatment.

It was demonstrated that by using a micro-Raman spectrometer equipped with 785 and 514.5 nm laser lines, it is possible to discriminate Gram-positive and Gram-negative plant bacteria [84]. Indeed, none of the studied Gram-negative bacteria exhibited the carotenoid bands, and all had the tyrosine peak at 1170–1175 cm^{-1}. However, the Gram-positive bacteria had strong ν_1 and ν_2 carotenoid bands and exhibited no tyrosine band. Moreover, the carotenoid bands in different species of Gram-positive bacteria exhibit different intensities and sensitivities for inducing the resonance spectrum by changing the exciting line from red to green. The bacteria of the genus *Xanthomonas* were selectively identified by an exclusively specific xanthomonadin carotenoid exhibiting ν_1 and ν_2 scattering at 1529–1531 cm^{-1} and at 1135–1136 cm^{-1}, respectively. Along with a discussion of other discriminative spectral features of *Xanthomonas*, It was concluded that Raman spectroscopy of bacteria may be a valuable method in understanding plant–bacteria interactions at the cellular level [84].

The structural analysis of single living cyanobacterial cells of *Thermosynechococcus elongatus*, which are too photolabile to be measured with visible laser excitation, was successfully executed using a multichannel near-infrared (NIR)–Raman microspectrometer using an incident beam of 1064 nm and an InP–InGaAsP multichannel detector [85]. Three basic pigments, β-carotene, chlorophyll *a*, and phycocyanin, were mapped *in vivo* in single living cells with lateral and depth resolutions of 0.7 μm and 3.1 μm, respectively, and no appreciable interference from autofluorescence or photodamage.

The CH combination Raman band range of 2750–2500 cm^{-1} was used to discriminate two types of flexirubins, natural non-isoprenoid aryl-polyene carboxylic acid esters, and carotenoids in colonies and cell extracts of *Flavobacterium johnsoniae* and *Flexibacter elegans* bacteria [86]. The colonies of bacteria containing flexirubrin-type pigments exhibit an immediate color shift from yellow to orange or red, purple, or brown, and revert to their initial color when flooded with acidic solution. However, such a color change is not specific to flexirubin pigments, whereas using Raman spectroscopy can be a more reliable test for chemotaxonomically relevant flexirubins.

Distinct bands obtained in coherent anti-Stokes Raman-scattering (CARS) spectra of cyanobacteria *Nostoc commune*, *Nostoc* sp. of cyanobacterias, and *Chlorella* sp. of green algae were assigned to carotenoids and used as spectral markers for imaging accumulation and the movement of chemical compounds at the subcellular level [87]. It was shown that despite the strength of the two-photon-excitation fluorescence signal generated by microalgae and cyanobacteria in CARS measurements, it can be effectively suppressed.

The Raman microspectroscopic imaging also served for the investigation of aggregation and biofilm development of *Rhodococcus* sp. [88]. It has been shown that as the biofilm develops, the intracellular concentration of carotenoids increases over threefold within a week and accumulates throughout the biofilm.

Carotenoids in red, extremely halophilic (salt-loving) Archaea prokaryotes (*Halobacterium salinarum*, *Halorubrum sodomense*, and *Haloarcula valismortis*) and *Salinibacter ruber* bacteria were investigated by Raman spectroscopy using a 514.5 nm excitation line [89]. Bacterioruberin, a 50-carbon carotenoid, was detected as the major carotenoid in all archaeal strains, whereas *Salinibacter* contains salinixanthin, a C_{40}-carotenoid acyl glycoside, for which the Raman bands assignments were given for the first time.

Selective *in vivo* detection of conformers of diadinoxanthin and diatoxanthin in intact *Cyclotella* cells has been performed using resonance Raman spectroscopy [90]. In addition, the discrimination between different pools of diadinoxanthin and their fate as a function of the illumination conditions is possible thanks to Raman spectronomy. Cells grown in high-light conditions adopt a more twisted diadinoxanthin conformation than those grown in low-light conditions. Thus, in high-light conditions, the pool of diadinoxanthin is most likely tightly bound to a protein-binding site.

6.3.1.2 Lichen Sixteen lichen, symbiotic organisms composed of a fungus and photosynthetic green algae or cyanobacteria (specimens growing on new basaltic lava fields and wood substrates), were analyzed by Raman spectroscopy [91]. Except for chlorophyll, the analysis indicated the presence of lutein or astaxanthin and a variety of other protective pigments, such as atranorin, usnic acid, gyrophoric acid, parietin, and pulvinic acid dilactone. Studies propose several survival strategies adopted by extremophile lichens to combat radiation insolation, desiccation, and high temperatures.

6.3.1.3 Algae Raman imaging was shown to be a selective and sensitive method for *in situ* and *in vivo* monitoring of astaxanthin distribution in the cyst form of *Haematococcus pluvialis* [92]. Also, the thermal stress on *H. pluvialis* can be analyzed *in situ* in a single cell as well as in a multicellular algal sample by Raman spectroscopy techniques (Figure 6.2, Color Supplement) [93]. The temperature change from −100 °C to 150 °C produces a significant shift of the ν_1 Raman band accompanied by intensity changes of several bands. These changes are in line with the discrete Fourier transform (DFT) predicted conformer population changes due to the mutual arrangement of the end rings. It was suggested that astaxanthin initially bound in the H-form aggregates in the *trans* arrangement of the end rings and that thermal stress on algae converts it into the more stable *gauche* form [93].

The Raman analysis combined with multivariate hyperspectral analysis provide enough information to successfully perform the Raman analysis of carotenoid pigments in algal species [94]. It was shown that even though the reference spectrum of carotenoids differed from the mixture of carotenoids present in the algae, the target orthogonal partial-least-squares method provides enough information to make a reliable imaging.

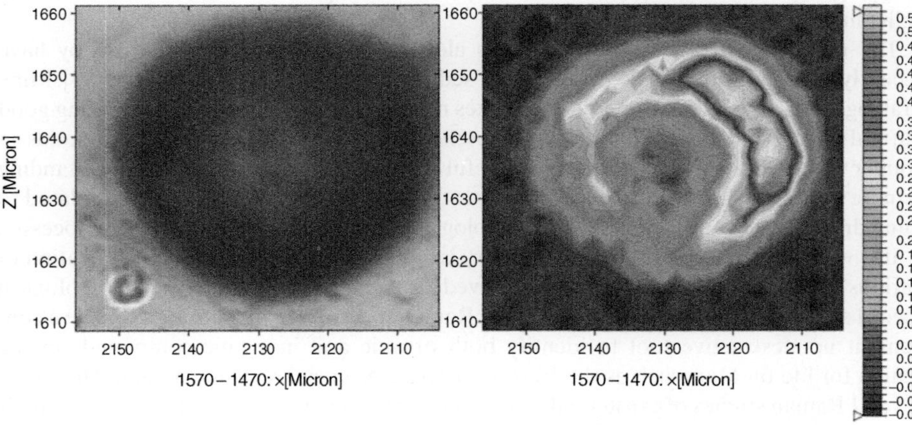

Figure 6.2 A visual image focused inside of the *Haematococcus pluvialis* cell with the collapsed cytoplasm (on the left, magnification 40×) and distribution of astaxanthin (AXT) in the sample (on the right) obtained by integration of the marker band at 1520 cm^{-1} (color code defined in the scale). The map was obtained by measuring 729 points (the distance between points on the *x* and *z* axes equals 2.0 μm). Reproduced from Ref. [93] with kind permission of Analyst Owner Societies. (*See insert for color representation of the figure.*)

The confocal Raman microscopy combined with multivariate analysis have been used for monitoring of astaxanthin and β-carotene in green *H. pluvialis* microalgae [95]. It was emphasized that, thanks to the chemometric techniques used, the resonance Raman bands of astaxanthin and β-carotene were resolved from the fluorescence of chlorophyll. Therefore, the simultaneous and separate monitoring of the two carotenoids was possible in various stages of the life cycle of the living cells. Interestingly, astaxanthin was identified within globular and punctuate regions of the cytoplasmic space, and β-carotene within both the chloroplast and astaxanthin in the cytosol.

The Raman microspectroscopic technique was used for assessing the β-carotene concentration in algal lipid bodies *in vivo*. It was demonstrated that the β-carotene concentration can be proportional to the volume of lipid bodies and light intensity during the cultivation [96]. The Raman microscopy can be useful to select rare natural mutants or genetically modified cells with desirable biotechnological characteristics.

Resonance Raman spectra of intact filamentous bodies in siphonous green algae, *Codium* (*C.*) *intricatum*, cultured under high- and low-light conditions to achieve high siphonaxanthin (a specific carotenoid) content, demonstrated an accumulation of all-*trans* neoxanthin (accompanied by the accumulation of violaxanthin and α-carotene) under high-irradiance conditions in addition to the normal 9'-*cis* neoxanthin form present in the whole-cell extract [97]. Based on variations of the concentrations of carotenes, a plausible model for cell adaptation to high-light conditions has been proposed.

6.3.1.4 Organisms in extreme environments Raman *in situ* chemical mapping demonstrated that in the extreme environments of the Arabian Gulf salt flats, dolomite is precipitated from microbial extracellular polymeric substances (EPS) [98]. The EPS bands at 1000, 1150, 1510, and 1130 cm^{-1} were widely distributed in the top 2 cm of the sediments. The former three bands were assigned to the $\nu_1 \div \nu_3$ Raman bands of astaxanthin, and the latter to polysaccharides. The mapping indicated dolomite clusters smaller than 2 μm embedded in a dense cyanobacterial EPS matrix. The study demonstrated the Raman mapping to be a robust and sensitive technique for the acquisition of *in situ* information on cell–mineral interactions.

The $\nu_1 \div \nu_3$ Raman bands of carotenoids along with luminescence spectroscopy have recently been used for the direct analysis of sediments from the Rio Tinto Basin [99]. Mine drainages can generate carotenoid complexes mixed with copper sulfates, presenting good natural models for the production of carotenoids from microorganisms. Carotenoids in copper sulfates have been shown to be useful biomarkers and proxies for understanding remote mineral formation as well as for terrestrial environmental investigations related to mine drainage contamination, including biological activity and photo-oxidation processes.

It is well known that Raman spectrometry is a powerful tool for the characterization of various biomarkers, organic minerals derived from biological activity in the geological record and minerals themselves. This is why Raman spectroscopy is considered to be a convenient nondestructive tool to identify both organic and inorganic compounds in the search for life on Mars such as the European Space Agency ExoMars mission. Therefore, several Raman studies of carotenoids have recently been performed in the context of their usefulness in identification of microbial life on Mars [100–103]. To this aim, the lowest β-carotene content detectable with Raman microspectrometry in experimentally prepared evaporitic gypsum, halite, and epsomite matrices was tested using laser beam resonant (514.5 nm) and nonresonant (785 nm) lines for carotenoids [100, 101]. The limit was found to be 0.1 to 10 mg/kg, depending on the particular mineral matrix and the excitation wavelength. Concentrations of β-carotene of circa one order of magnitude higher were identified when the matrices were analyzed through single crystals of gypsum and epsomite.

The objective of recent studies was also the optimization and development of the best measurement routines for the identification of β-carotene in cyanobacteria and various minerals with a Raman spectrometer under Mars analog conditions in different types of Martian soils [102].

Recently, in the context of astrobiological prospecting, the NIR–Raman spectra of carotenoids from fossilized microbes were analyzed [103]. The first Raman spectra were acquired from perhydro derivatives of β-carotene and lycopene formed by hydrogenation of the polyene chain during diagenesis (i.e., changes to the rock's original mineralogy and texture). This resulted in much less specific fossil hydrocarbons, such as chain-saturated β-carotene and lycopene. It has been proposed that diagenetically altered carotenoids formed by hydrogenation reactions during the fossilization processes also provide unique diagnostic spectra that can be interpreted as a biological signature.

The chemical compositions of four Middle Eocene iron ore types were investigated by means of micro-Raman spectroscopy [104]. The high spatial resolution and sensitivity of the method allowed for the identification of not only minerals but also the presence of carotenoids, demonstrating that the formation of some types of ironstone was biologically mediated. Raman spectroscopy is considered to be a powerful technique for the identification of both organic and inorganic substances in the studied iron ore deposits.

6.3.2 Corals and pearls

Vibrational spectroscopy has also found a wide application in geoscience and in particular in gemology [105]. Raman spectroscopy is especially useful in the identification of organic pigments such as carotenoids in corals and pearls that are of importance to mineralogy [106], biological sciences [107], and the jewelry market [108, 109]. Indeed, the potency of *in situ* resonance Raman spectroscopy for the identification of the polyenic origin of a large range of colors in shells and corals was already shown in the mid-1980s [110]. Studies found that the number of conjugated double bonds in the pigments of studied specimens varied from 7 to 17.

Raman and IR measurements were performed to explain the origin of the vivid red color in precious pink and red corals [50]. The DFT calculations demonstrated that at the location of the ν_1 Raman band, the Raman activities of the characteristic modes depend significantly on the number of double bonds in the *trans* configuration. This was the basis for the conclusion that two to three polyenes differing slightly in the number of double bonds are the sources of the color in pink and red corals.

The nature of the pigments found in three Brazilian octocorals, *Chromonephthea braziliensis*, *Leptogorgia punicea*, and *Leptogorgia violacea*, has been investigated by Raman spectroscopy using 632.8 and 1064 nm laser excitation lines [111]. Based on the observed positions of the ν_1 and ν_2 Raman polyene bands, it was suggested that the bands originate from a mixture of parrodienes (conjugated polyenes) rather than carotenoids.

Phyllogorgia dilatata, a Brazilian endemic gorgonian (an order of colonian coral known as sea whips or sea fans) with a natural color ranging from white to pale yellow, was studied by *in situ* Raman spectroscopy [112]. It was found that an unusual violet pigmentation surrounding tissue necrosis appeared in response to fungus infection and allelopathic interactions. The Raman analysis of the healthy white-cream tissues revealed the presence of the peridinin, typical of the endosymbiont that harbors this species. However, this pigment was not observed in the colorless sclerites that exclusively presented calcite bands. In contrast, the violet coloration of damaged tissue was assigned to psittacofulvins, which are lipid-soluble pigments usually present in parrots' feathers.

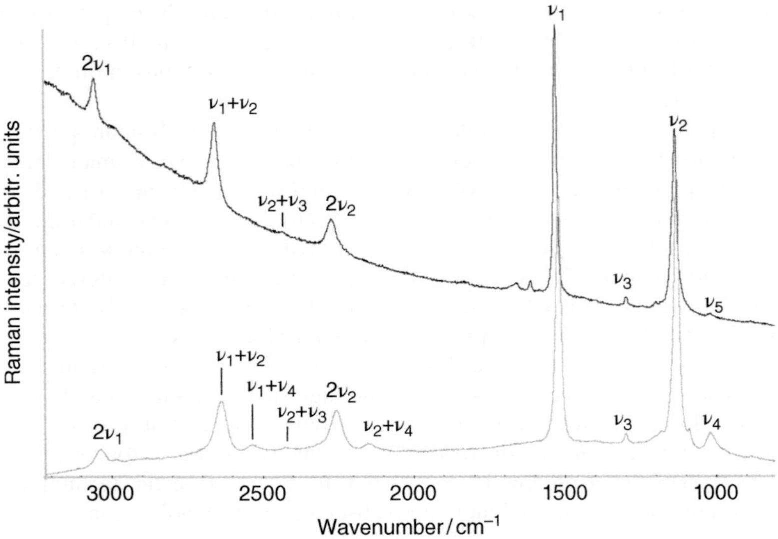

Figure 6.3 Raman spectra (lexc = 514.5 nm) of *Corallium rubrum* (black) and of a red feather of a parrot (grey scale). The assignments of fundamentals, overtones, and combination lines are labeled. The observation of the binary combinations $\nu_1 + \nu_4$ and $\nu_2 + \nu_4$ in the spectrum of *Corallium rubrum* indicates that the polyconjugated chain contains $-CH_3$ groups. Reproduced from Ref. [59] with kind permission of Wiley-Liss, Inc.

The observation of two ν_1, ν_2, and ν_3 Raman polyene bands using the 532, 785, and 1064 nm laser excitation lines allowed Maia *et al.* to distinguish between carotenoids and non-methylated conjugated polyenals in *Phyllogorgia dilatata*, *Leptogorgia punicea*, *Muricea atlantica*, and *Carijoa riisei* octocorals [113].

The Raman measurements of the $\nu_1 \div \nu_3$ Raman polyene bands of *in situ* and crude extracts of *Tubastraea coccinea* and *Tubastraea tagusensis* orange cup corals permitted the identification of astaxanthin, whereas the band at circa 1665 cm^{-1} to identify the imino-imidazolinone aplysinopsin alkaloid [114]. The crude extracts were demonstrated to have antioxidant activity that may protect corals against light-induced oxidative damage.

The $\nu_1 \div \nu_3$, but also ν_4 and ν_5, as well as overtone and combination Raman bands of *Corallium rubrum*, canthaxantin, and parrot feather pigments, were analyzed with the support of DFT calculations (Figure 6.3) [59]. It was demonstrated that because the main pigment of *Corallium rubrum* possessed neither a fully demethylated polyene chain nor a tetramethylated chain, as in carotenoids, the chain is partially methylated.

A comparison of the Raman spectra of synthetic (demethylated at the chain) analogs of natural conjugated polyenals found in octocorals has shown that in the resonance Raman spectra, the ν_1 and ν_2 bands were enhanced. However, the ν_2 band was only enhanced if the methyl groups were attached to the main chain, as is the case in carotenoids. The ν_2 band was absent in resonance condition if these groups were not attached to the chain as in parrodienes [60]. In the latter case, the methyl groups are, however, observed in the non-resonance Raman spectra. Moreover, in the synthetic polyene without methyls attached to the chain, the overtones and combination bands in carotenoids involving the ν_4 mode do not appear in resonance Raman spectra and are present at a slightly different position.

The Raman spectra for 30 untreated, freshwater-cultured pearls from the mollusk *Hyriopsiscumingi* were recorded using seven excitation lines (1064 nm, 676.44 nm,

647.14 nm, 514.53 nm, 487.98 nm, 457.94 nm, and 363.80 nm) [115]. Regardless of the specific hue of the pearls, aside from the white ones, the ν_1 and ν_2 polyene bands were observed. The position of the ν_1 band indicated, however, that the polyenes did not belong to the carotenoid family. Moreover, the shape and intensity of the ν_1 and ν_2 polyene bands also varied with the sample. Similar changes were observed upon changing the excitation lines. A band-fitting routine applied to the spectra obtained by changing excitation lines allowed to choose from four to nine different polyene pigments of the general formula R–(–CH=CH–)$_n$–R', where n=6 to 14, to be present in colorful pearls. Different colors corresponded to different mixtures of pigments rather than a single pigment change. Similar coloration mechanisms have been proposed to explain the origin of, for example, parrots' feathers. Similar results were obtained for pearls from *Hyriopsis schlegeli* [116], where the Raman spectra allowed assigning the pigments as noncarotenoids and also, supposedly, psittacofulvins. Importantly, a correspondence between Raman and diffuse reflectance spectra of freshwater-cultured pearls was also established.

Monitoring the effects on the accumulation of astaxanthin in the pearl oyster *Pinctada martensii*'s shells caused by its addition into the oyster's bait was performed using micro-Raman and HPLC methods [117]. The over-tenfold greater accumulation of astaxanthin (or astaxanthin esters) in the fed group than in the control not only provides the basis for colorful pearl cultivation via foodborne transmission, but also lays down a foundation for artificial regulation and control of pearl color.

Resonance and near-resonance micro-Raman spectroscopy was used to study organic pigments contained in carbonate polymorphs (vaterite and aragonite) present in freshwater-cultured pearls from Japan and China [118]. The use of four different excitation lines (487.9, 514.5, 532.2, and 632.8 nm) enabled one to identify 10 different pigments as unmethylated polyenes with chain lengths ranging from 8 to 12. Additionally, methylated polyenes were also detected for the first time together with unmethylated pigments in aragonite. Polyenes with chain lengths shorter than 8 or longer than 12 were not found in vaterite, whereas both shorter and longer pigment chains were observed in aragonite from the same pearls. Thus, pigments have lower concentrations, exhibit chain lengths from 8 to 12, and are distributed more homogeneously in vaterite than in aragonite, in which higher concentrations are arranged along the annual growth lines of the pearls, and pigments with shorter and longer chains are also present.

The nature of the coral and pearl pigments contained in calcite and aragonite was studied by means of Raman spectroscopy using a 473.1 nm excitation line and four basic polyene bands as well as overtones and combination modes [119]. Despite the meticulous analysis performed, it seems that the question of the relative importance of methylated and nonmethylated polyenes for the calcite- and aragonite-based organisms has remained unsolved.

Recently, a study on the coloration mechanism in cultured freshwater pearls from the mollusk *Hyriopsis cumingii* was performed by Raman scattering, IR spectroscopy, and plasma emission spectroscopy [120]. It was found that the pearls' colors are due to the presence of both pigments and trace elements. The concentration of polyenic pigments without methyl groups (of approximate CHO–(–CH=CH–)$_{10}$–OCH$_2$OH formula) and Ti, Ag, Mg, and Zn ions in the purple pearls is higher than in orange pearls.

Quite recently 60 precious gems, including pearls and corals, and colored glass fitted in a shield of silver Torah from the Jewish Museum in Prague have been unambiguously identified using portable Raman spectrometers equipped with lasers emitting 785 nm and 532 nm excitation lines [121]. The rather chaotic mixture of stones of various colors, cuts, and sizes as well as the total volume of imitation glass have supported a hypothesis that the gems were gathered from Jewish households and donated for the adornment of the shield.

The common portable Raman instruments are very convenient nondestructive tools for quick *in situ* identifications of gemstones mounted in historical artifacts in museums and collection sites.

6.3.3 Art and archeology

Dyes (including carotenoids) are among the most significant components in works of art and archaeological findings. Newly developed and improved analytical procedures and techniques for the characterization of organic dyes and their identification in microsamples have recently been reviewed [122]. The procedures, which describe both the chemical composition of natural organic dyeing materials used in the field of the cultural heritage and spectrometric and chromatographic techniques, have been hailed as the most valuable recent contribution to the study of organic dyes in works of art and archaeological findings.

The Raman and SERS analyses of Cape Jasmine (*Gardenia augusta* L.) at three different excitation wavelengths (633, 785, and 1064 nm), both with and without acid hydrolysis, had their effectiveness evaluated [123]. Raman bands at 1537, 1209, and 1165 cm^{-1} were selected as discriminating markers for the crocetin and crocin yellow colorants in dyed-on alum-mordanted wool, dyed-on nonmordanted and alum-mordanted silk, pigment precipitated on hydrated aluminum oxide, and extract mixed with a protein binder and painted on glass, and as a water-based glaze applied on a mockup of a typical Chinese wall painting. It was shown that in the case of Cape Jasmine dyes, the Raman spectroscopy offered a competitive alternative to the comparatively classical HPLC–photodiode array analytical protocols.

Twenty-five natural organic dyes used in antiquity, especially for dyeing textiles, and nine pure chromophores were analyzed by SERS spectroscopy on Ag colloids to build a wide database for the identification of dyes in archaeological fabric samples [124]. Spectra of 11 dyes—dragon's blood, sandalwood, annatto (containing bixin and crocetin carotenoids, dyes for cotton, silk, and wool), safflower yellow and red, old fustic, gamboge, catechu, kamala, aloe, and sap green—were never previously registered. The efficiency of the SERS analysis of organic dyes used in archaeological textiles has been remarkably improved.

The colonization of wall paintings by microorganisms is a serious problem in the field of art conservation. Confocal Raman microscopy (785 and 514 nm excitation lasers) was used to characterize the main carotenoids in brown stains or patinas on the wall painting in the atrium of Pompeian Marcus Lucretius House [125]. Raman imaging and depth profiling were also used to determine the distribution of biosynthesized carotenoids in the stains, as well as to determine the thickness of the brown patinas. Raman bands related to carotenoids ranging from 1000 cm^{-1} to 1600 cm^{-1} were also identified in the wall paintings of two Pompeian houses excavated 150 years ago that have since been mostly exposed outdoors [126]. This has provided a proof of biological activity on the walls.

The black stains threatening the rock-art paintings of Lascaux Cave were also analyzed by the SERS technique [127]. The stains were mainly composed of melanin from the fungus *Ochroconis* sp. and the fecal pellets of the collembolan *Folsomia candida*; however, the appearance of bands at 1534 and 1159 cm^{-1} also proved a presence of carotenoid compounds in the samples. It was concluded that SERS is a useful method for cultural heritage research.

The endolithic traces on stone monuments and natural outcrops, due to current and past biological colonizations in temperate and Mediterranean bioclimates, were identified by Raman spectroscopy to obtain biomarkers, such as scytonemin, anthraquinone compounds, and carotenoids, to help describe the strategies adopted by cyanobacteria, fungi, and lichens to wither strong UV radiation and dry conditions [128]. Importantly, the biological origin of these deterioration phenomena is often not recognized and is confused with abiotic damages. Indeed, different geomarkers, such as goethite and lepidocrocite, are caused by the mobilization of iron by lichen metabolic activity. Importantly, traces of endolithic microorganisms have not been heretofore discovered on stone monuments located in temperate and Mediterranean bioclimates, where climate conditions are extreme.

Recently, Raman, micro-FTIR, and X-ray fluorescence analyses allowed for the complex characterization of the pictorial palette, the inks, the support, and the material used in a previous restoration treatment of *Codex Rossanensis*, a sixth-century Byzantine illuminated manuscript written on purple parchment and conserved at the Museo Diocesano in Rossano Calabro, Italy [129]. The codex is one of the oldest surviving illuminated manuscripts of the New Testament. Out of four classes of dyes considered, the saffron dye containing crocetin carotenoid was detected in the manuscript. However, a novelty investigation has been the first experimental evidence for the use of the anthocyanines-containing elderberry lake in a sixth-century illuminated manuscript.

6.4 Perspectives

There are three main sources of progress in the use of vibrational spectroscopy methods to investigate carotenoids in diverse environments: the discovery of new and improvement of old vibrational spectroscopy techniques; steady improvements in computer hardware and chemometric methods and software; and the discovery of new carotenoids or examination of previously unexplored features of known carotenoids. Significant progress in quantum chemistry methods, development, and the accessibility of computational chemistry software, as well as improvements in tools for handling and processing computational data, have also significantly contributed to the progress of applied vibrational spectroscopy methods.

Advances in Raman spectroscopy have been recently reviewed by Nafie [130]. For perspectives in carotenoid studies, it is worth noting that the usage of SERS techniques and biological and biomedical application of Raman spectroscopy have increased significantly. The number of applications in art and archeology, pharmaceutical sciences, and forensic analyses, as well as the use of resonance, time-resolved, and nonlinear spectroscopy methods, have significantly increased over the last decade as well.

For carotenoids, the SERS technique has recently been used in art and archeology studies [123, 124], and in material chemistry for silica-encapsulated micro-algae [82]. Thus, the expansion of SERS applications will certainly herald an advance in its use in the analysis and mapping of carotenoids in various environments, including biological and biomedical applications [131]. Due to polyene chains, carotenoids exhibit a pronounced resonance Raman effect. Therefore, SERRS (surface-enhanced resonance Raman scattering), in which the scattering is enhanced by both a roughened metal surface and a resonance with visible chromophore, will likely be as successful in the analysis of carotenoids as it was for DNA samples [132]. Tip-enhanced Raman spectroscopy (TERS) was introduced one and a half decades ago [133]. TERS combines the structural information and signal enhancement of SERS with the high spatial resolution of atomic force microscopy (AFM) or scanning tunneling microscopy (STM). TERS was shown to perform well in characterizing different virus strains [134]. Hence, recent innovations increasing, *inter alia*, TERS reproducibility [135] make the use of this method in the study of carotenoids in biological or medical material quite likely.

The nonlinear Raman methods, such as CARS and stimulated Raman spectroscopy (SRS), have been successful in addressing biomedical challenges [136, 137]. In recent years, the CARS method was scarcely used in the analysis of carotenoids in plants, algae, and bacteria [87, 99], and the SRS technique has been mainly used to investigate carotenoids in photosynthetic light-harvesting processes [138]. It seems, however, that some work is still necessary to increase the reliability and reproducibility of CARS or SRS signals and to implement these techniques for massive investigations of carotenoids in biological and biomedical research [136].

A lot of newly synthesized [139] and isolated [140–144] carotenoids are chiral. Nevertheless, the chiroptic vibrational optical activity spectra [145], such as vibrational circular dichroism (VCD) [146] and Raman optical activity [147] (ROA), have never been applied in the investigation of chiral carotenoids. However, quite recently, the resonance ROA (RROA) spectra of conformers of astaxanthin, which as a monoestrified 3*S*,3'*S* isomer exists in *H. pluvialis* alga, have been calculated and served as a model for considering a pseudo-breakdown of the single electronic state paradigm of RROA [148]. With continuous improvement in the quality and reproducibility of VCD and ROA instrumentation, vibrational optical activity spectroscopy is a rapidly growing field of modern physicochemical techniques with great potential in pharmaceutical, biological, and biomedical applications. Therefore, an increase of vibrational optical activity spectroscopy in studies of carotenoids is likely.

Moore's law, describing a biennial doubling of chip capacity at a minimal cost, is expected to hold until at least 2020 [149, 150]. New and more efficient protocols, data analysis techniques, and (chemometric) software (e.g., [151–153]) facilitate the implementation of pre-processing techniques, improve the robustness and accuracy of spectroscopic analyzes, and, importantly, offer a user-friendly interface and functionality that make for easy graphical presentation of data. The miniaturization of Raman, IR, and NIR spectrometers has facilitated substantial progress, vastly broadening the range of the applications of vibrational spectroscopy methods [154]. These improvement factors are especially important for biomedical applications of spectroscopic methods such as Raman and IR imaging of diseased tissues (e.g., [155–158]) where the collected data must be reprocessed to provide unprecedented capability in measurement and scientific insight [159–164] into the role of carotenoids in human biochemistry, disease prevention, and human health.

Acknowledgments

This project was supported by the National Science Centre (DEC-2012/07/B/ST5/00889).

References

1. International Union of Pure and Applied Chemistry (IUPAC) and International Union of Biochemistry (IUB), issued by the IUPAC Commission on the Nomenclature of Organic Chemistry and the IUPAC–IUB Commission on Biochemical Nomenclature, Nomenclature of Carotenoids (Rules Approved 1974), London: Butterworth, 1974.
2. A. R. Moise, S. Al-Babili, and E. T. Wurtzel, "Mechanistic aspects of carotenoid biosynthesis," *Chem Rev.*, **114**, 164–93 (2014).
3. G. Britton, "Structure and properties of carotenoids in relation to function," *FASEB J.*, **9**, 1551–8 (1995).

4. T. G. Schmalz and L. L. Griffin, "How long are the ends of polyene chains?" *J. Chem. Phys.*, **131**, 224301 (2009).

5. J. L. Bredas, R. Silbey, D. S. Boudreaux, and R. R. Chance, "Chain-length dependence of electronic and electrochemical properties of conjugated systems: polyacetylene, polyphenylene, polythiophene, and polypyrrole," *J. Am. Chem. Soc.*, **105**, 6555–9 (1983).

6. H. E. Schaffer, R. R. Chance, R. J. Silbey, K. Knoll, and R. R. Schrock, "Conjugation length dependence of Raman scattering in a series of linear polyenes: Implications for polyacetylene," *J. Chem. Phys.*, **94**, 4161–70 (1991).

7. R. R. Chance, H. E. Schaffer, K. Knoll, R. R. Schrock, and R. J. Silbey, "Linear optical properties of a series of linear polyenes: implications for polyacetylene," *Synth. Met.*, **49**, 271–80 (1992).

8. C. Heller, G. Leising, C. Godon, S. Lefrant, W. Fischer, and F. Stelzer, "Raman excitation profiles of conjugated segments in solution, *Phys. Rev. B*, **51**, 8107–14 (1995).

9. D. Jacquemin and C. Adamo, "Bond length alternation of conjugated oligomers: wave function and DFT benchmarks," *J. Chem. Theory Comput.*, **7**, 369–76 (2011).

10. Q. Yu, S. Ghisla, J. Hirschberg, V. Mann, and P. Beyer, "Plant carotene cis-trans isomerase CRTISO: a new member of the FAD_{RED}-dependent flavoproteins catalyzing non-redox reactions," *J. Biol. Chem.*, **286**, 8666–76 (2011).

11. J. Vohlídal, "Mean-square end-to-end distance and characteristic ratio of polyvinylene (polyacetylene) chains of various configurations," *Macromol. Chem. Phys.*, **207**, 224–30 (2006).

12. G. E. Bartley, P. A. Scolnik, and P. Beyer, "Two *Arabidopsis thaliana* carotenedesaturases, phytoene desaturase and zeta-carotene desaturase, expressed in *Escherichia coli*, catalyse a poly-*cis* pathway to yield pro-lycopene," *Eur. J. Biochem.*, **259**, 396–403 (1999).

13. G. Britton, S. Liaaen-Jensen, and H. Pfander, *Carotenoids handbook*, Basel: Birkhäuser, 2004.

14. C. I. Cazzonelli, "Carotenoids in nature: insights from plants and beyond," *Functional Plant Biology*, **38**, 833–47 (2011).

15. T. W.-M. Boileau A. C. Boileau, and J. W. Erdman Jr., "Bioavailability of all-*trans* and *cis*-isomers of lycopene," *Exp. Biol. Med.*, **227**, 914–9 (2002).

16. D. B. Rodriguez-Amaya and M. Kimura, *HarvestPlus handbook for carotenoid analysis,* HarvestPlus Technical Monograph 2, Washington DC: HarvestPlus, 2004.

17. E. R. Schenk, V. Mendez, J. T. Landrum, M. E. Ridgeway, M. A. Park, and F. Fernandez-Lima, "Direct observation of differences of carotenoid polyene chain *cis/trans* isomers resulting from structural topology," *Anal. Chem.*, **86**, 2019–24 (2014).

18. W. Stahl, A. R. Sundquist, M. Hanusch, W. Schwarz, and H. Sies, "Separation of beta-carotene and lycopene geometrical isomers in biological samples," *Clin Chem.*, **39**, 810–14 (1993).

19. B. Honig, B. Hudson, B. D. Sykes, and M. Karplus, "Ring orientation in β-ionone and retinals," *Proc. Natl. Acad. Sci. USA*, **68**, 1289–93 (1971).

20. J. R. Thiel, C. J. Simmons, and R. S. H. Liu, "X-ray crystal structure of cis-mini-3 (a spiralene[3])," *Tetrah. Lett.*, **38**, 19–20 (1997).

21. R. Fujii, C.-H. Chen, T. Mizoguchi, and Y. Koyama, "^{1}H NMR, electronic-absorption and resonance-Raman spectra of isomeric okenone as compared with those of isomeric β-carotene, canthaxanthin, β-apo-8'-carotenal and spheroidene," *Spectrochim. Acta*, **54A**, 727–43 (1998).

22. H. Shirakawa, E. J. Louis, A. G. MacDiarmid, C. K. Chiang, and A. J. Heeger, "Synthesis of electrically conducting organic polymers: halogen derivatives of polyacetylene, $(CH)_x$," *J.C.S. Chem. Comm.*, 578–80 (1977).

23. W. Li, H. Huang, Y. Li, and J. Deng, "Particles of polyacetylene and its derivatives: preparation and applications," *Polym. Chem.*, **5**, 1107–18 (2014).

24. G. Colherinhas, T. L. Fonseca, H. C. Georg, and M. A. Castro, "Isomerization effects on chemical shifts and spin-spin coupling constants of polyacetylene chains: a GIAO-DFT study," *Int. J. Quant. Chem.*, **111**, 1616–25 (2011).

25. K. Schulten and M. Karplus, "On the origin of a low-lying forbidden transition in polyenes and related molecules," *Chem. Phys. Lett.*, **14**, 305–9 (1972).

26. B. S. Hudson and B. E. Kohler, "A low-lying weak transition in the polyene α,ω-diphenyloctatetraene," *Chem. Phys. Lett.*, **14**, 299–304 (1972).

27. R. L. Christensen, A. Faksh, J. A. Meyers, I. F. D. Samuel, P. Wood, R. R. Schrock, and K. C. Hultzsch, "Optical spectroscopy of long polyenes," *J. Phys. Chem. A*, **108**, 8229–36 (2004).

28. S. Prodhan, Z. G. Soos, and S. Ramasesha, "Model for triplet state engineering in organic light emitting diodes," *J. Chem. Phys.*, **140**, 214313 (2014).

29. M.Macernis, J. Sulskus, S. Malickaja, B. Robert, and L. Valkunas, "Resonance Raman spectra and electronic transitions in carotenoids: a density functional theory study," *J. Phys. Chem. A*, **118**, 1817–25 (2014).

30. J. L. Bredas, R. Silbey, D. S. Boudreaux, and R. R. Chance, "Chain-length dependence of electronic and electrochemical properties of conjugated systems: polyacetylene, polyphenylene, polythiophene, and polypyrrole," *J. Am. Chem. Soc.*, **105**, 6555–9 (1983).

31. T. Bally, K. Roth, W. Tang, R. R. Schrock, K. Knoll, and L. Y. Park, "Stable polarons in polyacetylene oligomers: optical spectra of long polyene radical cations," *J. Am. Chem. Soc.*, **114**, 2440–6 (1992).

32. A. Martínez, "Donator-acceptor map and work function for linear polyene-conjugated molecules: a density functional approximation study," *J. Phys. Chem. B*, **113**, 3212–7 (2009).

33. J. H. Starcke, M. Wormit, and A. Dreuw, "Nature of the lowest excited states of neutral polyenyl radicals and polyene radical cations," *J. Chem. Phys.*, **131**, 144311 (2009).

34. L. Piekara-Sady, A. S. Jeevarajan, and L. D. Kispert, "An ENDOR study of the canthaxanthin cation radical in solution," *Chem. Phys. Lett.*, **207**, 173–7 (1993).

35. L. Piekara-Sady, M. M. Khaled, E. Bradford, L. D. Kispert, and M. Plato, "Comparison of the INDO to the RHF-INDO/SP derived EPR proton hyperfine couplings for the carotenoid cation radical: experimental evidence," *Chem. Phys. Lett.*, **186**, 143–8 (1991).

36. A. S. Jeevarajan, L. D. Kispert, G. Chumanov, C. Zhou, and T. M. Cotton, "Resonance Raman study of carotenoid cation radicals," *Chem. Phys. Lett.*, **259**, 515–22 (1996).

37. V. Schettino, F. L. Gervasio, G. Cardini, and P. R. Salvi, "Density functional calculation of structure and vibrational spectra of polyenes," *J. Chem. Phys.*, **110**, 3241–50 (1999).

38. J. Y. Lee, S. J. Lee, and K. S. Kim, "Raman intensities of C5C stretching vibrational frequencies of polyenes: nodal mode analysis," *J. Chem. Phys.*, **107**, 4112–7 (1997).

39. J. Wang, X. Jing, and Z. Feng, "Normal vibrational analysis of *trans*-polyacetylene," *Chin. J. Polym. Sci.*, **5**, 316–24 (1987).

40. J. Wang, X. Jing, and Z. Feng, "Normal vibrational analysis of *cis*-polyacetylene," *Chin. J. Polym. Sci.*, **5**, 308–15 (1987).

41. H. Shirakawa and S. Ikeda, "Infrared spectra of poly(acetylene)," *Polymer J.*, **2**, 231–44 (1971).

42. H. Kuzmany, "Resonance Raman scattering from neutral and doped polyacetylene resonance Raman scattering from neutral and doped polyacetylene," *Phys. Status Solidi B*, **97**, 521–31 (1980).

43. P. Piaggio, G. Dellepiane, L. Piseri, R. Tubino, and C. Taliani, "Polarized infrared spectra of highly oriented polyacetylenes," *Solid State Commun.*, **50**, 947–56 (1984).

44. J. C. Merlin, "Resonance Raman spectroscopy of carotenoids and carotenoid-containing systems," *Pure Appl. Chem.*, **57**, 785–92 (1985).

45. M. M. Mendes-Pinto, D. Galzerano, A. Telfer, A. A. Pascal, B. Robert, and C. Ilioaia, "Mechanisms underlying carotenoid absorption in oxygenic photosynthetic proteins," *J. Biol. Chem.*, **288**, 18758–65 (2013).

46. Y. Koyama, T. Takii, K. Saiki, and S. Tsukida, "Configuration of the carotenoid in the reaction centers of photosynthetic bacteria .2. Comparison of the resonance Raman lines of the reaction centers with those of the 14 different *cis-trans* isomers of β-carotene," *Photobiochem. Photobiophys.*, **5**, 139–50 (1983).

47. I. Harada, Y. Furukawa, M. Tasumi, H. Shirakawa, and S. Ikeda, "Spectroscopic studies on doped polyacetylene and β-carotene," *J. Chem. Phys.*, **73**, 4746–57 (1980).

48. A. Painelli, L. del Freo, A. Girlando, and Z. G. Soos, "Polyacetylene oligomers: p-electron fluctuations, vibrational intensities, and soliton confinement," *Phys. Rev. B*, 8129–37.

49. A. Bianco, M. Del Zoppo, and G. Zerbi, "Experimental CC stretching phonon dispersion curves and electron phonon coupling in polyene derivatives," *J. Chem. Phys.*, **120**, 1450–7 (2004).

50. T. Kupka, H. Ming Lin, L. Stobiński, C.-H. Chen, W.-J. Liou R., Wrzalik, and Z. Flisak, "Experimental and theoretical studies on corals. I. Toward understanding the origin of color in precious red corals from Raman and IR spectroscopies and DFT calculations," *J. Raman Spectrosc.*, **41**, 651–8 (2010).

51. C. Sterling, "Crystal-structure analysis of β-carotene," *Acta Cryst.*, **17**, 1224–8 (1964).

52. W. G. Sly, "The crystal structure of 15,15′-dehydro-β-carotene," *Acta Cryst.*, **17**, 511–28 (1964).

53. C. H. Stam and C. H. MacGillavry, "The crystal structure of the triclinic modification of vitamin-A acid," *Acta Cryst.*, **16**, 62–8 (1963).

54. F. Mo, "X-ray crystallographic studies," in G. Britton, S. Liaaen-Jensen, and H. Pfander (eds.), *Carotenoids*, vol. 1B, Spectroscopy, Basel: Birkhäuser, 1995, pp. 321–42.

55. M. Helliwell, "Three-dimensional structures of carotenoids by X-ray crystallography," in G. Britton, S. Liaaen-Jensen, and H. Pfander (eds.), Basel: Birkhäuser, *Carotenoids*, vol. **4**, 2008, pp. 37–52.

56. G. Bartalucci, J. Coppin, S. Fisher, G. Hall, J. R. Helliwell, M. Helliwell, and S. Liaaen-Jensen, "Unravelling the chemical basis of the bathochromic shift in the lobster carapace; new crystal structures of unbound astaxanthin, canthaxanthin and zeaxanthin," *Acta Crystal. B*, **63**, 328–37 (2007).

57. M. Helliwell, S. Liaaen-Jensen, and J. Wilkinson, "Two polymorphs of 20-desmethyl-β-carotene," *Acta Crystal. C*, **64**, o252–6 (2008).

58. P. Qian, T. Mizoguchi, R. Fujii, and K. Hara, "Conformation analysis of carotenoids in the purple bacterium *Rhodobium marinum* based on NMR spectroscopy and AM1 calculation," *J. Chem. Inf. Comput. Sci.*, **42**, 1311–9 (2002).

59. L. Brambilla, M. Tommasini, G. Zerbi, and R. Stradi, "Raman spectroscopy of polyconjugated molecules with electronic and mechanical confinement: the spectrum of *Corallium rubrum*," *J. Raman Spectrosc.*, **43**, 1449–58 (2012).

60. R. F. Fernandes, L. F. Maia, M. R. Couri, L. A. Costa, and L. F. de Oliveira, "Raman spectroscopy as a tool in differentiating conjugated polyenes from synthetic and natural sources," *Spectrochim Acta A*, **134**, 434–41 (2015).

61. J. T. Landrum, D. C. Chatfield, A. M. Mebel, F. Alvarez-Calderon, and M. V. Fernandez, "The conformation of end-groups is one determinant of carotenoid topology suitable for high fidelity molecular recognition: a study of beta- and epsilon-end-groups," *Arch. Biochem. Biophys.*, **2493**, 169–74 (2010).

62. P. J. Spooner, J. M. Sharples, M. A. Verhoeven, J. Lugtenburg, C. Glaubitz, and A. Watts, "Relative orientation between the beta-ionone ring and the polyene chain for the chromophore of rhodopsin in native membranes," *Biochem.*, **41**, 7549–55 (2002).

63. Z. He, D. Gosztola, Y. Deng, G. Gao, M. R. Wasielewski, and L. D. Kispert, "Effect of terminal groups, polyene chain length, and solvent on the first excited singlet states of carotenoids," *J. Phys. Chem. B*, **104**, 6668–73 (2000).

64. V. Lukes, N. Christensson, F. Milota, H. F. Kauffmann, and J. Hauer, "Electronic ground state conformers of β-carotene and their role in ultrafast spectroscopy," *Chem. Phys. Lett.*, **506**, 122–7 (2011).

65. J. Y. Lee, B. J. Mhin, and K. S. Kim, "Roles of central and terminal carbon atoms in infrared and Raman intensities of polyenes: analysis of atomic polar and polarizability tensors," *J. Chem. Phys.*, **107**, 4881–5 (1997).

66. M.-M. Huo, W.-L. Liu, Z.-R. Zheng, W. Zhang, A.-H. Li, and D.-P. Xu, "Effect of end groups on the raman spectra of lycopene and β-carotene under high pressure," *Molecules*, **16**, 1973–80 (2011).

67. M. Macernis, J. Sulskus, S. Malickaja, A. Ruban, and L. Valkunas, "Resonance Raman spectra and electronic transitions in carotenoids: a density functional theory study," *J. Phys. Chem. A*, **118**, 1817–25 (2014).

68. B. Robert, "Resonance Raman spectroscopy," *Photosynth. Res.*, **101**, 147–55 (2009).

69. J. Lademann, M. C. Meinke, W. Sterry, and M. E. Darvin, "Carotenoids in human skin," *Exp. Dermatol.*, **20**, 377–82 (2011).

70. O. Howells, F. Eperjesi, and H. Bartlett, "Measuring macular pigment optical density *in vivo*: a review of techniques," *Graefes Arch. Clin. Exp. Ophthalmol.*, **249**, 315–47 (2011).

71. H. Abramczyk, B. Brozek-Pluska, J. Surmacki, J. Jablonska-Gajewicz, and R. Kordek, "Raman 'optical biopsy' of human breast cancer," *Prog. Biophys. Mol. Biol.*, **108**, 74–81 (2012).

72. B. Pacholczyk, A. Fabiańska, R. Kusińska, P. Potemski, R. Kordek, and S. Jankowski, "Analysis of cancer tissues by means of spectroscopic methods," *Contemp. Oncol. (Pozn.)*, **16**, 290–4 (2012).

73. D. Cvetković, L. Fiedor, A. Wisniewska-Becker, and D. Marković, "Organization of carotenoids in models of biological membranes: current status of knowledge and research," *Curr. Anal. Chem.*, **9**, 86–98 (2013).

74. M. Li, J. Xu, M. Romero-Gonzalez, S. A. Banwart, and W. E. Huang, "Single cell Raman spectroscopy for cell sorting and imaging," *Curr. Opin. Biotechnol.*, **23**, 56–63 (2012).

75. G. Rusciano, G. Pesce, M. Salemme, L. Selvaggi, C. Vaccaro, A. Sasso, and R. Carotenuto, "Raman spectroscopy of *Xenopus laevis* oocytes," *Methods*, **51**, 27–36 (2010).

76. S. M. Rivera and R. Canela-Garayoa, "Analytical tools for the analysis of carotenoids in diverse materials," *J. Chromatogr. A*, **1224**, 1–10 (2012).

77. N. D. T. Parab and V. Tomar, "Raman spectroscopy of algae: a review," *Nanomed. Nanotech.*, **3**, 1–7 (2012).

78. M. Barańska, M. Roman, J. Cz. Dobrowolski, H. Schulz, and R. Barański, "Recent advances in Raman analysis of plants: alkaloids, carotenoids, and polyacetylenes," *Curr. Anal. Chem.*, **9**, 99–118 (2013).

79. F. Schulte, J. Mäder, L. W. Kroh, U. Panne, and J. Kneipp, "Characterization of pollen carotenoids with *in situ* and high-performance thin-layer chromatography supported resonant Raman spectroscopy," *Anal. Chem.*, **81**, 8426–33 (2009).

80. E. H. Papaioannou, M. Liakopoulou-Kyriakides, D. Christofilos, I. Arvanitidis, and G. Kourouklis, "Raman spectroscopy for intracellular monitoring of carotenoid in *Blakeslea trispora*," *Appl. Biochem. Biotechnol.*, **159**, 478–87 (2009).

81. Y. Y. Huang, C. M. Beal, W. W. Cai, R. S. Ruoff, and E. M. Terentjev, "Micro-Raman spectroscopy of algae: composition analysis and fluorescence background behavior," *Biotechnol. Bioeng.*, **105**, 889–98 (2010).

82. C. Sicard, R. Brayner, J. Margueritat, M. Hémadi, A. Couté, C. Yéprémian, S. Djediat, J. Aubard, F. Fiévet-Vincent, J. Livage, and T. Coradin, "Nano-gold biosynthesis by silica-encapsulated micro-algae: a 'living' bio-hybrid material," *J. Mater. Chem.*, **20**, 9342–7 (2010).

83. P. Zhang, L. Kong, P. Setlow, and Y.-Q. Li, "Characterization of wet-heat inactivation of single spores of bacillus species by dual-trap Raman spectroscopy and elastic light scattering," *Appl. Environ. Microbiol.*, **76**, 1796–805 (2010).

84. M. L. Paret, S. K. Sharma, L. M. Green, and A. M. Alvarez, "Biochemical characterization of Gram-positive and Gram-negative plant-associated bacteria with micro-Raman spectroscopy," *Appl. Spectrosc.*, **64**, 433–41 (2010).

85. M. Ando, M. Sugiura, H. Hayashi, and H. O. Hamaguchi, "1064 nm deep near-infrared (NIR) excited Raman microspectroscopy for studying photolabile organisms," *Appl. Spectrosc.*, **65**, 488–92 (2011).

86. J. Jehlička, K. Osterrothová, A. Oren, and H. G. Edwards, "Raman spectrometric discrimination of flexirubin pigments from two genera of *Bacteroidetes*," *FEMS Microbiol. Lett.*, **348**, 97–102 (2013).

87. A. Dementjev and J. Kostkevičiene, "Applying the method of coherent anti-stokes Raman microscopy for imaging of carotenoids in microalgae and cyanobacteria," *J. Raman Spectrosc.*, **44**, 973–9 (2013).

88. Y.-T. Zheng, M. Toyofuku, N. Nomura, and S. Shigeto, "Correlation of carotenoid accumulation with aggregation and biofilm development in *Rhodococcus* sp. SD-74," *Anal. Chem.*, **85**, 7295–301 (2013).

89. J. Jehlička, H. G. M. Edwards, and A. Oren, "Bacterioruberin and salinixanthin carotenoids of extremely halophilic Archaea and bacteria: a Raman spectroscopic study," *Spectrochim. Acta A*, **106**, 99–103 (2013).

90. M. T. Alexandre, K. Gundermann, A. A. Pascal, R. van Grondelle, C. Büchel, and B. Robert, "Probing the carotenoid content of intact Cyclotella cells by resonance Raman spectroscopy," *Photosynth Res.*, **119**, 273–81 (2014).

91. S. E. Jorge-Villar and H. G. M. Edwards, "Lichen colonization of an active volcanic environment: a Raman spectroscopic study of extremophile biomolecular protective strategies," *J. Raman Spectrosc.*, **41**, 63–67 (2010).

92. A. J. Kaczor, K. Turnau, and M. Baranska, "*In situ* Raman imaging of astaxanthin in a single microalgal cell," *Analyst*, **136**, 1109–12 (2011).

93. A. J. Kaczor and M. Baranska, "Structural changes of carotenoid astaxanthin in a single algal cell monitored *in situ* by Raman spectroscopy," *Anal. Chem.*, **83**, 7763–70 (2011).

94. A. Abbas, M. Josefson, and K. Abrahamsson, "Characterization and mapping of carotenoids in the algae Dunaliella and Phaeodactylum using Raman and target orthogonal partial least squares," *Chemom. Intell. Lab. Syst.*, **107**, 174–7 (2011).

95. A. M. Collins, H. D. T. Jones, D. Han, Q. Hu, T. E. Beechem, and J. A. Timlin, "Carotenoid distribution in living cells of Haematococcus pluvialis (*Chlorophyceae*)," *PLoS ONE*, **6**, e24302 (2011).

96. Z. Pilát, S. Bernatová, J. Ježek, M. Šerý, O. Samek, P. Zemánek, L. Nedbal, and M. Trtílek, "Raman microspectroscopy of algal lipid bodies: β-carotene quantification," *J. Appl. Phycol.*, **24**, 541–6 (2012).

97. C. Uragami, D. Galzerano, A. Gall, Y. Shigematsu, M. Meisterhans, N. Oka, M. Iha, R. Fujii, B. Robert, and H. Hashimoto, "Light-dependent conformational change of neoxanthin in a siphonous green alga, *Codium intricatum*, revealed by Raman spectroscopy," *Photosynth Res.*, **121**, 69–77 (2014).

98. C. Paulo and M. Dittrich, "2D Raman spectroscopy study of dolomite and cyanobacterial extracellular polymeric substances from Khor Al-Adaid sabkha (Qatar)," *J. Raman Spectrosc.*, **44**, 1563–9 (2013).

99. J. Garcia-Guinea, M. Furio, S. Sanchez-Moral, V. Jurado, V. Correcher, and C. Saiz-Jimenez, "Composition and spectra of copper-carotenoid sediments from a pyrite mine stream in Spain," *Spectrochim. Acta A*, **135**, 203–10 (2015).

100. P. Vítek, J. Jehlicka, H. G. Edwards, and K. Osterrothová, "Identification of beta-carotene in an evaporitic matrix: evaluation of Raman spectroscopic analysis for astrobiological research on Mars," *Anal. Bioanal. Chem.*, **393**, 1967–75 (2009).

101. P. Vítek, K. Osterrothová, and J. Jehlicka, "Beta-carotene: a possible biomarker in the Martian evaporitic environment: Raman microspectroscopic study," *Planet. Space Sci.*, **57**, 454–9 (2009).

102. U. Böttger, J.-P. de Vera, J. Fritz, I. Weber, H.-W. Hübers, and D. Schulze-Makuch, "Optimizing the detection of carotene in cyanobacteria in a Martian regolith analogue with a Raman laser spectrometer on ExoMars," *Planet. Space Sci.*, **60**, 356–62 (2012).

103. C. P. Marshall and A. Olcott Marshall, "The potential of Raman spectroscopy for the analysis of diagenetically transformed carotenoids," *Philos. Trans. A Math. Phys. Eng. Sci.*, **368**, 3137–44 (2010).

104. V. Ciobotă, W. Salama, N. Tarcea, P. Rösch, M. El Aref, R. Gaupp, and J. Popp, "Identification of minerals and organic materials in Middle Eocene ironstones from the Bahariya Depression in the Western Desert of Egypt by means of micro-Raman spectroscopy," *J. Raman Spectrosc.* **43**, 405–10 (2012).

105. L. Kiefert, H. A. Hänni, and T. Ostertag, "Raman spectroscopic applications to gemmology," in I. R. Lewis and H. G. M. Edwards (eds.), Handbook of Raman *spectroscopy from the research laboratory to the process line*, Boca Raton, FL: CRC Press, chap. 11.

106. E. Fritsch, B. Rondeau, T. Hainschwang, and S. Karampelas, "Raman spectroscopy applied to gemmology," *Eur. Mineralog. Union Notes Mineralogy*, **12**, 455–89 (2012).

107. J. C. Merlin and M. L. Delé-Dubois, "Resonance Raman characterization of polyacetylenic pigments in the calcareous skeleton," *Compar. Biochem. Physiol. B*, **84**, 97–103 (1986).

108. C. P. Smith, S. F. McClure, S. Eaton-Magaña, and D. M. Kondo, "Pink-to-red coral: a guide to determining origin of color," *Gems and Gemology*, **43**, 4–15 (2007).

109. D. Bersani and P. P. Lottici, "Applications of Raman spectroscopy to gemology," *Anal. Bioanal. Chem.*, **397**, 2631–46 (2010).

110. L. Kiefert, H. A. Hanni, and T. Ostertag, "Applications of Raman spectroscopy to gemology," in I. R. Lewis and H. G. M. Edwards (eds.), *Handbook of Raman spectroscopy: from the research laboratory to the process line*, New York: Marcel Dekker, pp. 469–90.

111. L. F. Maia, B. G. Fleury, B. G. Lages, J. P. Barbosa, Â. C. Pinto, H. V. Castro, V. E. de Oliveira, H. G. Edwards, and L. F. de Oliveira, "Identification of reddish pigments in octocorals by Raman spectroscopy," *J. Raman Spectrosc.*, **42**, 653–8 (2011).

112. L. F. Maia, V. E. de Oliveira, M. E. R. de Oliveira, B. G. Fleury, and L. F. C. de Oliveira, "Polyenic pigments from the Brazilian octocoral *Phyllogorgia dilatata* Esper, 1806 characterized by Raman spectroscopy," *J. Raman Spectrosc.*, **43**, 161–4 (2012).

113. L. F. Maia, V. E. de Oliveira, M. E. R. de Oliveira, F. D. Reis, B. G. Fleury, H. G. M. Edwards, and L. F. C. de Oliveira, "Colour diversification in octocorals based on conjugated polyenes: a Raman spectroscopic view," *J. Raman Spectrosc.*, **44**, 560–6 (2013).

114. L. F. Maia, G. R. Ferreira, R. C. Costa, N. C. Lucas, R. I. Teixeira, B. G. Fleury, H. G. Edwards, and L. F. de Oliveira, "Raman spectroscopic study of antioxidant pigments from cup corals *Tubastraea* spp.," *J. Phys. Chem. A*, **118**, 3429–37 (2014).

115. S. Karampelas, E. Fritsch, J.-Y. Mevellec, J.-P. Gauthier, S. Sklavounos, and T. Soldatos, "Determination by Raman scattering of the nature of pigments in cultured freshwater pearls from the mollusk *Hyriopsis cumingi*," *J. Raman Spectrosc.*, **38**, 217–30 (2007).

116. S. Karampelas, E. Fritsch, J.-Y. Mevellec, S. Sklavounos, and T. Soldatos, "Role of polyenes in the coloration of cultured freshwater pearls," *Eur. J. Mineral.*, **21**, 85–97 (2009).

117. L. L. Ji, J. Liao, W. D. Song, J. S. Liu, and X. T. Ma, "Influence of astaxanthin on pearl oyster *Pinctada martensii*," *Adv. Mat. Res.*, 781–784, 889–94 (2013).

118. A. L. Soldati, D. E. Jacob, U. Wehrmeister, T. Häger, and W. Hofmeister, "Micro-Raman spectroscopy of pigments contained in different calcium carbonate polymorphs from freshwater cultured pearls," *J. Raman Spectrosc.*, **39**, 525–36 (2008).

119. L. Bergamonti, D. Bersani, D. Csermely, and P. P. Lottici, "The nature of the pigments in corals and pearls: a contribution from Raman spectroscopy," *Spectrosc. Lett.*, **44**, 453–8 (2011).

120. L. Shi, X. Liu, J. Mao, and X. Han, "Study of coloration mechanism of cultured freshwater pearls from mollusk *Hyriopsis cumingii*," *J. Appl. Spectrosc.*, **81**, 97–101 (2014).

121. K. Osterrothová, L. Minaříková, A. Culka, J. Kuntoš, and J. Jehlička, "*In situ* study of stones adorning a silver Torah shield using portable Raman spectrometers," *J. Raman Spectrosc.*, **45**, 830–7 (2014).

122. I. Degano, E. Ribechini, F. Modugno, and M. P. Colombini, "Analytical methods for the characterization of organic dyes in artworks and in historical textiles," *Appl. Spectrosc. Rev.*, **44**, 363–410 (2009).

123. M. V. Cañamares, M. Leona, M. Bouchard, C. M. Grzywacz, J. Wouters, and K. Trentelman, "Evaluation of Raman and SERS analytical protocols in the analysis of Cape Jasmine dye (*Gardenia augusta L.*)," *J. Raman Spectr.*, **41**, 391–7 (2010).

124. S. Bruni, V. Guglielmi, and F. Pozzi, "Historical organic dyes: a surface-enhanced Raman scattering (SERS) spectral database on Ag Lee-Meisel colloids aggregated by $NaClO_4$," *J. Raman Spectrosc.*, **42**, 1267–81 (2011).

125. M. Maguregui, U. Knuutinen, J. Trebolazabala, H. Morillas, K. Castro, I. Martinez-Arkarazo, and J. M. Madariaga, "Use of *in situ* and confocal Raman spectroscopy to study the nature and distribution of carotenoids in brown patinas from a deteriorated wall painting in Marcus Lucretius House (Pompeii)," *Anal. Bioanal. Chem.*, **402**, 1529–39 (2012).

126. M. Maguregui, U. Knuutinen, I. Martinez-Arkarazo, A. Giakoumaki, K. Castro, and J. M. Madariaga, "Field Raman analysis to diagnose the conservation state of excavated walls and wall paintings in the archaeological site of Pompeii (Italy)," *J. Raman Spectrosc.*, **43**, 1747–53 (2012).

127. P. M. Martin-Sanchez, S. Sanchez-Cortes, E. Lopez-Tobar, V. Jurado, F. Bastian, C. Alabouvette, and C. Saiz-Jimenez, "The nature of black stains in Lascaux Cave, France, as revealed by surface-enhanced Raman spectroscopy," *J. Raman Spectrosc.*, **43**, 464–7 (2012).

128. A. Casanova Municchia, G. Caneva, M. A. Ricci, and A. Sodo, "Identification of endolithic traces on stone monuments and natural outcrops: preliminary evidences," *J. Raman Spectrosc.*, **45**, 1180–85 (2014).

129. M. Bicchieri, "The purple Codex Rossanensis: spectroscopic characterization and first evidence of the use of the elderberry lake in a 6th century manuscript," *Environ. Sci. Pollut. Res. Int.*, **24**, 14146–57 (2014).

130. L. A. Nafie, "Recent advances in linear and nonlinear Raman spectroscopy. Part VII," *J. Raman Spectrosc.*, **44**, 1629–48 (2013).

131. S. Schlücker, "Surface-enhanced Raman spectroscopy: concepts and chemical applications," *Angew. Chem. Int. Ed.*, **53**, 4756–95 (2014).

132. K. S. McKeating, J. A. Dougan, and K. Faulds, "Nanoparticle assembly for sensitive DNA detection using SERRS," *Biochem Soc Trans.*, **40**, 597–602 (2012).

133. T. Schmid, L. Opilik, C. Blum, and R. Zenobi, "Nanoscale chemical imaging using tip-enhanced Raman spectroscopy: a critical review," *Angew. Chem. Int. Ed. Engl.*, **52**, 5940–54 (2013).

134. P. Hermann, A. Hermeling, V. Lausch, G. Holland, L. Möller, N. Bannert, and D. Naumann, "Evaluation of tip-enhanced Raman spectroscopy for characterizing different virus strains," *Analyst*, **136**, 1148–52 (2011).

135. N. Hayazawa, T.-A. Yano, and S. Kawata, "Highly reproducible tip-enhanced Raman scattering using an oxidized and metallized silicon cantilever tip as a tool for everyone," *J. Raman Spectrosc.*, **43**, 1177–82 (2012).

136. K. A. Antonio and Z. D. Schultz, "Advances in biomedical Raman microscopy," *Anal. Chem.*, **86**, 30–46 (2014).

137. M. Li, J. Xu, M. Romero-Gonzalez, S. A. Banwart, and W. E. Huang, "Single cell Raman spectroscopy for cell sorting and imaging," *Curr. Opin. Biotechnol.*, **23**, 56–63 (2012).

138. T. Takaya and K. Iwata, "Relaxation mechanism of β-carotene from S2 (1Bu(+)) state to S1 (2Ag(−)) state: femtosecond time-resolved near-IR absorption and stimulated resonance Raman studies in 900–1550 nm region," *J. Phys. Chem. A*, **118**, 4071–78 (2014).

139. C. L. Øpstad, H. Sliwka, and V. Partali, "New colours for carotenoids: synthesis of pyran polyenes," *Eur. J. Org. Chem.*, 435–9 (2010).

140. O. Mangoni, C. Imperatore, C. R. Tomas, V. Costantino, V. Saggiomo, and A. Mangoni, "The new carotenoid pigment moraxanthin is associated with toxic microalgae," *Mar. Drugs*, **9**, 242–55 (2011).

141. K. Shindo and N. Misawa, "New and rare carotenoids isolated from marine bacteria and their antioxidant activities," *Mar. Drugs*, **12**, 1690–8 (2014).

142. F. Zsila, J. Deli, and M. Simonyi, "Color and chirality: carotenoid self-assemblies in flower petals," *Planta*, **213**, 937–42 (2001).

143. F. Khachik, F. F. de Moura, D. Y. Zhao, C. P. Aebischer, and P. S. Bernstein, "Transformations of selected carotenoids in plasma, liver, and ocular tissues of humans and in nonprimate animal models," *Invest. Ophthalmol. Vis. Sci.*, **43**, 3383–92 (2002).

144. Y. Yamano, T. Maoka, and A. Wada, "Synthesis of (3*S*,3'*S*)- and meso-stereoisomers of alloxanthin and determination of absolute configuration of alloxanthin isolated from aquatic animals," *Mar. Drugs*, **12**, 2623–32 (2014).

145. L. A. Nafie, *Vibrational optical activity: principles and applications*, Hoboken, NJ: Wiley, 2011.

146. G. Yang and Y. Xu, "Vibrational circular dichroism spectroscopy of chiral molecules," in R. Naaman, D. N. Beratan, and D. H. Waldeck (eds.), *Electronic and magnetic properties of chiral molecules and supramolecular architectures*, Berlin: Springer-Verlag, 2011, pp. 189–236.

147. L. D. Barron, F. Zhu, L. Hecht, G. E. Tranter, and N. W. Isaacs, "Raman optical activity: An incisive probe of molecular chirality and biomolecular structure," *J. Mol. Struct.*, 7–16, 834–6 (2007).

148. G. Zając, A. Kaczor, K. Chruszcz Lipska, J. Cz. Dobrowolski, and M. Baranska, "Bisignate resonance Raman optical activity: a pseudo breakdown of the single electronic state model of RROA?" *J. Raman Spectrosc.*, **45**, 859–62 (2014).

149. S. Shankland, "Moore's law: the rule that really matters in tech," *CNET News*, 2012, http://www.cnet.com/news/moores-law-the-rule-that-really-matters-in-tech/

150. I. L. Markov, "Limits on fundamental limits to computation," *Nature*, **512**, 147–54 (2014).

151. Q. Yang, L. Zhang, L. Wang, and H. Xiao, "MultiDA: chemometric software for multivariate data analysis based on Matlab," *Chemom. Intell. Lab. Syst.*, **116**, 1–8 (2012).

152. P. Tosco and T. Balle, "Open3DQSAR: a new open-source software aimed at high-throughput chemometric analysis of molecular interaction fields," *J. Mol. Model.*, **17**, 201–8 (2011).

153. R. A. Viscarra Rossel, "ParLeS: software for chemometric analysis of spectroscopic data," *Chemomet. Intell. Lab. Syst.*, **90**, 72–83 (2008).

154. D. Sorak, L. Heberholz, S. Iwascek, S. Altinpinar, and H. W. Siesler, "New developments and applications of handheld Raman, mid-infrared, and near-infrared spectrometers," *Appl. Spectrosc. Rev.*, **47**, 83–115 (2012).

155. K. Majzner, A. Kaczor, N. Kachamakova-Trojanowska, A. Fedorowicz, S. Chlopicki, and M. Baranska, "3D confocal Raman imaging of endothelial cells and vascular wall: perspectives in analytical spectroscopy of biomedical research," *Analyst*, **138**, 603–10 (2013).

156. A. F. Palonpon, M. Sodeoka, and K. Fujita, "Molecular imaging of live cells by Raman microscopy," *Curr. Opin. Chem. Biol.*, **17**, 708–15 (2013).

157. J. V. Coe, Z. Chen, R. Li, R. Butke, B. Miller, C. L. Hitchcock, H. C. Allen, S. P. Povoski, and E. W. Martin Jr. "Imaging infrared spectroscopy for fixation-free liver tumor detection," *Proceedings of the SPIE, 8947, Imag. Manip. Anal. Biomol. Cells Tiss. XII*, 89470B 6 pp. (2014).

158. C. R. Flach and D. J. Moore, "Infrared and Raman imaging spectroscopy of ex vivo skin," *Int. J. Cosmet. Sci.*, **35**, 125–35 (2013).

159. H. Shinzawa, K. Awa, W. Kanematsu, and Y. Ozaki, "Multivariate data analysis for Raman spectroscopic imaging," *J. Raman Spectrosc.*, **40**, 1720–5 (2009).

160. R. Bhargava, "Infrared spectroscopic imaging: the next generation," *Appl. Spectrosc.*, **66**, 1091–120 (2012).

161. O. J. Old, L. M. Fullwood, R. Scott, G. R. Lloyd, L. M. Almond, N. A. Shepherd, N. Stone, H. Barr, and C. Kendall, "Vibrational spectroscopy for cancer diagnostics," *Anal. Methods*, **6**, 3901–17 (2014).

162. A. A. Bunaciu, Ş. Fleschin, and H. Y. Aboul-Enein, "Infrared microspectroscopy applications: review," *Curr. Anal. Chem.*, **10**, 132–9 (2014).

163. J. L. González-Solís, J. C. Martínez-Espinosa, J. M. Salgado-Román, and P. Palomares-Anda, "Monitoring of chemotherapy leukemia treatment using Raman spectroscopy and principal component analysis," *Lasers Med. Sci.*, **29**, 1241–9 (2014).

164. A. Largo-Gosens, M. Hernández-Altamirano, L. García-Calvo, A. Alonso-Simón, J. Alvarez, and J. L. Acebes, "Fourier transform mid infrared spectroscopy applications for monitoring the structural plasticity of plant cell walls," *Front Plant Sci.*, **5**, 303, 1–15 (2014).

7 Structural Studies of Carotenoids in Plants, Animals, and Food Products

Takashi Maoka

Research Institute for Production Development, Kyoto, Japan

7.1 Introduction

Since the first structural elucidation of β-carotene by Kuhn and Karrer in 1928–1930, about 750 naturally occurring carotenoids had been reported as of 2004 [1]. Improvements of analytical instruments such as nuclear magnetic resonance (NMR), mass spectroscopy (MS), high-performance liquid chromatography (HPLC), and so on have made it possible to perform the structural elucidation of very minor carotenoids in nature [2]. Annually, several new structures of carotenoids are being reported. Our research group has developed structural elucidation and analysis of naturally occurring carotenoids using NMR, MS, MS/MS, LC/MS [2], and so on over the last decade. Herein, I describe the techniques for structural elucidation and analysis of carotenoids in plants, animals, and food products.

7.2 Extraction and pre-preparation of carotenoids

Carotenoids are labile compounds for oxidation, heat, and light. Therefore, extraction and purification procedures should be carried out rapidly below 40 °C while taking care to avoid exposing them to strong light. Acetone is commonly used for extraction of

Carotenoids: Nutrition, Analysis and Technology, First Edition. Edited by Agnieszka Kaczor and Malgorzata Baranska.

carotenoid from biological materials, especially animal tissues. Methanol is also used for extraction of plant tissues. Mechanical, enzymatic, or alkaline disruption of the cell wall may be required for extraction of carotenoid from yeast and bacteria, which have rigid cell walls. For example, carotenoids in Phaffia yeast (*Xanthophyllomyces dendrorhrous*, formerly *Phaffia rhodozyma*), which has a rigid cell wall, were hardly extracted by acetone or methanol. They could effectively be extractable using dimethyl sulfoxide with heating to about 60 °C. In some cases, antioxidants are added to extracted solution to avoid oxidative degradation [3].

Acetone or methanol extracts of animal organs contain substantial amounts of water and polar lipid. They must be removed before evaporation to avoid bumping. For this purpose, the extracts are transferred to two-layer solution composed by diethyl ether–hexane (1:1) solution and water in a separating funnel. The organic epiphase, which contains carotenoids, was washed with water several times to remove acetone and water-soluble contaminants. After drying over Na_2SO_4 to remove water, the organic phase was evaporated to dryness below 40 °C. In the case of small volumes (about less than 2 ml) of sample solution, solvent can be evaporated directly by stream of nitrogen or inactive gas. Generally, steroids and neutral lipids (triglyceride, wax, etc.) are contained together with carotenoid in extract. These lipid impurities should be removed as much as possible before carotenoid analysis. These lipid contaminants are effectively removed through precipitation and filtration in cooled (below –20 °C) acetone or methanol solution.

Many carotenoids are stable toward base. Thus, saponification with KOH–methanol is commonly used on the carotenoid extracts to remove triglyceride from a lipid-rich sample. Saponification is also available for hydrolysis of carotenoid ester. However, saponification causes several side reactions for alkaline unstable carotenoids [3]. The following reactions were typically reported:

1. Astaxanthin is oxidized to astacen. This reaction occurs for all carotenoids having a 3-hydroxy-4-keto-β-end group.
2. Saponification also causes dehydration on carotenoids with a 2-hydroxy-4-keto-β-end group, such as 2-hydroxy-canthaxanthin.
3. Fucoxanthin and it derivatives are converted to corresponding hemiketal compounds by base.
4. Peridinin also decomposes under base.
5. Seco-carotenoids, such as tobiraxanthns, are converted to carotenoids having unique five-member rings by alkaline medium [2, 4].

To avoid these side reactions, enzymatic hydrolysis using cholesterol esterase [5] or lipase [6, 7] has been employed for hydrolysis of alkaline labile carotenoid esters.

Carotenoid esters and triglycerides possess almost similar polarity in many cases. Therefore, it is difficult to separate these compounds using normal and/or reverse-phase chromatography. In these cases, gel filtration chromatography (GPC) using polystyrene gel can effectively separate them because the molecular size of carotenoid esters is larger than that of triglycerides. For example, fucoxanthin ester in clams [8] and astxanthin esters in crustaceans [9] were successively isolated by HPLC using this GPC column.

Purified carotenoids should be submitted to spectral analysis as soon as possible, and they were stored below –20 °C, or preferably at –80 °C, under inactive gas.

7.3 Chromatography and separation of carotenoids

7.3.1 Column chromatography and thin-layer chromatography

Column chromatography is commonly used for the first separation procedure of carotenoid from crude extract. Silica gel is exclusively used as an adsorbent of carotenoid separation now, whereas magnesium oxide, calcium carbonate, cellulose powder, and aluminum oxide were once used as adsorbents of carotenoid separation.

Thin-layer chromatography (TLC) is the simplest and quickest method for analysis of carotenoids. Most carotenoid showed yellow, orange, and red color. Therefore, many carotenoid spots are easily observed without detection procedures such as fluorescent monitoring and spraying of dying agents. From the retention factor (Rf) values and spot color on TLC, many carotenoids can be tentatively identified. Precoated silica gel 60 G plate is most frequently used for analysis of carotenoids. Reversed-phase TLC is also available now. Preparative TLC is employed in the separation of natural carotenoids. This is the simplest and quickest procedure for separation of carotenoids.

7.3.2 High-performance liquid chromatography

HPLC is widely used for not only qualitative and qualitative analysis but also preparative separation of carotenoids. Normal-phase HPLC using a silica gel column is conveniently used for separation of carotenoids. Carotenoids are eluted according to their polarity. This method is powerful for the separation of xanthophylls, but carotenes are poorly resolved on this method.

Reverse-phase HPLC using C_8, C_{18} (ODS), and C_{30} bonded-phase columns are also used for separation of carotenoids. Reverse-phase HPLC with a gradient mobile-phase system is applicable to carotenoids of all levels of polarity. The C_{30} column is effective for separation of carotenes, including their geometrical isomers. A nitrile-phase column is also used for separation of geometrical isomers of carotenoids. Recently, an ultra-high-performance liquid chromatography (UPLC) system, which used a C_{18} microparticle size column (1.7 μm), was developed. Compared with an ordinary HPLC system, the UPLC system afforded finer separation and sensitivity, and a reduction of analytical time. Figure 7.1 showed a chromatogram of carotenoids in human erythrocytes using the UPLC system. Eleven carotenoids were detected within 8 min [10].

GPC and ion exchange columns also use carotenoid separation. Chiral-phase columns are used for separation of optical isomers of carotenoids. We achieved the separation of optical isomers of carotenoids using chiral-phase columns: Sumichiral OA-2000 for carotenoids with a 3-hydroxy-4-oxo-β-end group [11] and 3-hydroxy-β-end group [12], and Chiral cell OD for carotenoids with a 4-hydroxy-β-end group [13]. Chiral pack AD [14] and Chiral pack IC [15] were also used for separation of the optical isomers of zeaxanthin and astaxanthin, respectively. Recently, three optical isomers of alloxanthin were also achieved using the Chiral pack AD-H column [16].

Semipreparative HPLC using columns that are 25–50 cm long with an internal diameter of 6–10 cm are used on the milligram scale for carotenoid separation, which was required for NMR analysis. In my experience, it is difficult to obtain pure carotenoids for single-system HPLC. Therefore, I recommend using both normal and reverse-phase HPLC systems for purification of carotenoids.

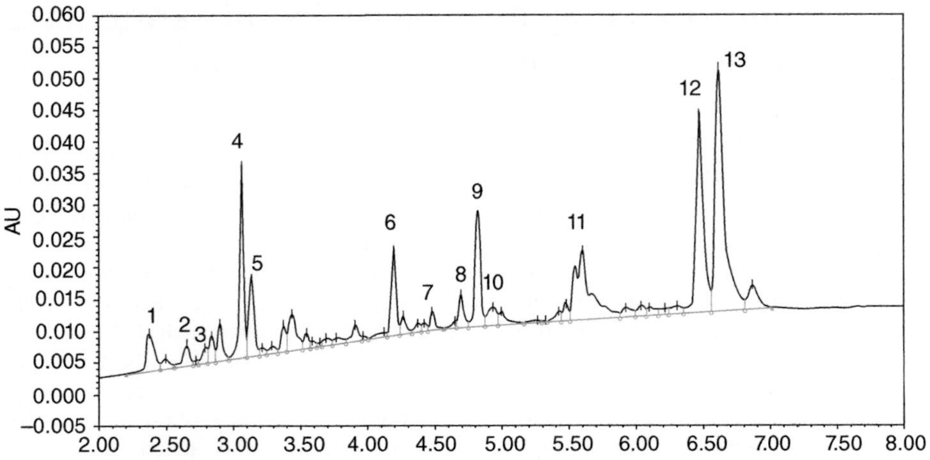

Figure 7.1 UPLC of carotenoids in astaxanthin-supplemented human erythrocyte using the UPLC system. Peak 1: astaxanthin; Peak 2: 9-*cis*-astaxanthin; Peak 3: 13-*cis*-astaxanthin; Peak 4: lutein; Peak 5: zeaxanthin; Peak 6: anhydrolutein I; Peak 7: anhydrolutein II; Peak 8: α-cryptoxanthin; Peak 9: β-cryptoxanthin; Peak 10: 9-*cis*-β-cryptoxanthin; Peak 11: lycopene; Peak 12: α-carotene; and Peak 13: β-carotene. For a HPLC condition ACQUITY UPLC system (Waters): column, BEH Shield RP18 (1.7 μm, 2.1×150 mm); mobile phase, AcCN/H_2O (85:15) → AcCN/MeOH (65:35); column temperature, 40 °C; flow rate, 0.4ml/min; and detection, 452 nm.

7.4 Quantification of carotenoids

Many carotenoids have a strong visible-light (Vis) absorption band around 400~500 nm. There are a few compounds with the same absorption band. Therefore, carotenoid absorption maxima around 400~500 nm are selective and sensitive. Carotenoid content in crude extract can be calculated from the absorption coefficient. Carotenoid content in crude extract can be calculated using the coefficient $E^{1\%}_{cm} = 2500$ for mainly β-carotene and lutein samples, $E^{1\%}_{cm} = 2100$ (in hexane) for mainly astaxanthin samples, and $E^{1\%}_{cm} = 1600$ (in hexane), 1060 (in acetone), 1140 (in ethanol) for mainly fucoxanthin samples [3, 17]. Individual carotenoid content is calculated by HPLC using a Vis absorption chromatogram or selective ion mass (MS) chromatogram.

7.5 Identification and structural elucidation of carotenoids

Identification of carotenoids needs aligning Rf values on TLC, retention time of HPLC with two different detection systems, and UV-Vis and MS spectral data with authentic samples. An LC/MS instrument coupled with a photodiode array detector (DAD) is a powerful tool for identification of natural carotenoids. Favorably, ^{1}H-NMR spectral data were needed for the identification of complex structural carotenoids, such as carotenoid glycosides and geometric isomers. The identification of optical isomers of carotenoids needs CD spectral data and/or chiral HPLC analysis.

Structural elucidation of natural carotenoids needs UV-Vis; high-resolution MS; ^{1}H and ^{13}C NMR, including two-dimensional (2D) NMR analysis; and CD spectral data in the case of chiral carotenoids [2]. Chemical dramatization also provides valuable information for structural data.

7.5.1 Chemical dramatization

Chemical dramatizations such as reduction with $NaBH_4$ or $LiALH_4$, acetylation, trimethyl siliylation, methylation, and epoxide–furanoxide rearrangement have been employed for detection of functional groups such as hydroxy groups, carbonyl groups, and epoxides in carotenoids [18]. However, this structural information can be provided from NMR, MS, infrared (IR) spectrometry, and so on. Therefore, chemical dramatizations are not used often now.

However, acetylation is still useful to improve HPLC and NMR analyses. Although it is difficult to separate the related carotenoids that contain rhamnoside and fucoside in their original structure in HPLC analysis, the acetylated derivatives elute separately in HPLC analysis. In general, ^{1}H NMR signals of sugar moiety in carotenoid glycosides are severely overlapped. Acetylation can resolve this problem by its lower-field shift effect.

7.5.2 UV-Vis, IR, and Raman spectrometry

UV-Vis absorption spectra comprise very simple and essential spectrometry for carotenoid analysis. Absorbance max (λmax) values in the UV-Vis spectra provide information on conjugated double-bond numbers in carotenoids. The shape of the UV-Vis spectra is analyzed using the parameters of %III/II and $\%D_B/D_{II}$ values. Values of %III/II provide information on the end groups (β-, ε-, γ-end groups, etc.) in carotenoids. Values of $\%D_B/D_{II}$ provide information on the presence of *cis* double bonds in carotenoids [17]. Carotenoids having conjugated carbonyl groups at C-4 in the β-end group, such as canthaxanthin and astaxanthin, show broad bell-shaped UV-Vis spectra. Although carotenoids having no conjugated carbonyl group such as β-carotene show triplet-shaped UV-Vis spectra, DAD coupled with HPLC provide online UV-Vis spectra during HPLC analysis.

The IR spectrum affords information on functional groups such as hydroxy, carbonyl, allene, acetylene, and other groups in carotenoids [19]. Fourier transform (FT) IR enables one to measure the IR spectrum with a sub-microgram sample. But the information from the IR spectrum is complicated and not confirmatory in many cases. Thus, IR spectrometry is not used often now.

Like IR spectroscopy, Raman spectroscopy provides detailed information on molecular vibration. Resonance Raman spectroscopy can be obtained at very low concentrations (to 10^{-8} M) even if the chromophore is included in a complex biological medium. Therefore, resonance Raman spectrometry is used for analysis of carotenoids with a protein complex in biological materials. Resonance Raman spectroscopy is a very useful method to study the structures and interaction of pigments such as chlorophylls and carotenoids in photosynthetic protein. Characteristic resonance Raman bands of carotenoids are 1600–1500 cm^{-1} (C=C stretching vibration), 1300–1100 cm^{-1} (CC stretching/in-plane C–H vending vibration), 1000 cm^{-1} (CH_3 vending vibration), and 960 cm^{-1} (out-of-plane C–H vending vibration). The E/Z geometry of the polyene chain in carotenoids can be characterized in the 1300–1100 cm^{-1} region of spectra [20]. Furthermore, resonance Raman spectrometry can detect carotenoids in living organisms. Recently, Uragami *et al.* succeeded in detecting astaxanthin in astaxanthin-administered rat skin using 3D mapping of the Raman spectrum [21].

7.5.3 Mass spectrometry

7.5.3.1 Instruments and high-resolution MS MS is a most sensitive tool for analysis of organic compounds. Double-focusing magnetic-field instruments and time-of-flight (TOF) instruments can provide high-resolution mass (so-called mil mass) data. Molecular formulas can be determined by comparison of observed high-resolution masses of molecular ions or quasi-molecular ions with possible composition using accurate masses of individual isotopes ($^{12}C=12$,$^{1}H=1.007825$,$^{16}O=15.994915$, etc.). If measured accurate mass was observed within the error of 5 ppm or 3 mmu from the predicted (calculated) value, the molecular formula of this compound can be judged "correct." High-resolution MS data are essentially required to determine new carotenoids.

7.5.3.2 Ionization and observed ions Electro-ionization (EI) MS of carotenoids provides not only molecular ions [M^+] but also several fragment ions such as elimination of water [$M\text{-}H_2O]^+$, elimination of the acetyl group $[M\text{-}AcOH]^+$, $[M\text{-}80]^+$ (a characteristic ion observed in epoxy carotenoids), elimination of toluene from the polyene chain $[M\text{-}92]^+$, elimination of xylene from the polyene chain $[M\text{-}106]^+$, elimination of end groups from the polyene chain, and so on. These fragment ions give important information on the carotenoid structure. Enzell and Back compiled typical fragment ions of carotenoids in EI MS [22]. However, molecular ions of polar carotenoids, such as carotenoid glycoside and sulfate, were hardly observed by EI MS.

On the other hand, soft ionization of mass spectrometry, such as field desorption (FD), fast atom bombardment (FAB), atmospheric pressure chemical ionization (APCI), electrospray ionization (ESI), and matrix-associated laser desorption (MALDI), provides molecular ions or molecular-related ions predominantly. Figure 7.2 showed the EI, FAB, FD, and ESI mass spectra of violaxanthin. The molecular ion $[M]^+$ was predominantly observed in EI, FD, FAB, and MALDI MS. On the other hand, in the APCI MS, the protonated molecular ion $[M+H]^+$ was mainly observed as a molecular-weight-related ion for both carotenes and xanthophylls. ESI ionization provided several molecular-weight-related ions of carotenoids. For example, the molecular ion [M^+] was predominantly observed in carotenes. Both M^+ and $[M+H]^+$ ions were predominantly observed in hydroxy carotenoids such as β-cryptoxanthin and zeaxanthin. In our experience, $[M+H]^+$ was predominant when more than 1 ng of sample was injected. On the other hand, M^+ was predominant when less than 1 ng of sample was injected. In the case of lutein, fragment ions at *m/z* 550 (elimination of water from M^+) and/or *m/z* 551 (elimination of water from $[M+H]^+$) were observed predominantly instead of M^+ and/or $[M+H]^+$. Keto-carotenoids such as astaxanthin predominantly provided sodium adduct ion [M+Na]+ along with $[M+H]^+$. ESI MS of violaxanthin provides alkaline metal adduct ions $[M+Na]^+$ and $[M+K]^+$, predominantly along with protonated molecular ion $[M+H]^+$, as shown in Figure 7.2.

7.5.3.3 MS/MS spectrometry Generally, soft ionization of mass spectrometry provides a fragmentation-less spectrum. Therefore, MS/MS techniques were employed to observed several product ions (fragment ions) in soft ionization of mass spectrometry.

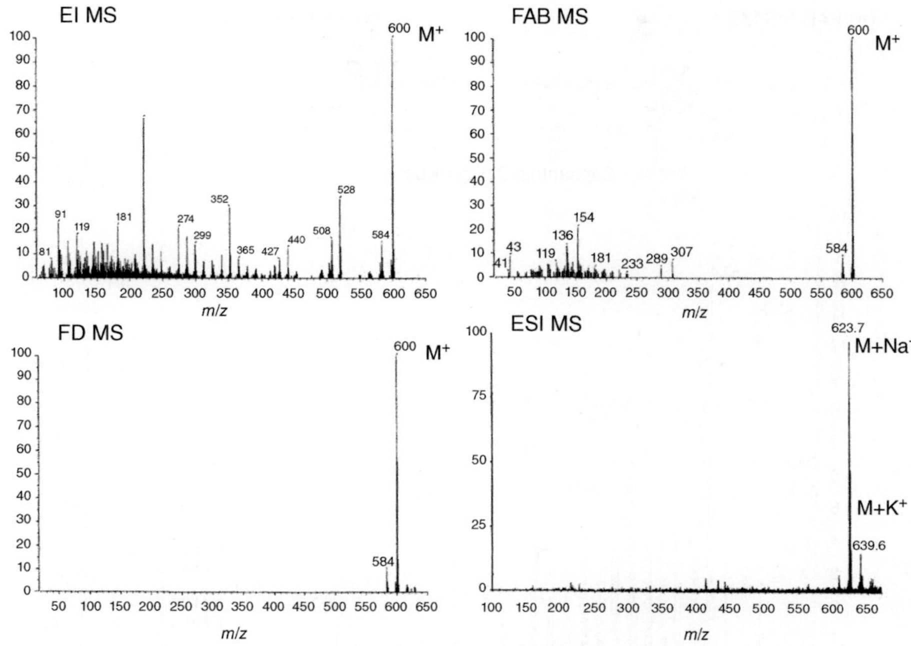

Figure 7.2 Positive ion EI, FAB, FD, and ESI MS spectra of violaxanthin.

FAB collision-induced dissociation (CID) MS/MS using a two-sector mass spectrometer has been used for the structural analysis of natural products. Therefore, we have applied a high-energy FAB MS/MS technique for structural analysis of carotenoids. The FAB MS/MS of carotenoids, using the molecular ion $[M]^+$ as a precursor ion, provides EI MS–like fragmentation [23–25]. The FAB MS/MS spectra of more than 100 natural carotenoids are available on the Mass Bank website [26]. Figure 7.3A showed the FAB MS/MS of capsanthin 3,6-epoxide using a molecular ion at *m/z* 600 as a precursor ion. Capsanthin 3,6-epoxide showed the characteristic product ions at *m/z* 582 $[M–H_2O]^+$ and *m/z* 520 $[M–80]^+$, indicating the presence of a hydroxy group and epoxy group, respectively. Elimination of toluene moiety from the polyene chain at m/z 508 $[M–92]^+$ was also observed as weak intensity. Furthermore, a series of product ions resulting from cleavage of C–C bonds in the polyene chain from the epoxy end group (i.e., *m/z* 181, 221, 286, 455, and 473) was observed. The product ions at *m/z* 473 $[M–127]^+$ (cleavage between C-6′ and C-5′) and *m/z* 445 $[M–155]^+$ (cleavage between C-7′ and C-6′) indicated the presence of 3-hydroxy-κ-end group. Recently, quadrupole–quadrupole (Q-Q) and quadrupole-TOF (Q-TOF) instruments with ESI or APCI ionization were widely used for MS/MS measurement of several natural products. Figure 7.3B showed ESI Q-TOF MS/MS of capsanthin 3,6-epoxide using protonated molecular ion $[M+H]^+$ at *m/z* 601 as a precursor ion. As same as FAB MS/MS, product ions elimination of water at *m/z* 583 $[M+H–H_2O]^+$ and at *m/z* 565 $[M+H–2H_2O]^+$, and elimination of toluene moiety at *m/z* 509 $[M+H–92]^+$, were observed. However, product ions' elimination of the epoxy group $[M+H–80]^+$, product ions resulting from cleavage between C-6′ and C-5′, and cleavage between C-7′ and C-6′, which were predominantly observed in FAB MS/MS, were not observed in ESI Q-TOF MS/MS. However, ESI Q-TOF MS/MS of sodium adduct ion $[M+Na]^+$ of xanthophylls provided

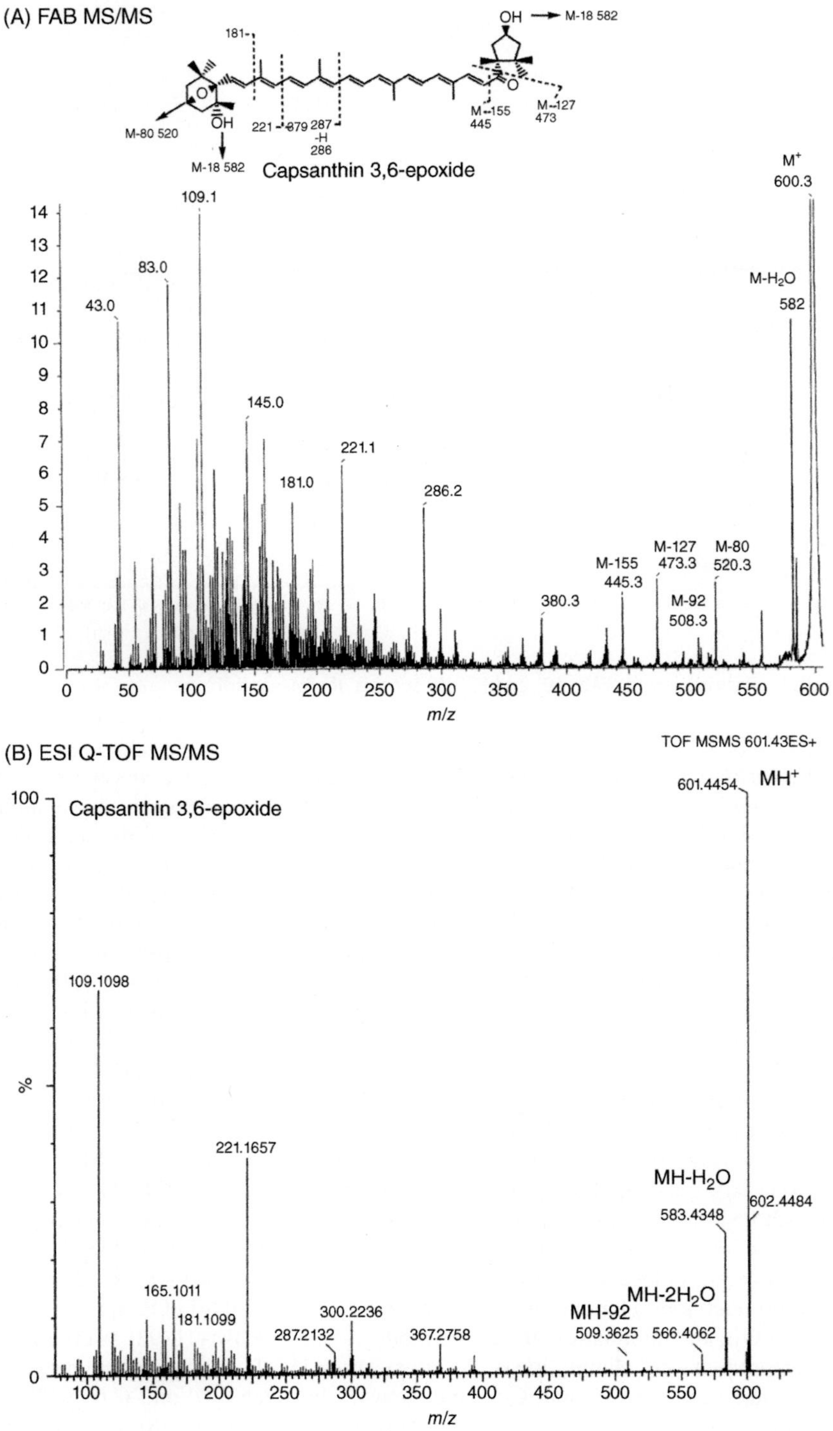

Figure 7.3 MS/MS spectrum of capsanthin 3,6-epoxide, (upper) FAB MS/MS and (lower) ESI Q-TOF MS/MS.

elimination of toluene moiety $[M+Na-92]^+$ and elimination of xylene moiety $[M+Na-106]^+$, which were diagnostic fragments in EI MS of carotenoids [27–28].

7.5.3.4 LC/MS and LC/MS/MS LC/MS is a powerful technique for the identification and quantification of carotenoids in various biological samples with high sensitivity [29–31]. Several ionizations such as FAB have been employed for ionization of LC/MS. APCI and ESI ionization tools are a conveniently combined LC system. Therefore, APCI and ESI ionization is now exclusively used for ionization of LC/MS. LC/APCI mass spectra of carotenoids provide not only $[M+H]^+$ but also characteristic fragment ions such as $[M+H\text{-}nH_2O]^+$, $[M+H\text{-}AcOH]^+$, and $[M+H\text{-}sugar]^+$ [32]. In ESI ionization, xanthophylls provided alkaline metal adduct ions, $[M+Na]^+$, and $[M+K]^+$ predominantly.

The detection limit of LC/APCI MS is several nanograms [29, 30]. LC/ESI MS is the most highly sensitive, and its detection limit is at the *sub*-nanogram level [31]. We found the following detection limits of carotenoids in an LC/ESI MS DAD system using a Waters Xevo G2S Q TOF mass spectrometer equipped with an Acquity UPLC system. Full-scan ESI MS (*m/z* 100–1500) and PDA (200–600 nm) spectra could be measured even with 0.5 ng of astaxanthin and α-carotene. Using the selective ion monitoring (SIM) method, the detection limit for $[M+H]^+$ of astaxanthin and M^+ of α-carotene on chromatograms was approximately 0.05 ng.

The reverse-phase HPLC system is exclusively used for LC/MS, although we found that APCI LC/MS could be performed with a normal-phase HPLC system by using tetrahydrofuran as a polar solvent in hexane [32]. LC/MS/MS is a powerful tool for the identification and quantification of carotenoids. Even in the presence of contaminant, the MS/MS spectrum can provide accurate carotenoid structural information. An LC/Q-TOF MS instrument combined with DAD is a very powerful tool for identification and quantification of carotenoids. Retention time in HPLC, UV-Vis spectrum from DAD, molecular ion $[M]^+$ or quasi-molecular ions ($[M+H]^+$, $[M+K]^+$, $[M+Na]^+$, etc.) from the MS spectrum, and the same product ions from the MS/MS spectrum provide accurate structural information on natural carotenoids from online HPLC. Furthermore, carotenoids were quantified with both UV-Vis and MS chromatograms.

Although LC/MS is a high-sensitivity tool, lipid contamination sometimes prevents detection of carotenoids. It is important to remove lipid impurities as much as possible during pre-preparation of samples. In my experience, the sensitivity of carotenoid detection could be increased about 10–100 times by removing lipid impurities during pre-preparation.

7.5.4 NMR spectrometry

7.5.4.1 Instruments and sensitivity NMR spectroscopy has become the most efficient spectroscopic tool for structural elucidation of organic compounds. In the 1960s, more than 10 mg sample was required for an ordinary ^{1}H NMR measurement with 60 MHz continuous-wave instruments. In the 1970s, the advent of pulsed FT NMR spectrometry and the increase of measuring frequencies (100–200 MHz) strongly improved the sensitivity and also enabled the routine measurement of ^{13}C NMR. Since then, the development of high-magnetic-field instruments (300–900 MHz) and the progress of pulse sequence techniques have enabled the structural elucidation of carotenoids with less than a *sub*-milligram of sample. Today, using a 400–500 MHz instrument with a 5 mm internal diameter sample tube (sample solution volume 600 μl), about 50 μg, 500 μg, and 2 mg of samples are generally required to measure 1D ^{1}H NMR, ^{1}H detected heteronuclear-correlated 2D NMR, and ^{13}C NMR, respectively. Furthermore, ^{1}H NMR of a few micrograms of sample can be measured within 30 min of acquisition by using a SHIGEMI

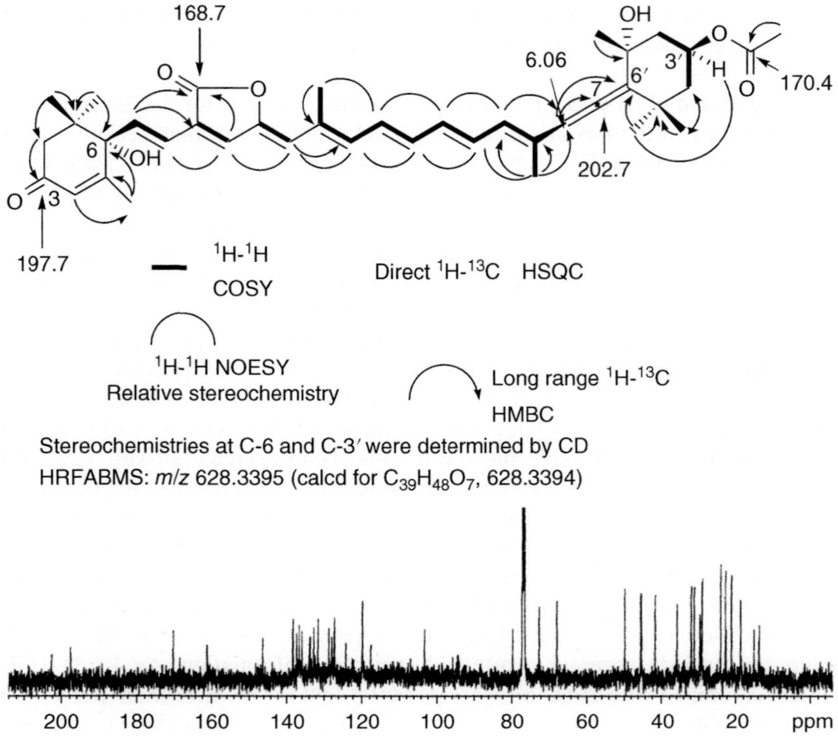

Figure 7.4 Structure of new carotenoid from oyster and ^{13}C NMR (500 μg sample in 30 μg in $CDCl_3$, using a Nano probe for 18 h acquisition).

microtube (sample solution volume 200 μl). Moreover, the Nano Probe (Agilent Technologies, formerly Varian, sample solution volume 30 μl) enables one to measure the complete decoupled ^{13}C NMR of several hundred micrograms of carotenoids for overnight acquisition, as shown in Figure 7.4 [33].

7.5.4.2 Sample preparation for carotenoids In order to obtain a high-quality spectrum, special attention should be devoted to the sample preparation. Signals of water and residual solvents appear as very high-intensity peaks and overlap on the carotenoid signals, when less than 10 μg sample measurements are used. Therefore, samples should be dried carefully in high vacuum or under the stream of nitrogen to remove moisture and residual solvents before dissolving the NMR measurement solvent.

Chloroform-d_1 ($CDCl_3$) is commonly used as a solvent for various carotenoids. We recommend using $CDCl_3$ with silver foil as a stabilizer, because $CDCl_3$ without a stabilizer gradually generates hydrochloric acid (HCl), and carotenoids are degraded by HCl during measuring time. Especially, 5,6-epoxy carotenoid is immediately converted to the corresponding 5,8-epoxide in degenerate $CDCl_3$ solution.

Benzene-d_6 (C_6D_6) is a useful solvent for NMR measurement of carotenoids. Contrary to $CDCl_3$, carotenoids are stable in C_6D_6. In addition, due to the anisotropic effect of benzene, signals of olefinic protons of carotenoids are well resolved. In $CDCl_3$ solution, a water signal appears at 1.56 ppm and sometimes overlaps with methyl or methylene signals of carotenoids. On the other hand, a water signal appears at 0.5 ppm in C_6D_6. Therefore, a water signal is not overlapped with carotenoid signals in C_6D_6 solution. However, C_6D_6 shows less solubility for xanthophylls than $CDCl_3$.

Methanol-d_4 (CD_3OD), acetone- d_6 ($(CD_3)_2CO$), and a mixture of $CDCl_3$ with CD_3OD are used for polar carotenoids, such as carotenoid glycoside and sulfate. Tetramethylsilane (TMS) is commonly used for internal standards (0 ppm) of NMR spectra. Residual solvent signals of $CDCl_3$ (7.26 ppm for ^1H NMR and 77.0 ppm for ^{13}C NMR) are also used for internal standard signals.

7.5.4.3 Identification of carotenoids by NMR Carotenoids have a long polyene chain in the central part of the molecule. Therefore, the chemical sift and coupling constant of both end groups are not influenced by each other [34]. Thus, identification of the known carotenoid could be accomplished by comparison of NMR data of end groups and the polyene chain with published data. ^1H NMR chemical shifts of 140 end groups and ^{13}C NMR chemical shifts of more than 90 end groups of carotenoids in $CDCl_3$ are available in the literature [34]. Geometry of the polyene chain was also elucidated in the isomerization shift of ^1H and ^{13}C signals of the polyene part [34]. Furthermore, we and Japanese research groups [35, 36] newly assigned the ^1H NMR signals of 44 end groups (Figure 7.5) and the ^{13}C NMR signals of 28 end groups of carotenoids (Figure 7.6). They are shown in Figure 7.5 and Figure 7.6.

7.5.4.4 NMR experimental techniques for structural elucidation of carotenoids 1D NMR experimental techniques such as ^1H-^1H decoupling and ^1H-^1H NOE (nuclear Overhauser effect) difference spectra are classical methods, but they are still important because these techniques provide fine-resolution spectra with high sensitivity [37, 38]. 2D NMR spectra are routinely used for structural analysis now [34]. ^1H-^1H COSY (correlated spectroscopy) and TOCSY (total correlation spectroscopy) elucidate proton–proton (^1H-^1H) chemical-shift connections. COSY detects the connections of geminal or vicinal coupling protons. TOCSY elucidates the continuous coupling of ^1H-^1H connections. 1D TOCSY provides fine-resolution spectra and can reveal ^1H-^1H connections in strongly crowded signals.

NOE is observed at both proton pairs, which locate at within 3.5 Å. Both NOESY (nuclear Overhauser enhancement and exchange spectroscopy) and ROESY (rotation frame nuclear Overhauser effect spectroscopy) spectra provide information on the distance geometry of the protons in organic compound. The intensity and phase (positive or negative signal) of NOE are dependent on the measuring frequency of the NMR instrument and the molecular weight of the sample. When measuring frequencies in the range of a 400–600 MHz instrument, NOE is observed as a strong and positive signal for the small molecules below 700 Da, and it becomes small or even completely vanishes for the molecular masses around 800 Da. NOE is observed as a strong and negative signal for the large molecules higher than 1000 Da. From the above reason, carotenoid glycosides or fatty acid esters having molecular masses 800–1000 Da show very weak NOE in 1D NOE difference and NOESY spectra. Transverse or rotating-frame NOE (ROE) show always-positive and strong NOE in the medium molecular mass range. Therefore, ROESY is encouraged for NOE measurement of compounds that have molecular masses 800–1000 Da. Recently, gradient-assisted 1D NOE spectroscopy (GOESY), a new technique of NOE experiment using a pulse field gradient (PFG), has also been applied to NOE experiments on carotenoids, and it showed very highly sensitive results.

Connection of a proton–carbon chemical shift (^1H-^{13}C) is elucidated by ^{13}C-^1H COSY, ^{13}C-^1H long-range COSY, HSQC (heteronuclear singlet-quantum coherence), and HMBC (heteronuclear multiple-bond coherence). ^{13}C detected spectroscopy (^{13}C-^1H COSY and ^{13}C-^1H long-range COSY) is low sensitivity and requires samples larger than 10 mg. Therefore,

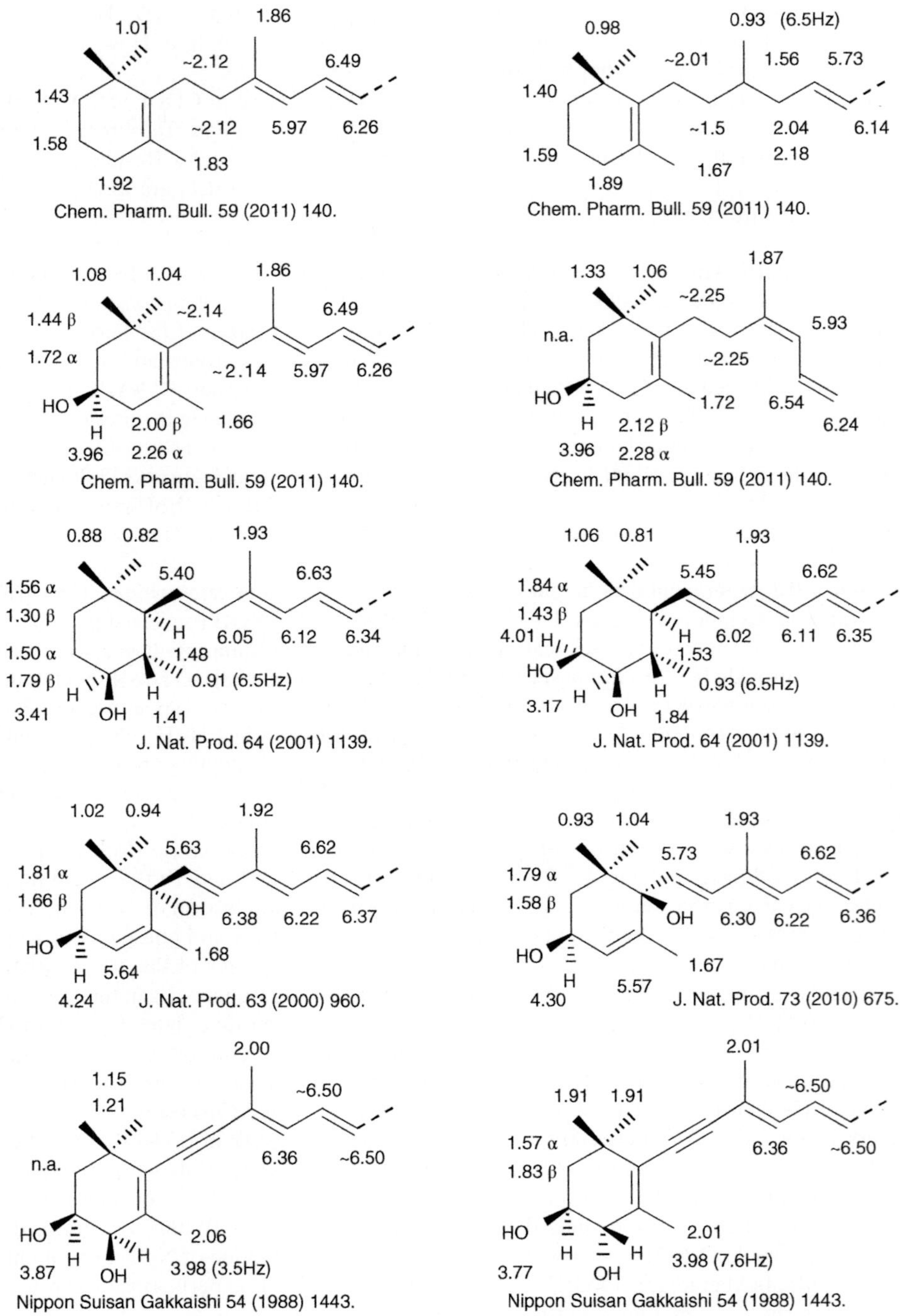

Figure 7.5 ^{1}H NMR chemical shifts of carotenoid end groups.

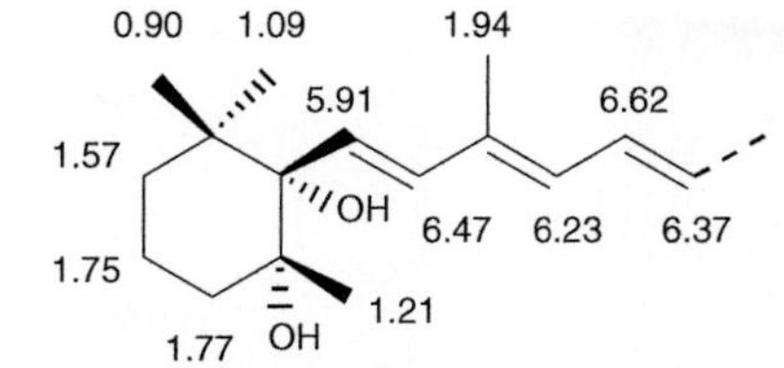

Phytochemistry 68 (2007) 1744.

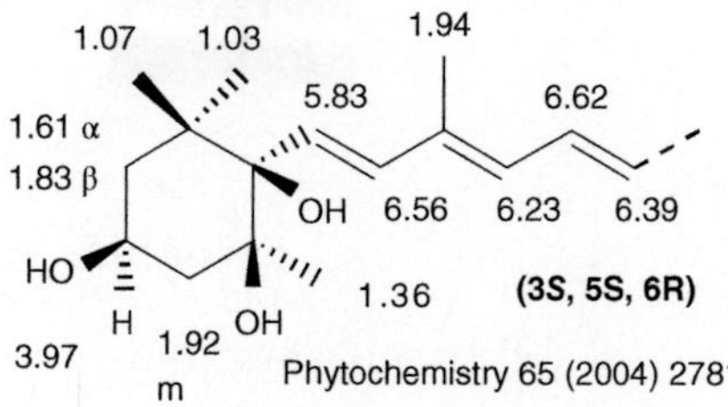

Phytochemistry 65 (2004) 2781.

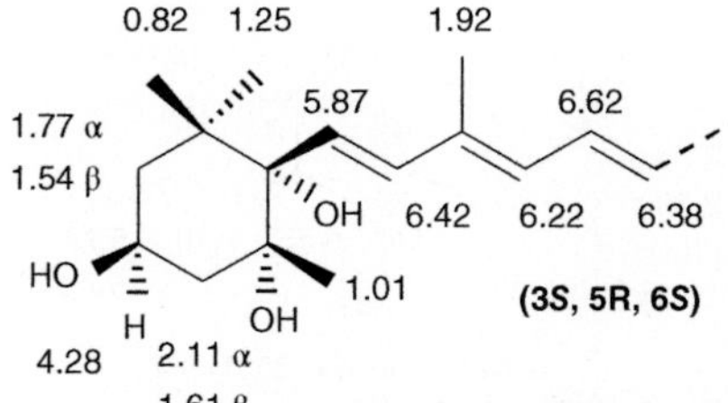

J. Nat. Prod. 68 (2005) 1371.

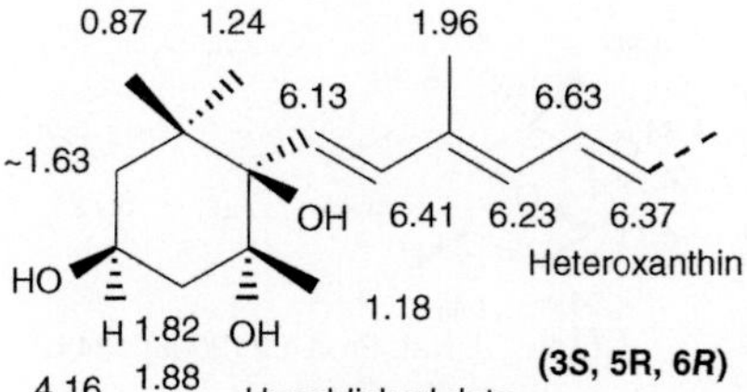

Unpublished data

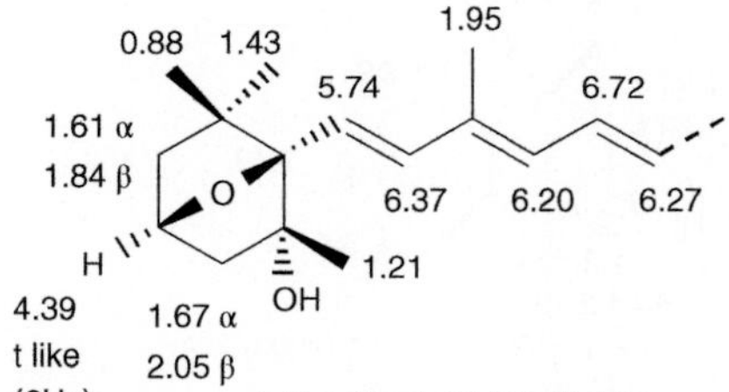

J. Nat. Prod. 67 (2004) 115.

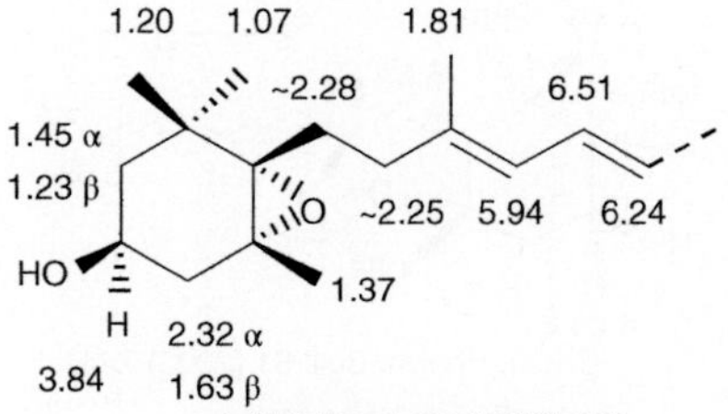

J. Nat. Prod. 73 (2010) 675.

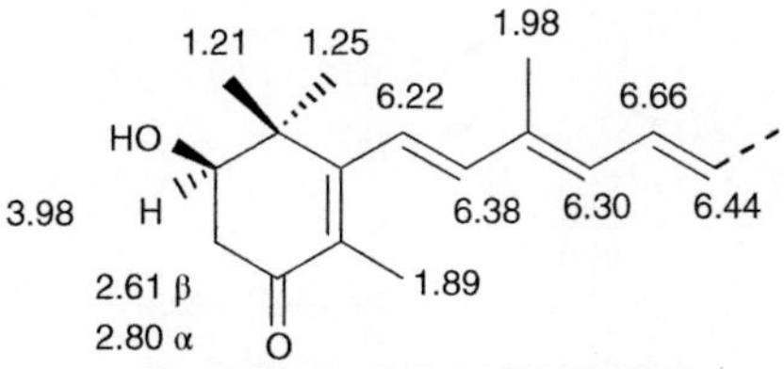

Chem. Phram. Bull. 54 (2006) 1462.

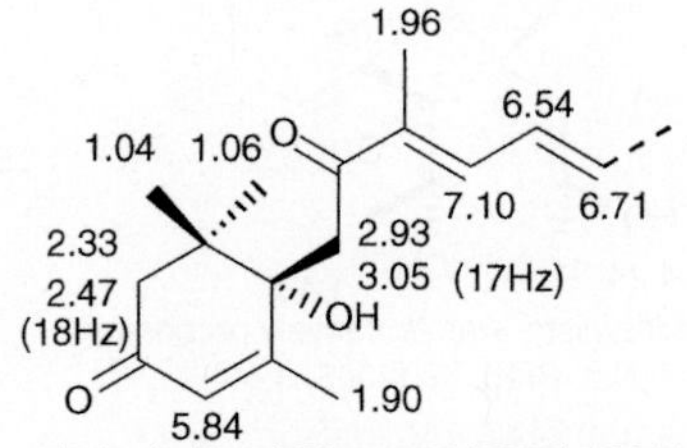

J. Agric. Food Chem. 56 (2008) 12069.

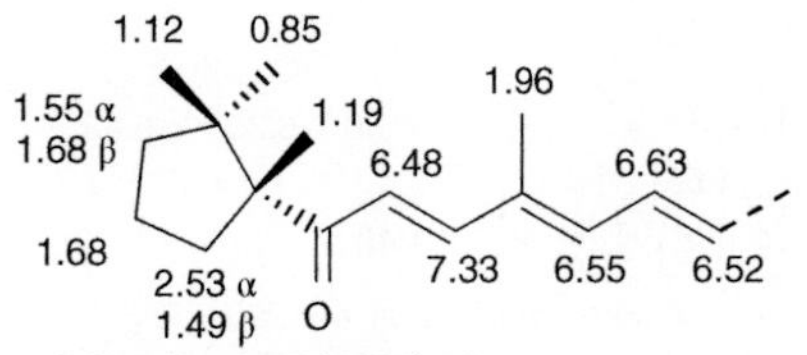

J. Nat. Prod. 67 (2004) 115.

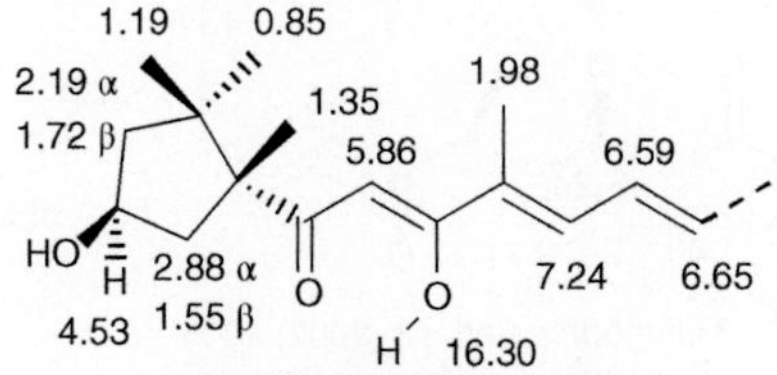

J. Nat. Prod. 64 (2001) 578.

Figure 7.5 (*Continued*)

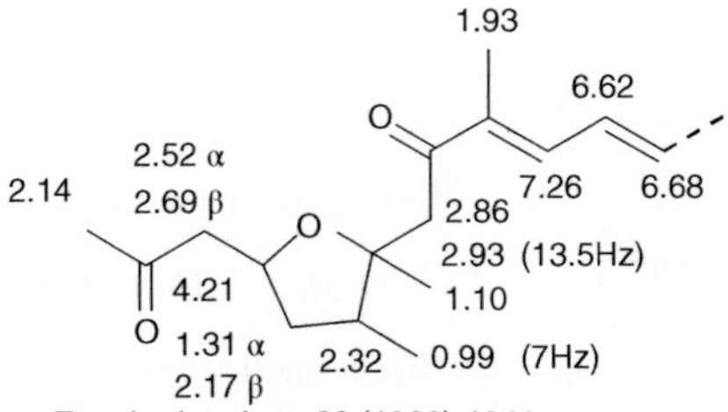

Tetrahedron Lett. 33 (1922) 4941.

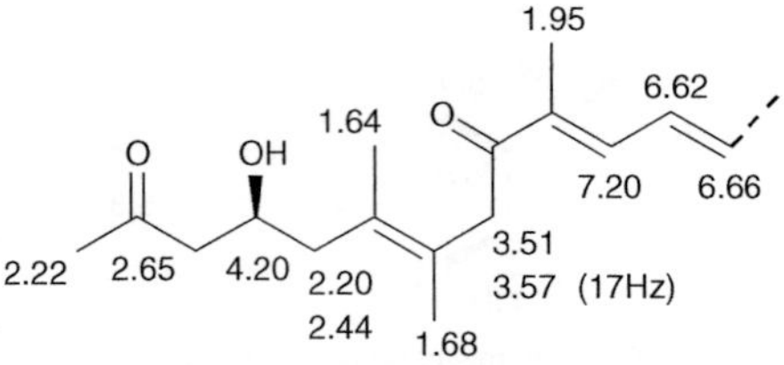

Tetrahedron Lett. 33 (1922) 4941.

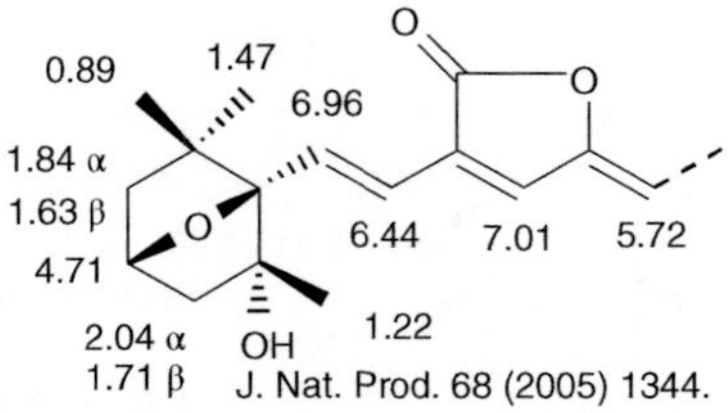

J. Nat. Prod. 68 (2005) 1344.

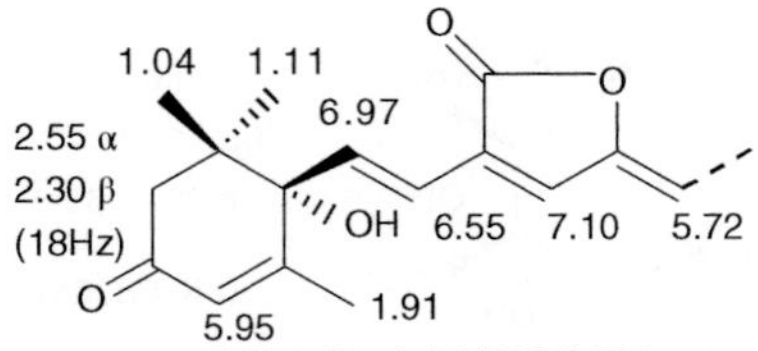

J. Nat. Prod. 64 (2001) 578.

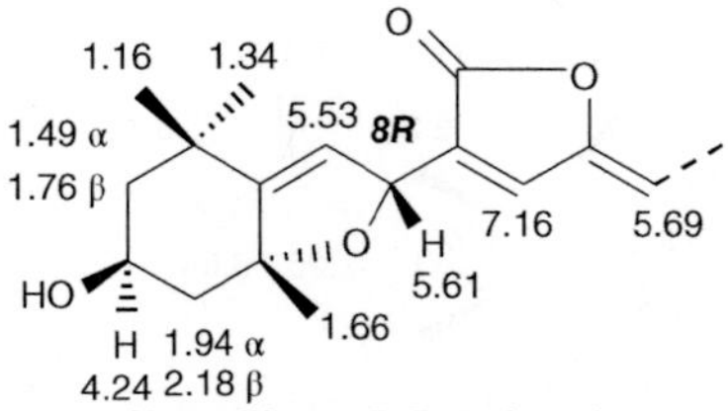

Chem. Pharm. Bull. 51 (2003) 724.

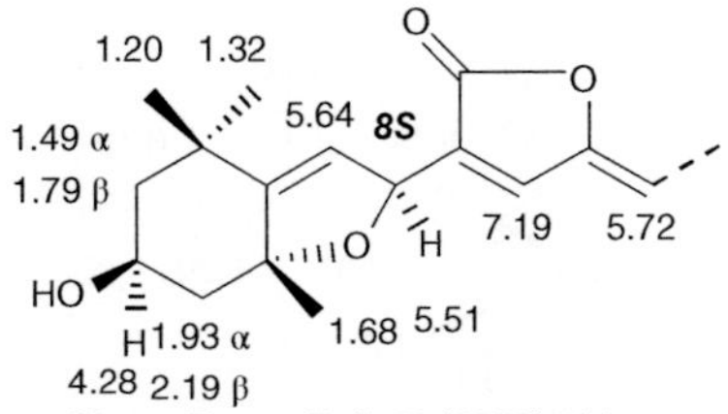

Chem. Pharm. Bull. 51 (2003) 724.

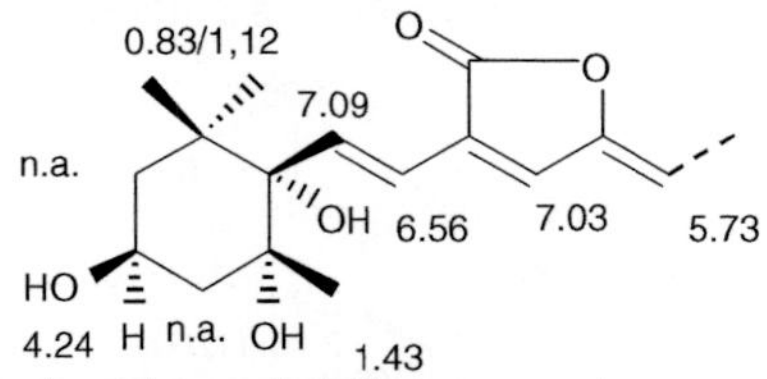

Stereochemistry was tentatively proposed
J. Nat. Prod. 68 (2005) 1344.

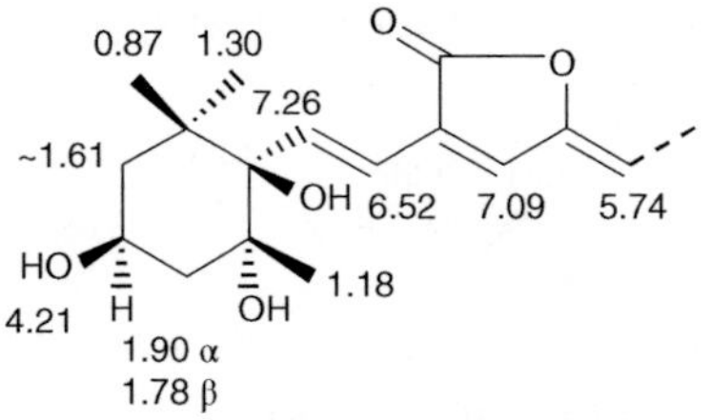

J. Agric. Food Chem. 56 (2008) 12069.

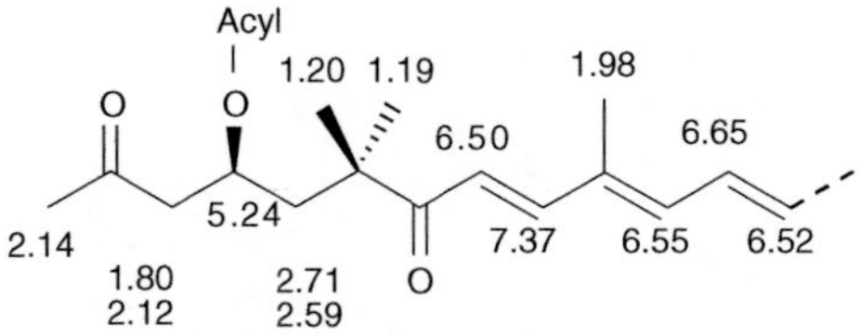

Tetrahedron Lett. 43 (2002) 4385.

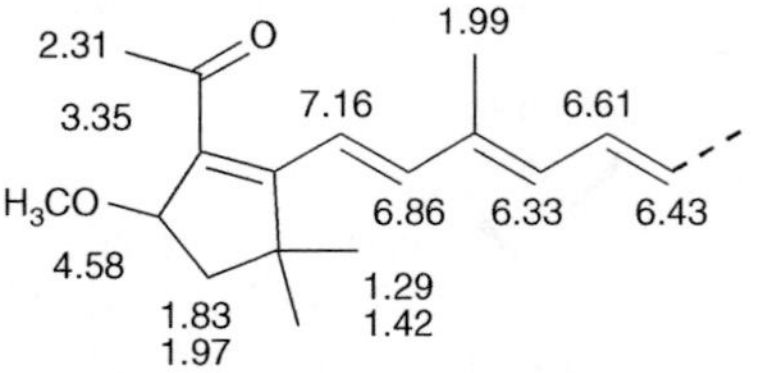

Chem. Pharm. Bull. 49 (2001) 985.

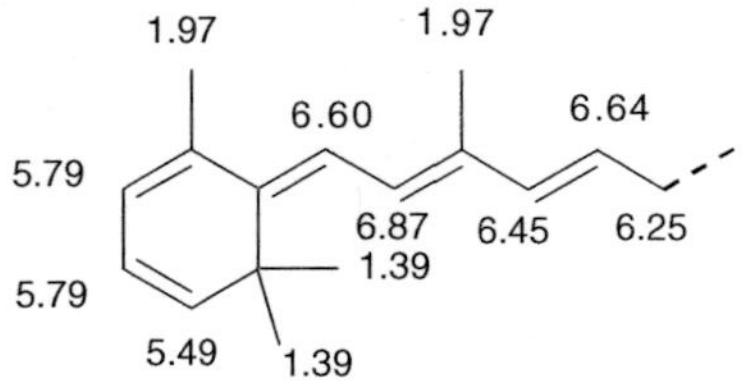

J. Plant Res. 108 (1995) 369.

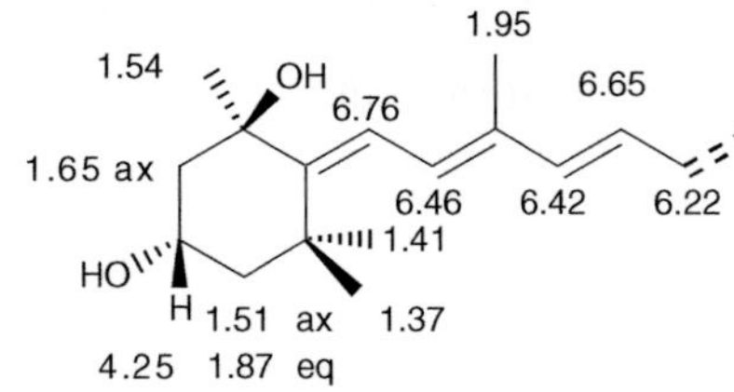

J. Nat. Prod. 63 (2000) 1288.

Figure 7.5 (*Continued*)

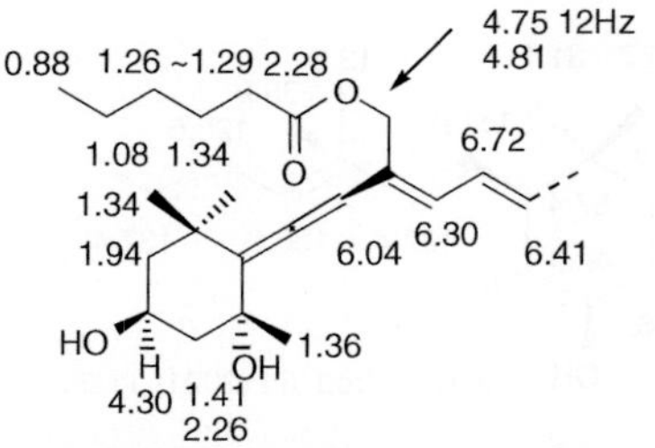

J. Agric. Food Chem. 59 (2011) 13059.

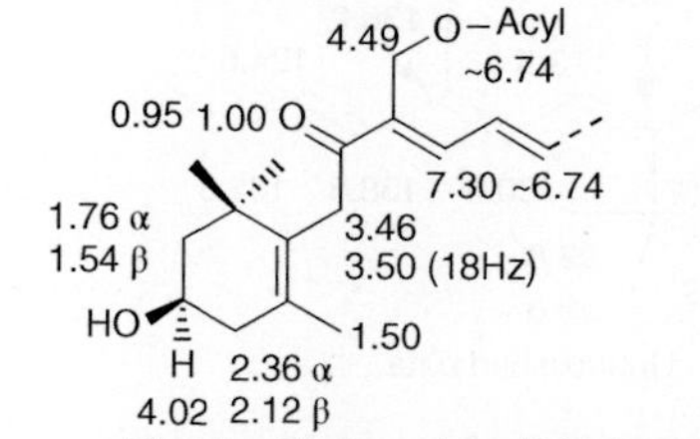

Biochim. Biophys. Acta 1810 (2011) 497.

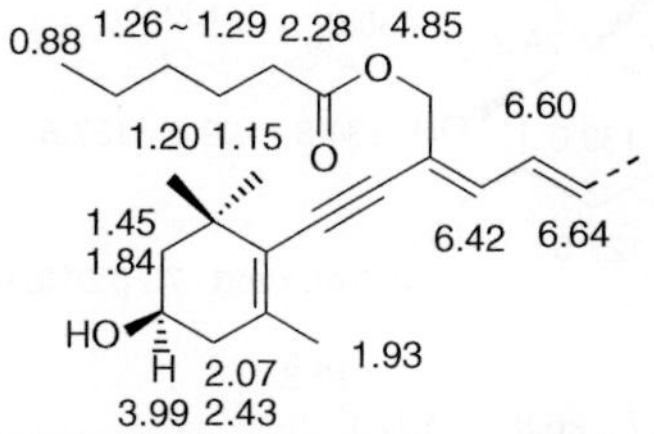

J. Agric. Food Chem. 59 (2011) 13059.

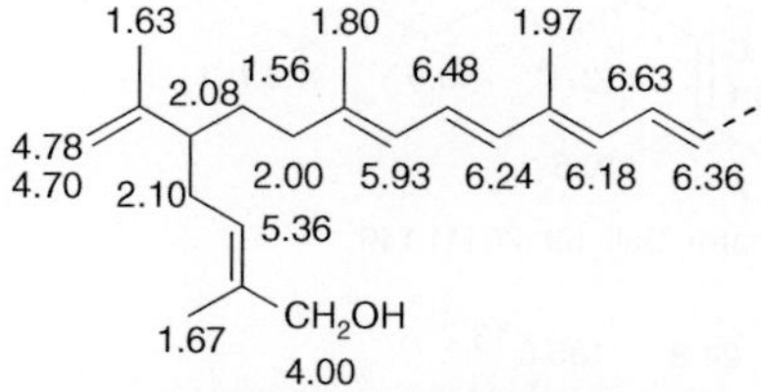

Arch. Microbiol. 176 (2001) 217.

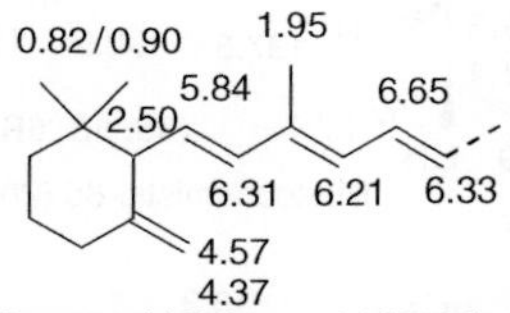

Carotenoid Science 14 (2009) 46.

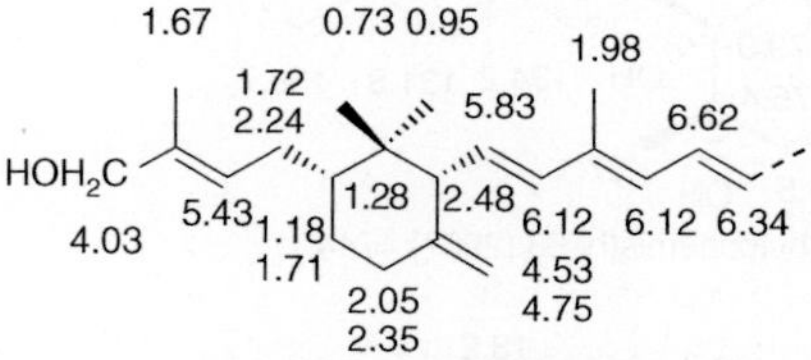

J. Oleo Sci. 59 (2010) 653.

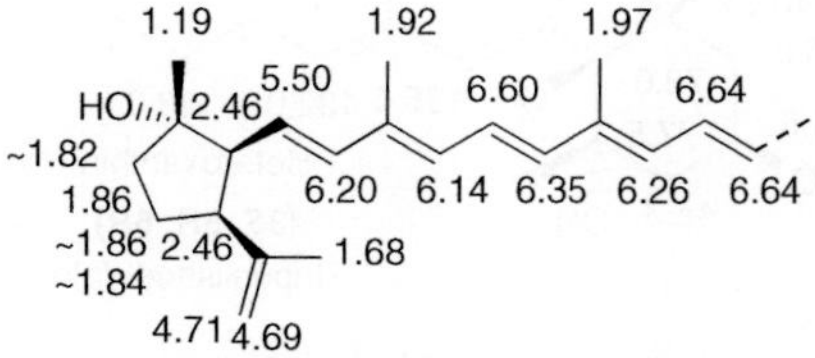

J. Agric. Food Chem. 63 (2015) 1622.

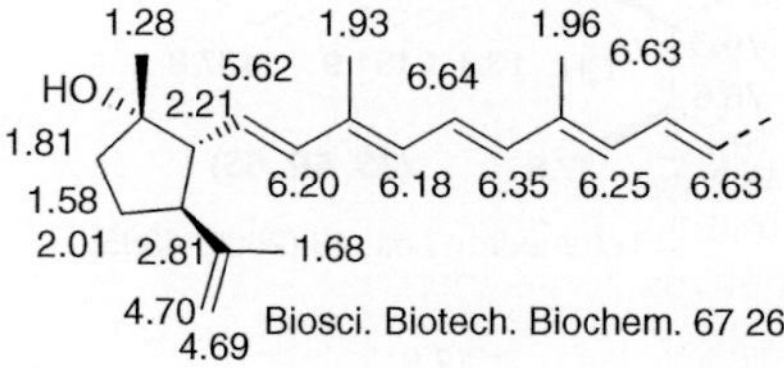

Biosci. Biotech. Biochem. 67 2644 (2003)

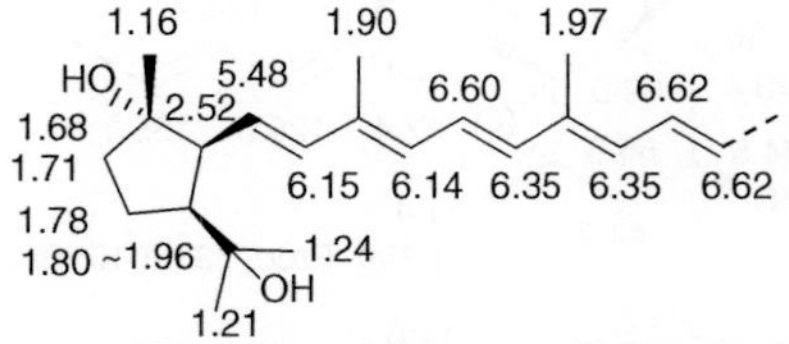

Biosci. Biotech. Biochem. 67 2644 (2003)

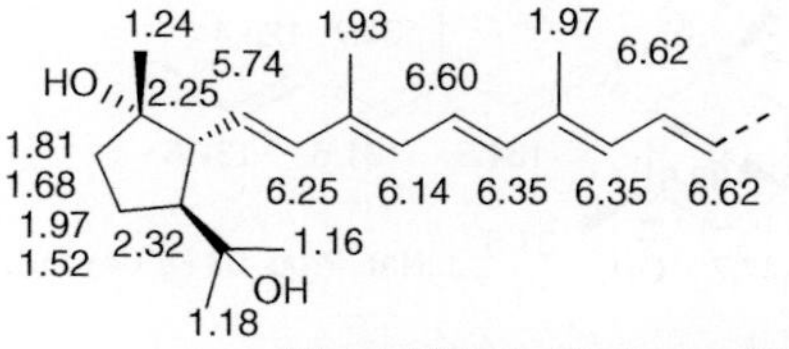

Biosci. Biotech. Biochem. 67 2644 (2003)

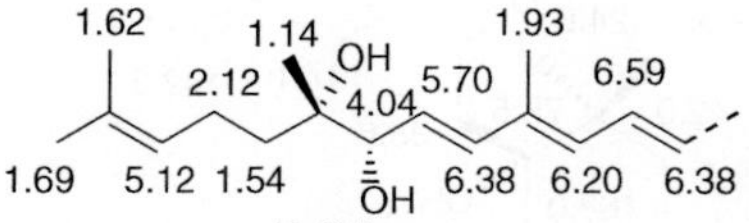

5, 6 threo

J. Agric. Food Chem. 63 (2015) 1622.

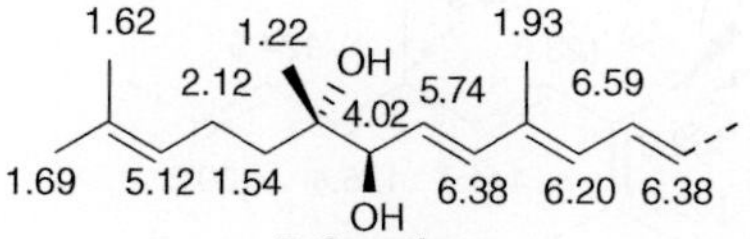

5, 6 erythro

J. Agric. Food Chem. 63 (2015) 1622.

Figure 7.5 (*Continued*)

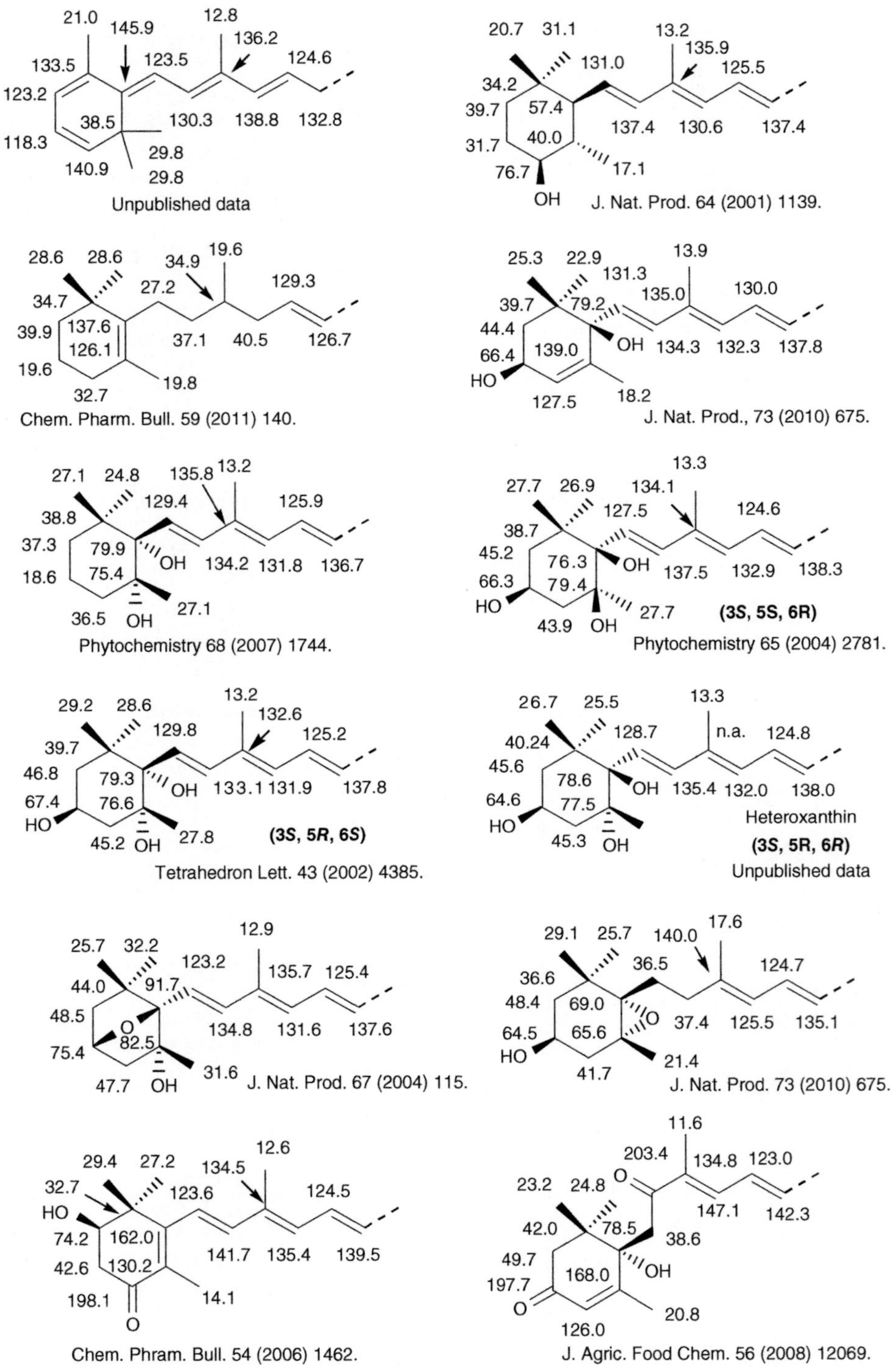

Figure 7.6 ^{13}C NMR chemical shifts of carotenoid end groups.

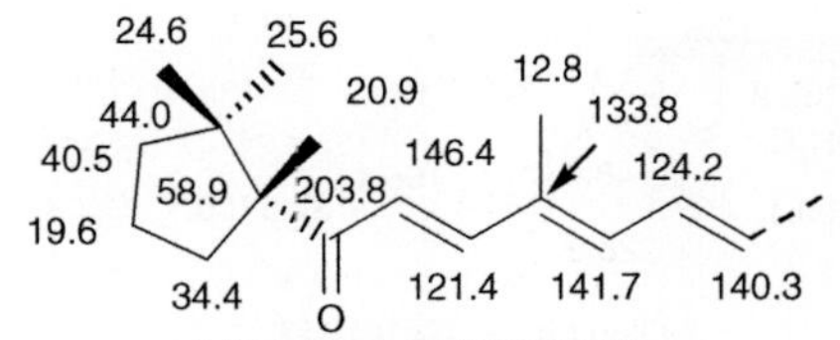

J. Nat. Prod. 67 (2004) 115.

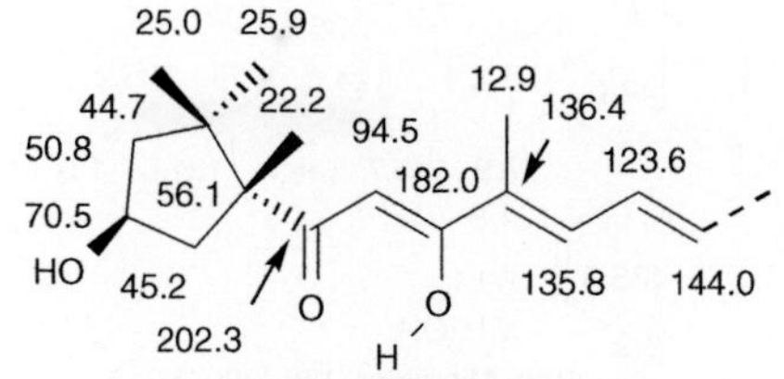

J. Nat. Prod. 64 (2001) 578.

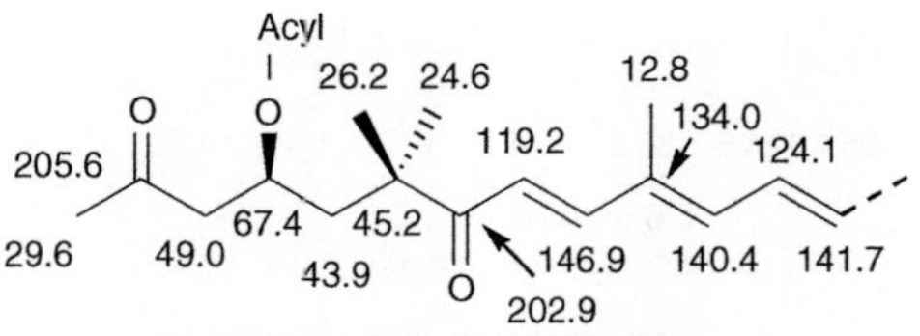

Tetrahedron Lett. 43 (2002) 4385.

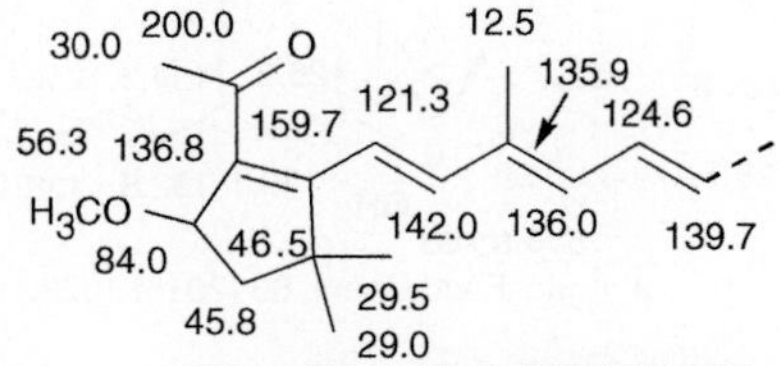

Chem. Pharm. Bull. 49 (2001) 985.

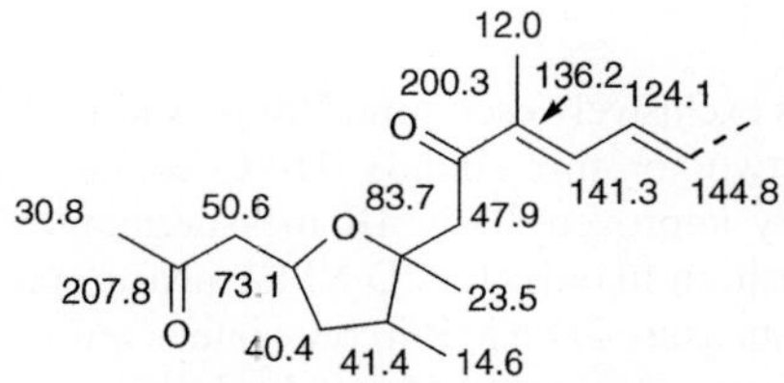

Tetrahedron Lett. 33 (1922) 4941.

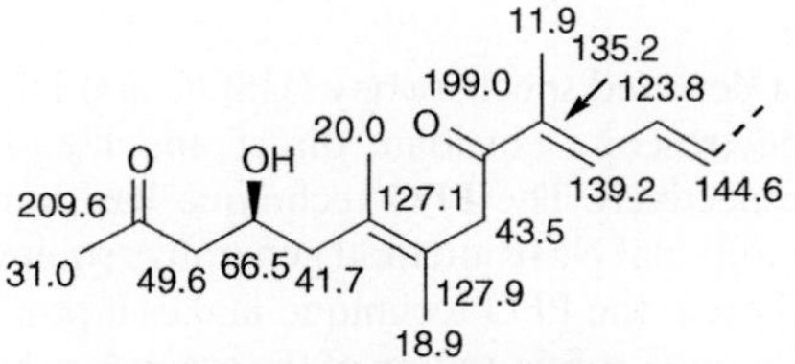

Tetrahedron Lett. 33 (1922) 4941.

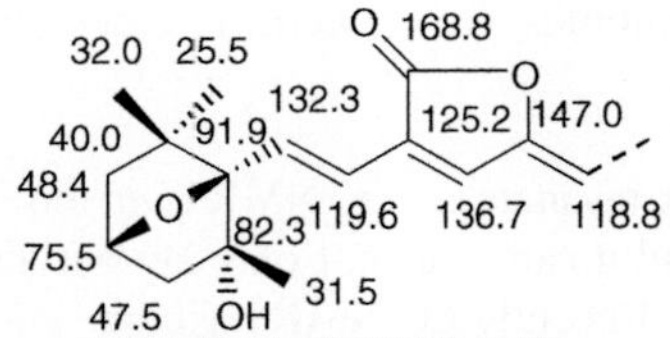

J. Nat. Prod. 68 (2005) 1344.

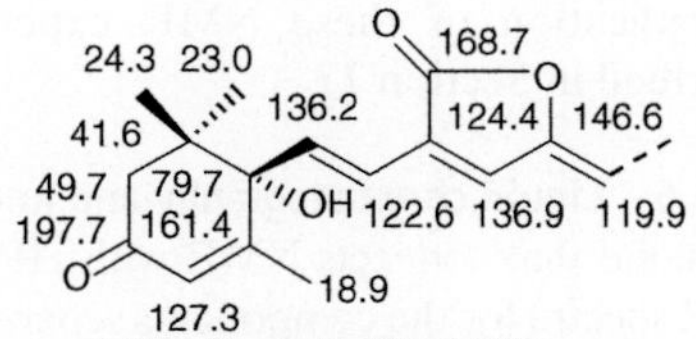

J. Nat. Prod. 64 (2001) 578.

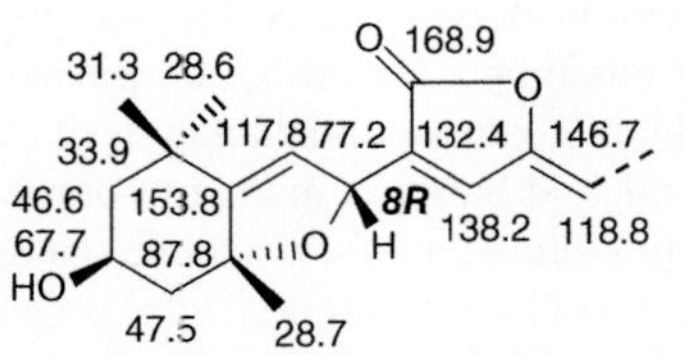

Chem. Pharm. Bull. 51 (2003) 724.

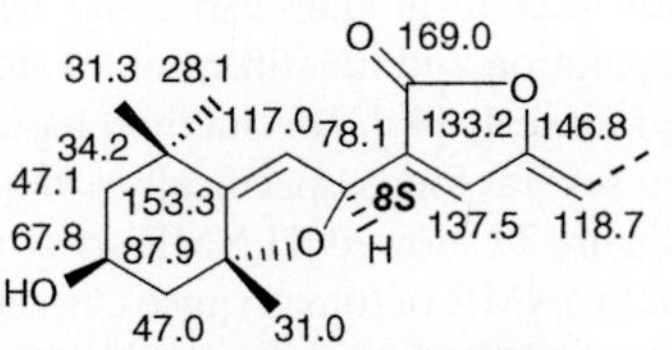

Chem. Pharm. Bull. 51 (2003) 724.

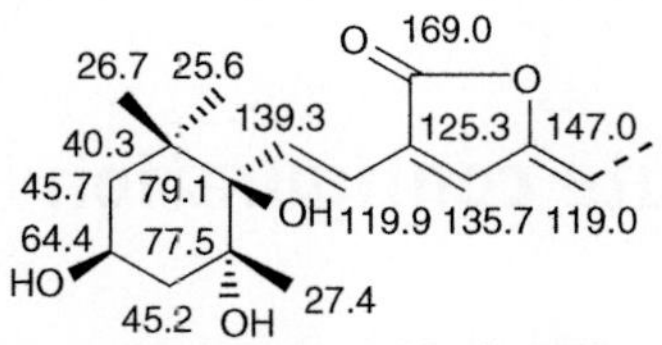

J. Agric. Food Chem. 56 (2008) 12069.

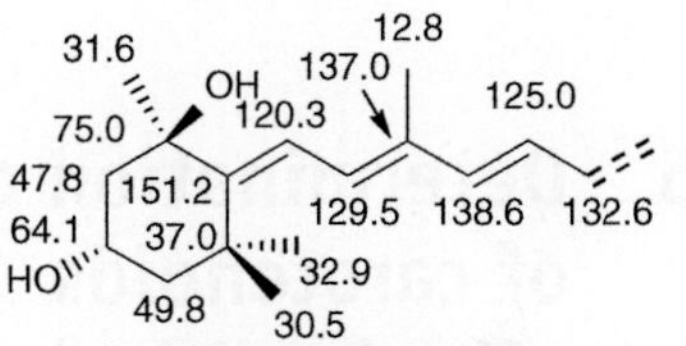

J. Nat. Prod. 63 (2000) 1288.

Figure 7.6 (*Continued*)

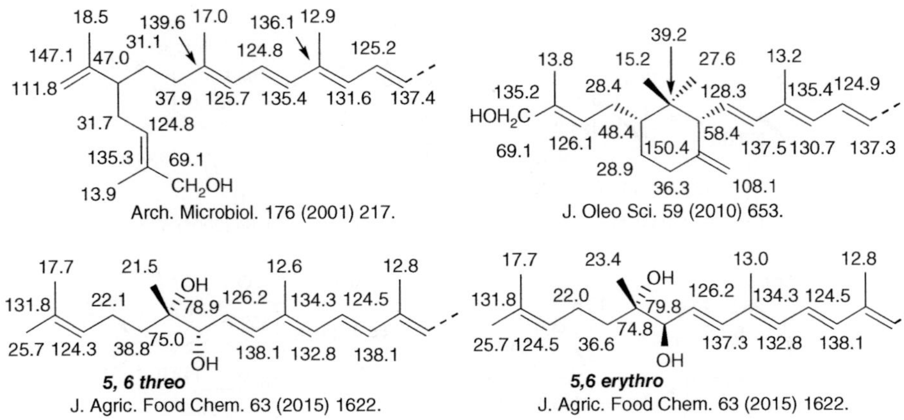

Figure 7.6 *(Continued)*

^{1}H detected spectroscopy (HSQC and HMBC) is exclusively used now. HSQC and HMBC spectroscopy elucidate direct and long-range (two- or three-bond) ^{1}H-^{13}C connections, respectively. The PFG technique has dramatically improved 2D NMR measurement. The traditional NMR method generally requires acquisition 16 times for 2D NMR measurement, whereas the PFG technique makes it possible to measure 2D NMR in only one acquisition. Absolute configuration of the secondary hydroxy group in carotenoids can be determined by NMR using the modified Mosher method [39]. Details are described in Section 6.2.

Application of these NMR experimental techniques for structural elucidation is described in Section 7.7.

7.5.4.5 Liquid chromatography and nuclear magnetic resonance LC/NMR is an innovative technique that connects NMR with HPLC online, and it can offer not only 1D but also 2D NMR spectra for the components separated by HPLC. Recently, LC/NMR has come into wide use because of improved sensitivity due to higher magnetic fields of superconductive magnets and advanced techniques, especially the solvent suppression method. LC/NMR was applied for the separation and identification of stereoisomers of lutein and zeaxanthin in spinach at the nanogram scale [40]. This method has also been applied to componential analysis of carotenoids in several foods, specifically tomato juice, palm oil, and Satsuma mandarin orange juice [41]. Figure 7.7 showed ^{1}H NMR spectra of lycopene, phytofuluene, and phytoene obtained by online LC/NMR of tomato juice extract. ^{1}H NMR spectra of each carotenoid were obtained by the stopped-flow mode with water suppression enhanced through the T1 effect (WET) technique. COSY spectra were also obtained using a WETgCOSY pulse sequence [41].

7.6 Determination of absolute configuration of carotenoids

7.6.1 Circular dichroism (CD) spectroscopy

Most naturally occurring carotenoids possess at least one asymmetric carbon and occur in nature in an optical active form. CD spectroscopy is generally used for determination of the absolute stereochemistry of carotenoids. Many carotenoids showed CD absorbance

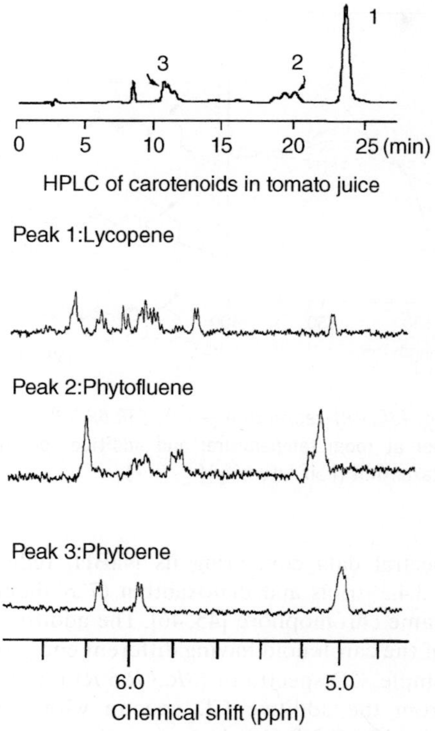

Figure 7.7 HPLC chromatogram of tomato juice extract (detected at 300 nm) and ^1H NMR spectra of lycopene, phytofuluene, and phytoene obtained by online LC/NMR. Chromatographic separation was carried out on a COSMOSIL 5C18-AR-II column (150 mm × 4.6 mm; particle size, 4.5 μm) with the mobile phase of 5% $CDCl_3$ and 95% CD_3CN (start) to 10% $CDCl_3$ and 90% CD_3CN (15 min, linear gradient) at the flow rate of 1 mL/min. LC-NMR experiments were performed on a Varian UNITY INOVA-500 spectrometer equipped with a 60 μL microflow NMR probe at room temperature. ^1H NMR spectra were obtained in the stopped-flow mode with water suppression enhanced through the T1 effect (WET) method to suppress the peak of the residual CH_3CN in CD_3CN, and the residual $CHCl_3$ in $CDCl_3$.

around 200–400 nm at room temperature. Most CD spectra of carotenoids exhibit strong temperature dependence. The intensity of the CD spectrum ($\Delta\varepsilon$) increases significantly in low temperatures due to stabilization of the conformation. CD spectral data of some natural carotenoids were compiled by Buchecker and Noack [42].

Generally, the absolute configuration cannot be determined unequivocally by only CD spectra data. Absolute configuration of the new carotenoid can be determined by comparison with CD spectra of similarly structured carotenoids with known chirality. For example, the absolute configuration of deepoxysalmoxanthin, (3*R*,3′*S*,6′*R*)-β,ε-carotene-3,6,3′-triol was determined by comparison with CD data of known stereoisomers of lutein, (3*R*,3′*S*,6′*S*)-β,ε-carotene-3,3′-diol with the same chromophore system [43]. Later, the validity of this proposed stereochemistry was confirmed by a synthetic method [44]. Reduction of the carbonyl group in carotenoids is sometimes employed for analysis of the absolute configuration of carotenoids with the 3-hydroxy-4-keto-β-end group and 2-hydroxy-4-keto-β-end group by CD spectra. For example, absolute configuration of pectenolone (3,3′-dihydroxy-7′,8′-didehydro-β,β-caroten-4-one) was

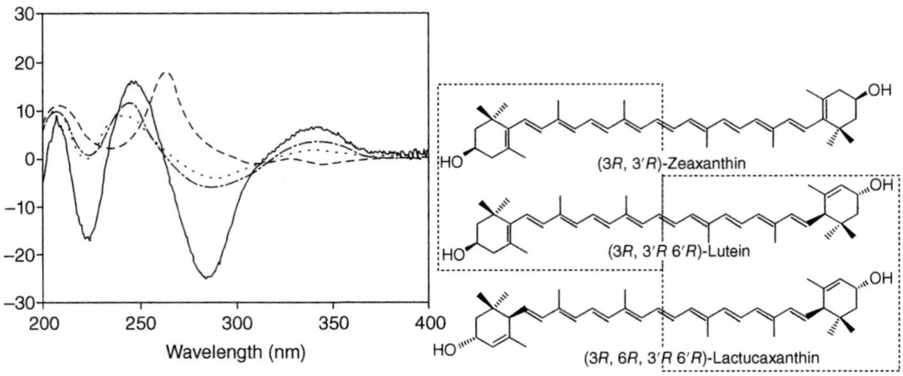

Figure 7.8 CD spectrum of *(3R,3′R)*-zeaxanthin(——), *(3R,6R,3′R,6′R)*-lactucaxanthin(- - -), and *(3R,3′R,6′R)*-lutein in ether at room temperature; and additive spectrum of *(3R,3′R)*-zeaxanthin and *(3R,6R,3′R,6′R)*-lactucaxanthin (half intensity)(- · · - ·).

determined by CD spectral data comparing its $NaBH_4$ reduction products of 7′,8′-didehydro-β,β-carotene-3,4,3′-triols and diatoxanthin (7′,8′-didehydro-β,β-carotene-3,3′-diol), which have the same chromophore [45, 46]. The additivity rule of CD is used to estimate the chirality of the carotenoid having different end groups in both sides of the polyene chain. For example, CD spectra of *(3R,3′R,6′R)*-lutein (β,ε-carotene-3,3′-diol) could be simulated from the additive CD spectra with *(3R,3′R)*-zeaxanthin (β,β-carotene-3,3′-diol) and *(3R,6R,3′R,6′R)*-lactucaxanthin (ε,ε-carotene-3,3′-diol) with half intensity. Therefore, the absolute configuration of *(3R,3′R,6′R)*-lutein could be postulated with additive CD spectra with *(3R,3′R)*-zeaxanthin and *(3R,6R,3′R,6′R)*-tunaxanthin, as shown in Figure 7.8. In the same manner, *(3R,3′S,6′S)*-, *(3R,3′R,6′S)*-, and *(3S,3′R,6′S)*-luteins were determined by CD spectrometry [47]. Benzoylation was applied for determination of absolute configuration of allylic hydroxy group. In order to confirm the postulated absolute configuration, a synthetic approach or chemical derivatizations are necessary.

7.6.2 NMR spectrometry using the modified Mosher method

The absolute configuration of the hydroxy group in a saturated end group such as 5,6-hydro-β-end group and κ-end group, lacking chromophore neighbors of asymmetric carbon, cannot be determined by CD spectrometry. Chiralities of these compounds can be determined by the modified Mosher method using NMR spectrometry [39].

NMR is not able to determine the absolute configuration of an organic compound directly, whereas relative stereochemistry can be elucidated by NMR. Therefore, the absolute configuration of an organic compound is determined by diastereomeric derivatization with a known optical active compound by NMR. The modified Mosher method can be determined by absolute configuration of a secondary hydroxy group in an organic compound unequivocally by diastereomeric esterification with asymmetrical methoxytrifluoromethylphenylacetic acid (MTPA) [39]. This method is based on the anisotropic effect that the phenyl group of the chiral auxiliary MTPA exerts on both the right and left

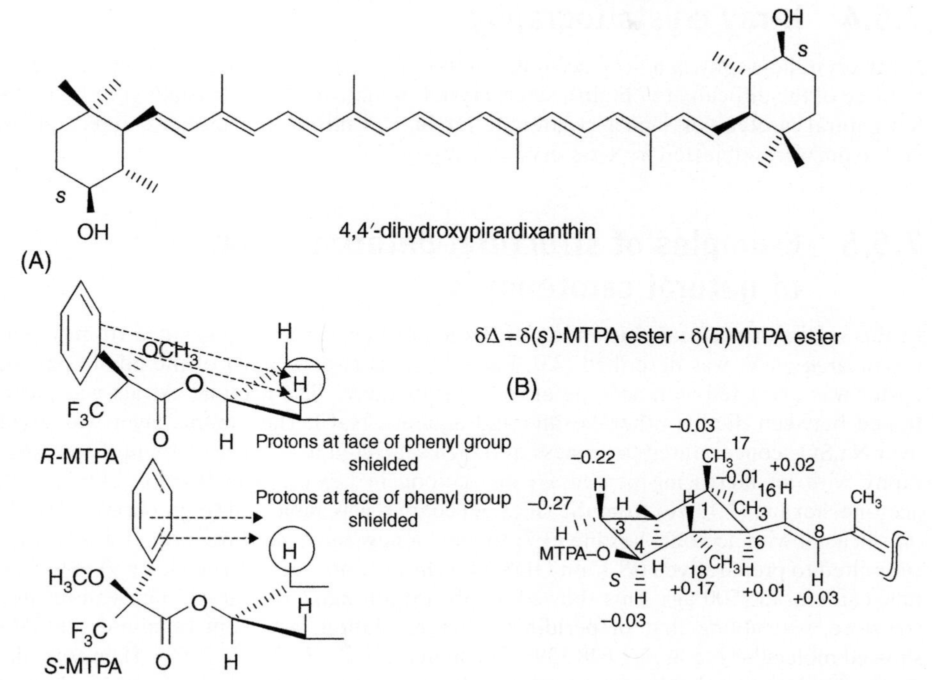

Figure 7.9 Determination of absolute configuration of 4,4′-dihydroxypiraridixanthin by the modified Mosher method. The absolute configuration at C-4 was determined by the difference values of ^{1}H NMR signals of (*S*) and (*R*) MTPA esters Δδ (=δS-δR) of each protons in the 4-hydroxy-5,6-didehydro-β-end group. The positive Δδ values for the protons oriented on the right side of the MTPA plane and negative Δδ values for the protons located on the left side of the MPTA plane in the 4-hydroxy-5, 6-didehydro-β-end group disclosed the *S* configuration at C-4 according to the Mosher model.

sides of nearby protons at the chiral center of the secondary hydroxy group, as shown in Figure 7.9A. Absolute configurations of the hydroxy group at C-4 and C-4′ in 4,4′-dihyd roxypiraridixanthin were determined by this modified Mosher method, as shown in Figure 7.9. The first (*R*)- and (*S*)- MTPA esters of 4,4′-dihydroxypiraridixanthin were prepared. Next, the different values of ^{1}H NMR signals of (*S*) and (*R*) MTPA esters [Δδ (=δS–δR)] of each proton in the 4-hydroxy-5,6-didehydro-β-end group were evaluated. The positive Δδ values for the protons oriented on the right side of the MTPA plane and negative Δδ values for the protons located on the left side of the MPTA plane in the 4-hydroxy-5,6-didehydro-β-end group disclosed the *S* configuration at C-4 according to the Mosher model as shown in Figure 7.9B [48].

7.6.3 Synthetic approach

A synthetic approach needs determination of the absolute configuration of more complex carotenoids. Absolute configuration of crassostreaxanthin B, which has novel a cyclic tetra substituted olefinic end group, could be determined by only synthetic study [49].

7.6.4 X-ray crystallography

X-ray crystallography is a very accurate method for structural determination. However, because of the difficulty to obtain a single crystal suitable for X-ray crystallography, only a few natural carotenoids, such as β-carotene, lutein, zeaxanthin, astaxanthin, canthaxanthin, and so on, were subjected to X-ray crystallography [50].

7.6.5 Examples of structural determination of natural carotenoids

In this section, structural elucidation of the minor new carotenoid isolated from oyster, *Crassostrea gigas*, was described [33]. Ten kilograms (wet weight) of the edible part of oyster was extracted with acetone at room temperature. The acetone extract was partitioned between diethyl ether–hexane and aqueous NaCl. The organic layer was dried over Na_2SO_4, concentrated to dryness, and then subjected to silica gel column chromatography with an increasing percentage of acetone in hexane. The fraction eluted with acetone–hexane (1:1, v/v) from the silica gel column was subjected to preparative HPLC on silica gel with acetone–hexane (3:7) to yield a new carotenoid fraction. It was further submitted to preparative HPLC on ODS with chloroform–acetonitrile (1:9, v/v) to yield a new carotenoid (500 μg). This showed an absorption maximum at 457 nm without fine structure, resembling that of peridinin. High-resolution fast atom bombardment MS showed molecular ion at *m/z* 628.3395 (calculated for $C_{39}H_{48}O_7$ 628.3394). Therefore, the molecular formula of this compound was determined to be $C_{39}H_{48}O_7$ ^1H NMR showed that this carotenoid has a peridinin-type structure. A complete decoupled ^{13}C NMR spectrum could be observed by using the Nano Probe for 18 h acquisition. From these NMR spectral data and high-resolution MS, the presence of 39 carbons, including 14 quaternary carbons and 46 carbon-bonded protons, in this carotenoid was confirmed. The noticeable signals due to three carbonyl carbons (δ C 170.4, 168.7, and 197.7 ppm) and allene groups (δC 202.7 ppm and δH 6.06 ppm) were observed. The ^1H-^1H and direct-bonding ^1H-^{13}C connections were elucidated by COSY and HSQC spectra, respectively. The assignments of the remaining 14 quaternary carbons were made by long-range ^1H-^{13}C connections obtained by HMBC experiment. From these accumulated spectral data, the planer structure of this carotenoid could be determined as shown in Figure 7.4. The relative stereochemistry was confirmed by NOE obtained by NOESY spectrum. The absolute configuration of this compound was determined by CD spectrum by comparison with those of related carotenoids such as amarouciaxanthin A. The strategy of structural elucidation by NMR is shown in Figure 7.4. Furthermore, the absolute configuration was determined by comparison of CD data of known carotenoids with similar structures. MS/MS data also confirmed this structure. In this case, about several hundred micrograms of sample were required for structural elucidation.

The second example described structural elucidation of novel carotenoid pyropheophorbide A esters (Figure 7.10A and 7.10B) from abalone, *Haliotis diversicolor aquatilis* [51]. Viscera of abalone (100 g from 50 specimens) were extracted with acetone. The acetone extract was partitioned with diethyl ether–hexane (1:1, v/v) and water. The diethyl ether–hexane layer was evaporated to dryness and chromatographed on silica gel using an increasing percentage of diethyl ether in hexane. The fraction eluted with diethyl ether–hexane (6:4, v/v) was subjected to HPLC on silica gel with acetone–hexane (3:7, v/v) to yield a series of brown pigments. This brown pigment showed absorption maxima at 411, 447, and 666 nm. This UV-Vis spectrum resembled the additive UV-Vis spectra of

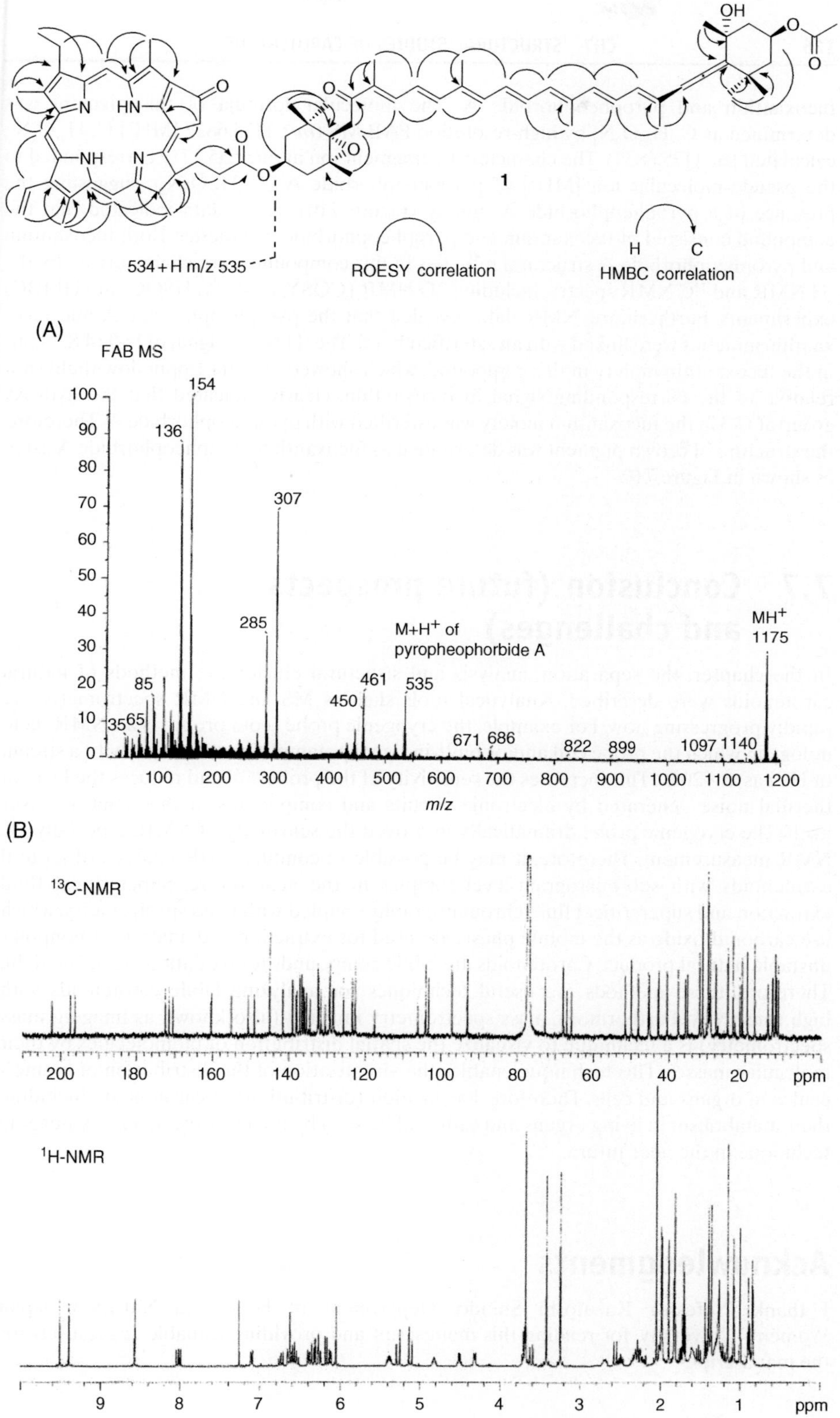

Figure 7.10 Key ROESY and HMBC correlations and FAB MS fragmention of 1, and FAB MS and NMR spectra of fucoxanthin pyropheophorbide A ester.

fucoxanthin and pyropheophorbide A. The molecular formula of this pigment was determined as $C_{75}H_{90}O_8N_4$ by high-resolution FAB MS (*m/z* 1175.6827 [MH^+] $C_{75}H_{91}O_8N_4$, calculated for 1175.6837). The characteristic fragment ion at *m/z* 535.2719 corresponded to the pseudo-molecular ion [MH^+] of pyropheophorbide A ($C_{33}H_{35}O_3N_4$), suggesting the presence of a pyropheophorbide A moiety (Figure 7.10). These data indicated that the compound consisted of fucoxanthin and pyropheophorbide A moieties. Both fucoxanthin and pyropheophorbide A structural moieties in this compound were characterized by the ^1H NMR and ^{13}C NMR spectra, including 2D NMR (COSY, ROESY, HSQC, and HMBC) experiments. Furthermore, NMR data revealed that the pyropheophorbide A and fucoxanthin moieties were linked with an esterified bond. The ^1H NMR signal of H-3 (4.82 ppm) in the fucoxanthin moiety in this compound, which showed about a 1 ppm downfield shift relative to the corresponding signal in fucoxanthin, clearly indicated that the hydroxy group at C-3 in the fucoxanthin moiety was esterified with pyropheophorbide A. Therefore, the structure of brown pigment was determined as fucoxanthin pyropheophorbide A ester, as shown in Figure 7.10.

7.7 Conclusion (future prospects and challenges)

In the chapter, the separation, analysis and structural elucidation methods of natural carotenoids were described. Analytical tools such as MS and NMR spectrometry are rapidly progressing now. For example, the cryogenic probe (cold probe) is an NMR technology in which the probe coil and/or built-in signal preamplifier are cooled with a stream of He gas at ~20 K. This increases the sensitivity of the probe coil and reduces the level of thermal noise generated by electronic circuits and components of the signal receiver itself. The cryogenic probe dramatically improved the sensitivity of NMR, especially ^{13}C NMR measurement. Therefore, it may be possible to conduct NMR analysis of natural carotenoids with sub-microgram-level samples in the near future. Supercritical fluid extraction and supercritical fluid chromatography coupled with mass spectrometry, which use carbon dioxide as the mobile phase, are used for extraction and analysis of nonpolar unstable natural product. Carotenoids are labile compounds for oxidation, heat, and light. Therefore, these methods are useful techniques for analyzing labile carotenoids with high sensitivity. Furthermore, mass spectrometry imaging (also known as imaging mass spectrometry) is a technique to visualize the spatial distribution of biomolecules by their molecular masses. This technique enables the visualization of the distribution of biomolecules in organs and cells. Therefore, localization (distribution) of carotenoids, including their metabolism in living organs and cells, will be seen by the mass spectrometry imaging technique in the near future.

Acknowledgments

I thank Professor Kazutoshi Shindo, Department of Food and Nutrition, Japan Women's University, for reading this manuscript and providing valuable suggestions for the manuscript.

References

1. G. Britton, S. Liaaen-Jensen, and H. Pfander (eds.), *Carotenoids hand book*, Basel: Birkhäuser, 2004.
2. T. Maoka, "Recent progress in structural studies of carotenoids in animals and plants," *Archiv. Biochem. Biophys.*, 2009, **483**, 191–5.
3. K. Schiedt and S. Liaaen-Jensen, "Isolation and analysis," in G. Britton, S. Liaaen-Jensen, and H. Pfander (eds.), *Carotenoids*, vol. **1A**, Basel: Birkhäuser, 1995, pp. 81–108.
4. Y. Fujiwara, K. Hashimoto, K. Manabe, and T. Maoka, "Structures of tobiraxanthins A1, A2, A3, B, C and D, new carotenoids from the seeds of *Pittosporum tobira*," *Tetrahedron Lett.*, **43**, 4385–8 (2002).
5. P. B. Jacobs, R. D. LeBoeut, S. A. McCommas, and J. D. Tauber, "The cleavage of carotenoid esters by cholesterol esterase," *Comp. Biochem. Physiol.*, **72B**, 157–60 (1982).
6. T. Matsuno, M. Ookubo, T. Nishizawa, and I. Shimizu, "Carotenoids of sea squirt-1. New marine carotenoids, halocynthiaxanthin," *Chem. Pharm. Bull.*, **32**, 4309–15 (1984).
7. T. Matsuno, M. Katsuyama, T. Hirono, T. Maoka, and T. Komori, "The carotenoids of tilapia *Tilapia nilotica*," *Bull. Jap. Scoc. Sci. Fish.*, **52**, 115–19 (1986).
8. T. Maoka, Y. Fujiwara, K. Hashimoto, and N. Akimoto, "Characterization of fucoxanthin and fucoxanthinol esters in the Chinese surf clam, *Mactra chinensis*," *J. Agric. Food Chem.*, **55**, 1563–7 (2007).
9. T. Maoka and N. Akimoto, "Carotenoids and their fatty acid esters of spiny lobster *Panulirus japonicus*," *J. Oleo Science*, **57**, 3, 145–52 (2008).
10. T. Nakajima, T. Wada, N. Tarui, S. Ito, Y. Yuasa, and T. Maoka, "Analysis of carotenoids in human serum and erythrocyte by ultra performance liquid chromatography (UPLC)," *Carotenoid Science*, **14**, 46–9 (2009).
11. T. Maoka, T. Komori, and T. Matsuno, "Direct resolution of diastereomeric carotenoid-I. 3-oxo-β-end group," *J. Chromatography*, **318**, 122–4 (1985).
12. T. Maoka, A. Arai, M. Shimizu, and T. Matsuno, "The first isolation of enantiomeric and meso-zeaxanthin in nature," *Comp. Biochem. Physiol.*, **83B**, 121–4 (1986).
13. T. Maoka and T. Matsuno, "Diastereomeric resolution of carotenoids: IV. Carotenoids with a 4-hydroxy-β-end group," *J. Chromatography*, **482**, 189–95 (1989).
14. F. Khachik, F. F. de Moura, D.-Y. Zhao, C.-P. Aebischer, and P. S. Bernstein, "Transformations of selected carotenoids in plasma, liver, and ocular tissues of humans and in nonprimate animal models," *Invest. Ophthalm. Visual Sci.*, **43**, 3383–92 (2002).
15. C. Wang, D. W. Armstrong, and C. D. Chang, "Rapid baseline separation of enantiomers and a mesoform of all-trans-astaxanthin, 13-cis-astaxanthin, adonirubin, and adonixanthin in standards and commercial supplements," *J. Chromatogr. A*, **1184**, 172–7 (2008).
16. Y. Yamano, T. Maoka, and A. Wada, "Synthesis of (3S,3'S)- and meso-stereoisomers of alloxanthin and determination of absolute configuration of alloxanthin isolated from aquatic animals," *Marine Drugs*, **12**, 2623–32 (2014).
17. G. Britton, "UV/visible spectroscopy," in G. Britton, S. Liaaen-Jensen, and H. Pfander (eds.), *Carotenoids*, vol. **1A**, Basel: Birkhäuser, 1995, pp. 13–62.
18. C. H. Eugster, "Chemical derivatization: microscale tests for the presence of common functional groups in carotenoids," in G. Britton, S. Liaaen-Jensen, and H. Pfander (eds.), *Carotenoids*, vol. **1A**, Basel: Birkhäuser, 1995, pp. 71–80.

19. K. Bernhard and M. Grosjean, "Infrared spectroscopy," in G. Britton, S. Liaaen-Jensen, and H. Pfander (eds.), *Carotenoids*, vol. **1B**, Basel: Birkhäuser, 1995, pp. 117–34.
20. J. C. Merlin, "Resonance Raman spectroscopy of carotenoids and carotenoid-containing systems," *Pure Appl. Chem.*, **57**, 785–92 (1985).
21. C. Uragami, E. Yamashita, A. Gall, B. Robert, and H. Hashimoto, "Application of resonance raman microscopy to in vivo carotenoid," *Acta Biochim. Pol.*, **59**, 53–6 (2012).
22. C. R. Enzell and S. Bach, "Mass spectrometry of carotenoids," in G. Britton, S. Liaaen-Jensen, and H. Pfander (eds.), *Carotenoids*, vol. **1B**, Basel: Birkhäuser, 1995, pp. 261–320.
23. R. B. van Breemen, H. H. Schmitz, and S. J. Schwartz, "Fast atom bombardment tandem mass spectrometry of carotenoids," *J. Agric. Food Chem.,* **43**, 384–9 (1995).
24. N. Akimoto, T. Maoka, Y. Fujiwara, and K. Hashimoto, "Analysis of carotenoids by FAB CID-MS/MS," *J. Mass Spectrom. Soc. Jpn.*, **48**, 32–41 (2000).
25. T. Maoka, Y. Fujiwara, K. Hashimoto, and N. Akimoto, "Characterization of epoxy carotenoids by fast atom bombardment collision-induced dissociation MS/MS," *Lipids*, **39**, 179–83 (2004).
26. Mass Bank, Japan, http://www.massbank.jp/index.html
27. R. Frassantio, M. Cantonati, G. Flaim, I. Manchini, and G. Guella, "A new method for the identification and the structural characterisation of carotenoid esters in freshwater microorganisms by liquid chromatography/electrospray ionisation tandem mass spectrometry," *Rapid Commun Mass Spectrom.*, **22**, 3531–9 (2008).
28. Y. Weesepoel, J-.P. Vincken, P. M. Pop, K. Liu, and H. Gruppen, "Sodiation as a tool for enhancing the diagnostic value of MALDI-TOF/TOF-MS spectra of complex astaxanthin ester mixtures from *Haematococcus pluvialis*," *J. Mass Spectrom.*, **48**, 862–74 (2013).
29. R. B. van Breemen, C. R. Huang, Y. Tan, L. C. Sander, and A. B. Schilling, "Liquid chromatography/mass spectrometry of carotenoids using atmospheric pressure chemical ionization," *J. Mass Spectrom.*, **31**, 975–81 (1996).
30. P. A. Clarke, K. A. Barner, J. R. Stain, F. I. Ibe, and M. J. Shepherd, "High performance liquid chromatography/atmospheric pressure chemical ionization-mass spectrometry for the determination of carotenoids," *Rapid Comm. Mass Spectrom.,* **10**, 1781–5 (1996).
31. R. B. van Breemen, "Electrospray liquid chromatography-mass spectrometry of carotenoids," *Anal. Chem.*, **67**, 2004–6 (1995).
32. T. Maoka, Y. Fujiwara, K. Hashimoto, and N. Akimoto, "Rapid identification of carotenoids in a combination of liquid chromatography / UV-visible absorption spectrometry by photodiode-array detector and atomospheric pressure chemical ionization mass spectrometry (LC/PAD/APCI-MS)," *J. Oleo Sciences*, **51**, 1–9 (2002).
33. T. Maoka, K. Hashimoto, N. Akimoto, and Y. Fujiwara, "Structures of five new carotenoids from the oyster *Crassostrea gigas*," *J. Natur Prod.*, **64**, 578–81 (2001).
34. G. Englert, "NMR spectroscopy," in G. Britton, S. Liaaen-Jensen, and H. Pfander (eds.), *Carotenoids*, vol. **1B**, Basel: Birkhäuser, 1995, pp. 147–262.
35. M. Suzuki, K. Watanabe, S. Fujiwara, T. Kurasawa, T. Wakabayashi, M. Tsuzuki, K. Iguchi, and T. Yamori, "Isolation of peridinin-related norcarotenoids with cell growth-inhibitory activity from the cultured dinoflagellate of *Symbiodinium* sp., a symbiont of the Okinawan soft coral *Clavularia viridis*, and analysis of fatty acids of the dinoflagellate," *Chem Pharm. Bull.*, **51**, 724–7 (2003).
36. T. Yokota, H. Etoh, S. Oshima, K. , "Oxygenated lycopene and dehydrated lutein in tomato puree," *Tetrahedron Lett.*, **33**, 4941–4 (1992).
37. Y. Fujiwara, T. Maoka, M. Ookubo, and T. Matsuno, "Crassostreaxanthins A and B: novel marine carotenoids from the oyster *Crassostrea gigas*," *Tetrahedron Lett.*, **33**, 4941–4944 (1992).

38. T. Maoka and Y. Fujiwara, "Absolute configuration of mytiloxanthin and 9-*E*-mytiloxanthin," *J. Jpn. Oil. Chem., Soc.*, **45**, 667–70 (1996).

39. I. Ohtani, T. Kusumi, Y. Kashman, and K. Kakisawa, "High-field FT NMR application of Mosher's method: the absolute configurations of marine terpenoids," *J. Am. Chem. Soc.*, **113**, 4092–6 (1991).

40. M. Dachtler, T. Glaser, K. Kohler, and K. Albert, "Combined HPLC-MS and HPLC-NMR on-line coupling for the separation and determination of lutein and zeaxanthin stereoisomers in spinach and in retina," *Anal. Chem.*, **73**, 667–74 (2001).

41. C. Tode, T. Maoka, and M. Sugiura, "Application of LC-NMR to analysis of carotenoids in foods," *J. Sep. Sci.*, **32**, 3659–62 (2009).

42. R. Buchecker and K. Noack, "Circular dichroism," in G. Britton, S. Liaaen-Jensen, and H. Pfander (eds.), *Carotenoids*, vol. **1B**, Basel: Birkhäuser, 1995, pp. 63–116.

43. T. Matsuno, M. Tsushima, and T. Maoka, "Salmoxanthin, deepoxysalmoxanthin and 7,8-dideepoxysalmoxanthin from the salmon *Oncorynchus keta*," *J. Nat. Prod.*, **64**, 507–10 (2001).

44. Y. Yamano, K. Endo, Y. Hirata, H. Kurimoto, and A. Wada, "Stereocontrolled first total syntheses of salmoxanthin and deepoxysalmoxanthin," *Curr. Org. Synth.*, **12**, 180–8 (2015).

45. K. Hiraoka, T. Matsuno, M. Ito, K. Tsukida, Y. Shichida, and T. Yoshizawa, "Absolute configuration of pectenolone," *Bull. Jap. Soc. Sci. Fish.*, **48**, 215–17 (1982).

46. T. Maoka and T. Matsuno, "Isolation and structural elucidation of three new acetylenic carotenoids from the Japanese sea mussel *Mytilus coruscus*," *Nippon Suisan Gakkaishi*, **54**, 1443–7 (1988).

47. T. Matsuno, T. Maoka, M. Katsuyama, T. Hirono, Y. Ikuno, M. Shimizu, and T. Komori, "Comparative biochemical studies of carotenoids in fishes: XXIX isolation of new luteins, lutein F and lutein G from marine fishes," *Comp. Biochem. Physiol.*, **85B**, 77–80 (1986).

48. M. Tsushima, T. Maoka, and T. Matsuno, "Structure of carotenoids with 5,6-dihydro-β-end groups from the spindle shell *Fushinus perplexus*," *J. Nat. Prod.*, **64**, 1139–42 (2001).

49. C. Tode, Y. Tamano, and Y. Ito, "Carotenoids and related polyenes. Part 7. Total synthesis of crassostreaxanthin B Applying the stereoselective rearrangement of tetrasubstituted epoxides," *J. Chem. Soc. Perkin Trans.*, **1**, 3338–45 (2001).

50. M. Helliwell, "Three-dimensional structures of carotenoids by X-ray crystallography," in G. Britton, S. Liaaen-Jensen, and H. Pfander (eds.), *Carotenoids*, vol. **4**, Basel: Birkhäuser, 2008, pp. 37–52.

51. T. Maoka, T. Etoh, N. Akimoto, and H. Yasui, "Novel carotenoid pyropheophorbide A esters from abalone," *Tetrahedron Lett.*, **52**, 3012–15 (2011).

8

In Situ Studies of Carotenoids in Plants and Animals

Malgorzata Baranska[a,b], Jan Cz. Dobrowolski[c,d], and Grzegorz Zajac[a,b]

[a]*Faculty of Chemistry, Jagiellonian University, Krakow, Poland*
[b]*Jagiellonian Centre for Experimental Therapeutics (JCET), Jagiellonian University, Krakow, Poland*
[c]*Institute of Chemistry and Nuclear Technology, Warsaw, Poland*
[d]*National Medicines Institute, Warsaw, Poland*

8.1 Introduction

In this chapter, we present the Raman spectroscopy *in situ* analysis of carotenoids measured in various plants and animals, as well as in humans, at the tissue and cellular levels. Although these natural pigments occur *in vivo* as minor components, resonance Raman spectroscopy can achieve a sensitive detection in the visible (Vis) region when the wavenumber of the laser excitation coincides with an electronic transition of the individual carotenoid. Near-infrared (NIR) Fourier transform (FT)–Raman spectroscopy also strongly enhances carotenoids' Raman spectra thanks to the pre-resonance effect. Furthermore, it avoids the disturbing fluorescence effect of biological material usually observed when laser excitation is performed in the Vis wavelength range. Carotenoids are identified in the Raman spectra by strong bands within the 1500–1550 and 1150–1170 cm^{-1} ranges due to in-phase C=C (ν_1) and C–C stretching (ν_2) vibrations of the polyene chain. Additionally, in-plane rocking modes of CH_3 groups (ν_4) attached to the polyene chain and coupled with C–C bonds are seen as a peak of medium intensity in the 1000–1020 cm^{-1} region.

8.2 Plants

Several papers gathered in reviews have demonstrated the special advantages of FT–Raman spectroscopy for *in situ* studies of various carotenoids that occur all over the plant kingdom [1, 2]. Spectra obtained from various tissues of a range of plant species indicate

Carotenoids: Nutrition, Analysis and Technology, First Edition. Edited by Agnieszka Kaczor and Malgorzata Baranska.

that the location of the C=C stretching vibrations is mainly influenced by the length as well as the terminal substituents of the polyene chain of carotenoids and by their interactions with other plant constituents (Table 8.1).

The usefulness of Raman spectroscopy in the investigation of *cis–trans* isomerization of carotenoids has been demonstrated. The individual distribution of carotenoids in the intact plant tissue can be studied using 2D Raman mappings (i.e., the different 7-, 8-, and 9-double-bond conjugated carotenoids can be analyzed independently in the same sample). The application of Raman spectroscopy for *in situ* detection of unstable substances such as epoxycarotenoids has also been demonstrated.

Based on a range of standard extracts and FT–Raman measurements of natural carotenoids present in over 50 specimens of plant tissue, it has been shown that there may be a serious problem in the interpretation of the spectroscopic data because of significant wavenumber shifts caused by carotenoid interactions with organic tissue [3]. Therefore, because of the progressive shift in the wavenumber of the ν_1 Raman band as the number of the conjugated C=C bonds is increased, an individual carotenoid in biological samples cannot be unambiguously identified and determined.

The size, shape, density, and location of different types of carotenoid bodies in orange-fleshed sweet potatoes, carrots, and mangoes have been quantified and mapped using the ν_1 Raman band to register coherent anti-Stokes Raman scattering (CARS) microscopy [4]. The data have also been related to the plant–matrix morphology by a simultaneous second-harmonic generation microscopy of starch granules. Whereas potatoes and carrots showed heterogeneous CARS signals coming from bodies with high carotenoid densities, the carotenoid-filled lipid droplets in mangoes were homogeneous. Interestingly, the β-carotene density and morphology after the potato was thermally processed showed that the carotene-containing bodies remained intact despite significant changes to the surrounding starch granules.

Raman mapping supported by cluster analysis was used for *in situ* discrimination of flavonoids, anthocyanins, and carotenoids that determine the colors of the flower petals of different pansy cultivars *Viola x wittrockiana* [5]. Hierarchical cluster analysis based on the TLC extracts and the reference spectra taken from the flower petals allowed for discriminating the three groups of pigments against each other and drawing Raman maps of the distributions of carotenoids, anthocyanins, and flavonols reflecting the relative concentrations of these compounds.

A direct *in situ* Raman microspectroscopy detection of carotenoids has been shown to also be possible at the subcellular level [6]. Indeed, single carotenoid crystals sequestered in a carrot cell, predominantly formed from β-carotene, were identified using ν_1 and ν_2 Raman bands and an FT–Raman spectrometer equipped with a microscope and a 40× magnification objective. However for a more detailed *in situ* study of single carotenoid crystals present in the carrot root cells, a dispersive Raman microscope with 532 nm and 488 nm excitations was applied [7]. Three categories of roots differing in both β/α-carotene ratio and in total carotenoid content were selected for the study, based on high-performance liquid chromatography (HPLC) measurements. The results showed that, independently from the carotenoid composition of the root, carotenoid crystals are composed of more than one compound (Figure 8.1, Color Supplement). Individual spectra extracted from Raman maps every 0.2–1.0 μm had similar shapes in the 1500–1550 cm^{-1} region, indicating that different carotenoid molecules were homogeneously distributed within the whole crystal volume.

Surface-enhanced resonance Raman scattering (SERRS) measurements were carried out for a "sandwich" system composed of β-carotene embedded in the membrane proteins of Photosystem I placed between a roughened silver slice and single silver particles [8]. A high signal-to-noise ratio and a fairly good reproducibility for very low carotene

Table 8.1 Wavenumber positions of ν_1, ν_2, and ν_4 modes of the predominant carotenoids that occur in various plant tissues and standards in the spectra obtained by Fourier transform (FT)–Raman spectroscopy. The number of double bonds in the conjugated system is shown in brackets. Adopted from Ref. [1].

Plant name	Sample	ν_1 [cm^{-1}]	ν_2 [cm^{-1}]	ν_4 [cm^{-1}]	Predominant Carotenoids
Saffron *Crocus sativus* L.	Stigma	1536	1165	1020	Crocetin (7)
Marigold *Calendula officinalis* L.	Petal	1536	1157	1007	Auroxanthin (7)
Marigold *Calendula officinalis* L.	Petal/pollen	1531–1529	1157	1004	Flavoxanthin (8) Luteoxanthin (8)
Chamomille *Chamomilla recutita L.*	Pollen	1529	1157	1006	Carotenoid (8)
Marigold *Calendula officinalis* L.	Pollen	1524	1157	1004	Lutein (9) Antheraxanthin (9)
Nectarine *Prunus perica* L. var. *nucipersica* (Sucrow) C. Schneid	Fruit	1527	1157	1005	β-cryptoxanthin (9)
Carrot *Daucus carota* L.	Yellow root	1527	1157	1006	Lutein (9)
Carrot *Daucus carota* L.	Leaf	1526	1157	1004	Lutein (9) β-carotene (9)
Ivy *Hedera helix* L.	Leaf	1526	1157	1004	Lutein (9) β-carotene (9)
Euonymus fortunei Turcs. 'Canadale Gold'	Leaf	1525	1156	1004	Lutein (9) β-carotene (9)
Basil *Ocimum basilicum* L.	Leaf	1525	1158	1005	Lutein (9) β-carotene (9)
Begonia *Begonia x semperflorens-cultorum* Hort.	Leaf	1525	1157	1005	Lutein (9) β-carotene (9)
Broccoli *Brassica oleracea* var. *italica* L.	Flower	1524	1157	1005	Lutein (9) β-carotene (9)
French bean *Phaseolus vulgaris* L.	Green pod	1524	1157	1005	Lutein (9) β-carotene (9)
Corn *Zea mays* L.	Seed	1522	1157	1005	Zeaxanthin (9)
Pumpkin *Cucurbita pepo* L.	Fruit	1524	1157	1009	β-carotene (9)
Apricot *Prunus armeniaca* L.	Fruit	1524	1156	1003	β-carotene (9)
Carrot *Daucus carota* L.	Orange root	1520	1156	1007	β-carotene (9)
Annatto	Seed	1518	1154	1011	*cis*-Bixin (9)
Bixa orellana L.		1523	1155	1008	*trans*-Bixin (9)
Pepper *Capsicum annuum* L.	Red fruit	1517	1158	1004	Capsanthin (9)
Watermelon *Citrullus lanatus* Thumb.	Fruit	1510	1158	1008	Lycopene (11)
Tomato *Lycopersicon esculentum* Mill.	Fruit	1510	1156	1004	Lycopene (11)
Standard	Powder	1522	1157	1008	Lutein (9)
Standard	Powder	1521	1157	1006	α-carotene (9)
Standard	Powder	1515	1156	1007	β-carotene (9)

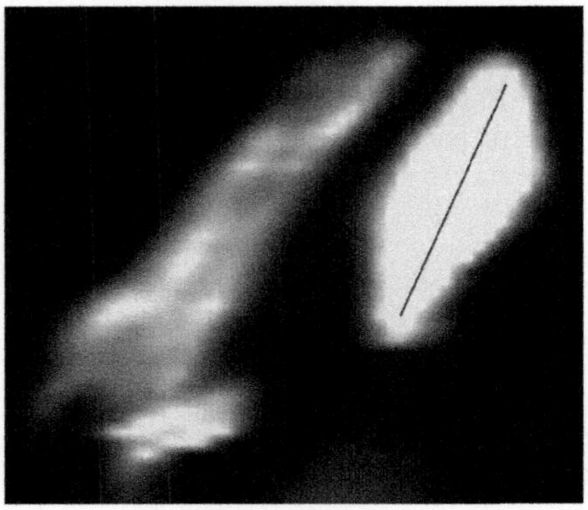

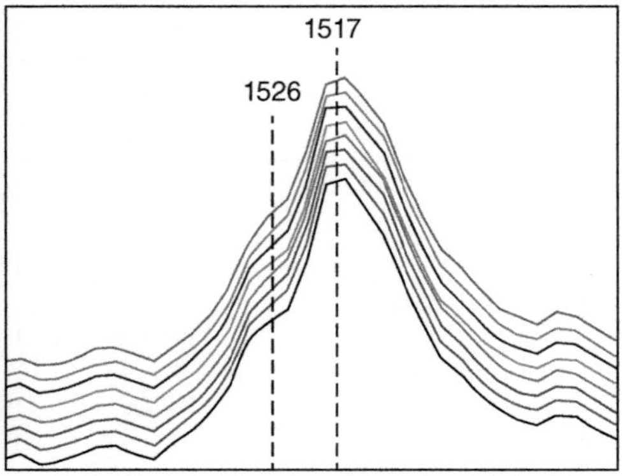

Figure 8.1 An example of a carotenoid crystal located in a cell of the high α and β root. Left: Raman map obtained by the integration of the ν_1 band. Right: Raman spectra (532 nm) in the range of the ν_1 band extracted every 0.2 μm along a marked line. Reprinted with permission from M. Roman, K. M. Marzec, E. Grzebelus, P. W. Simon, M. Baranska, and R. Baranski, "Composition and (in)homogeneity of carotenoid crystals in carrot cells revealed by high resolution Raman imaging," *Spectrochimica Acta Part A: Molecular and Biomolecular Spectroscopy*, **136**, 1395–1400 (2015) [7]. Copyright (2015) Elsevier. (*See insert for color representation of the figure.*)

concentrations in membrane proteins isolated from spinach (*Spinacia oleracea* L.) leaves were achieved in such a sampling method in SERRS experiments. It was found that the β-carotene in the complex was predominantly in the all-*trans* configuration.

The study focused on the effectiveness of minimizing fluorescence in the analysis of Cape Jasmine (*Gardenia augusta* L.) by applying dispersive Raman spectroscopy (at three different excitation wavelengths: 633, 785, and 1064 nm) and surface-enhanced Raman spectroscopy (SERS). During it, two carotenoid colorant components were identified [9]. Raman bands at 1537, 1209, and 1165 cm^{-1} were assigned as discriminating markers for all-*trans*-crocetin and all-*trans*-crocin. It has also been shown that both vibrational techniques offer an alternative analytical approach for natural organic dyes and pigments in reference to the more classical HPLC–photodiode array (HPLC–PDA) analytical protocols.

8.3 Animals

Raman maps of the distribution of astaxanthin in living aquatic animals have demonstrated that its distribution is tissue specific [10]. The differing Raman signatures of astaxanthin present in various tissues are caused by differences in astaxanthin intermolecular interactions and conformational changes.

The micro-Raman spectra of seven species of bivalve larvae were analyzed to assess the types of pigments present in the shells of each species and the inorganic versus organic material changes [11]. The Raman spectra of 1-day-old larvae were differentiable when the larvae were reared in waters with different organic signatures. The differences in spectra and pigments between most species and the neural network algorithm allowed for the classification of five out of seven species with an accuracy greater than 85%. Thus, using micro-Raman spectroscopy makes the identification of some unknown species and their natal origin possible.

Raman imaging supported by mass spectroscopy measurements has shed light on the putative physiological functions of carotenoids in an archaic photosynthetic mechanism in insects [12]. Using a 488 nm laser wavelength corresponding to the maximum of carotene ultraviolet (UV)-Vis absorption, the carotene signature corresponding to the $\nu(1)$, $\nu(2)$, and $\nu(4)$ resonance Raman bands was always registered in living aphids. The carotenoid crystals that formed spontaneously after crushing adult orange aphids were also mapped. Moreover, Raman imaging was carried out on the reddish/brown aphid eyes containing a heavy concentration of retinal. A higher intensity of the three peaks was consistently found with the green phenotype compared to the orange one. Moreover, the method was able to follow carotene synthesis in developing embryos where the signals were correlated with the appearance of orange pigmentation. A substantial increase in the concentrations of *trans-β* and *trans-γ* carotene was observed in the green variant compared to the orange one. At the opposite end, the *cis*-torulene drastically increased in the orange phenotype, whereas the *trans*-torulene (a precursor metabolite) was roughly unchanged. The abundant carotenoid synthesis in aphids strongly suggests that carotenoids have a major and unknown physiological role beyond their canonical antioxidant properties.

Pigments in waterbears (Tardigrades, *Echiniscus blumi*) have been identified as carotenoids by applying Raman microspectroscopy on living specimens [13]. The distribution of carotenoids within the animal's body was visualized—its dietary origin, its presence in eggs and eye spots, and its absence in the cuticle and epidermis. A decrease in carotenoid content was detected after inducing oxidative stress, demonstrating that *in vivo* Raman microspectroscopy can be used for studying the role of carotenoids in oxidative stress–related processes in tardigrades.

The carotenoids and psittacofulvins (mostly recognized in parrot plumage) have been identified (based on ν_1 and ν_2 Raman bands and the CH=CH in-plane rocking mode band at 1293 cm^{-1}, respectively) and found to be responsible for mollusk shells' colorations [14]. The Raman characterizations of limnic (freshwater) and gastropod (terrestrial) shell specimens exhibited no differences between the two phyla, suggesting similarities in the chemical structures of the polyene pigments contained in their shells.

Raman spectra have also been registered from the oocyte cytoplasm of the African clawed frog (*Xenopus laevis*) using 785 nm and 532 nm laser lines [15]. The red 785 nm line showed the nonresonant contribution (from molecules such as phenylalanine and metalloproteins that are present inside the cell) to the Raman spectrum, whereas the green 532 nm probe enabled detecting β-carotene through the resonant Raman scattering and mapping its distribution along a diameter of a single oocyte.

Reflectance and resonance Raman spectroscopies were used to investigate the induced molecular structural changes and carotenoid–protein interactions responsible for different colorations in the plumage of the brilliant red scarlet ibis (*Eudocimus ruber*, Threskiornithidae), the orange-red summer tanager (*Piranga rubra*, Cardinalidae), and the violet-purple feathers of the white-browed purpletuft (*Iodopleura isabellae*, Tityridae) [16]. Feathers of these three species contain canthaxanthin as their primary pigment. A significant variation of the ν_1 Raman band frequency between the species has been reported. The most significant variation is found in *I. isabellae* feathers and is correlated with a red shift in canthaxanthin absorption that results in violet reflectance. The head-to-tail molecular alignment (i.e., J-aggregation) of the protein-bound carotenoid molecules is thought to be an additional factor of the color shift.

Rhodoxanthin, one of a few retrocarotenoids in nature, has been characterized *in situ* in the plumage of fruit doves (*Ptilinopus*, Columbidae) and cotingas (*Phoenicircus*, Cotingidae), and was subsequently compared with the isolated pigment in a solution and in thin solid films using resonance Raman spectroscopy and UV-Vis reflectance [17]. The coloration associated with the rhodoxanthin-containing plumage ranges from brilliant red to magenta or purple. The vibrational signatures of rhodoxanthin, supported by discrete Fourier transform (DFT) calculations of the Raman spectra of three isomers, have been used to distinguish rhodoxanthin from more common carotenoids and to propose various mechanisms that change the electronic absorption, including the structural distortion of the chromophore and the enhanced delocalization of π-electrons in the ground state.

The Raman analysis of the carotenoids contained in ventral feathers confirmed reports from earlier video recordings made at the nests of the great tit, which claimed that the biomass of leaf-eating insects during the first nesting cycle was three times higher than during the second cycle [18].

Raman spectroscopy, coupled with multivariate statistics, has been used to identify the most abundant carotenoid within a single feather barb of 36 avian species [19]. Feathers rich with adoradexanthin, astaxanthin, canary xanthophylls, canthaxanthin, cotingin, or lutein were discriminated by subtle shifts in Raman spectral band positions, and by novel bands associated with particular carotenoids. The Raman data on pigment presence have been compared with HPLC results. It has been shown that α-doradexanthin is present in the plumage of *Petroica robins* from Australia, whereas *Petroica* immigrants to New Zealand display a yellow carotenoid that is likely lutein.

It has recently been shown that discovering plumage carotenoids in fossil feathers could provide insight into the ecology of ancient birds and nonavian dinosaurs [20]. Using a modern feather as reference, the chemical evidence of carotenoids in six feathers preserved in amber (Miocene to mid-Cretaceous) and in a feather preserved as a compression fossil (Eocene) was detected without sample destruction through an amber matrix using confocal Raman spectroscopy. Using principal component analysis, it was established that, depending on the feather's color, the primary pigment was methoxy-keto-carotenoid (cotingin), canthaxanthin, α-doradexanthin, lutein, zeaxanthin, or a combination of these carotenoids.

With confocal Raman microspectroscopy at 660 nm, pig ear skin was investigated and compared with abdominal human skin (Transkin). A difference between the samples was found in the content of carotenoids, besides other components (e.g., lipids and hyaluronic acid) [21]. The comparison was made at the level of the stratum corneum (SC), the SC–epidermis junction, and the viable epidermis. A significant difference in carotenoid content was observed for the SC. The study was done on pig's ear skin because it is usually used as a substitute for human skin for active-ingredient assessments in the dermatological and cosmetics fields.

The other aspect of the dermatological study was focused on astaxanthin and its specific antioxidant activities (i.e., anti-photoaging). Confocal Raman microscopy was used to detect *in vivo* the three-dimensional distribution of astaxanthin in rat skin [22]. The study demonstrated that, when swabbed onto the outer surface of the skin, astaxanthin can very quickly penetrate into the inner skin.

It has previously been shown that the carotenoid content of human skin *in vivo* is directly influenced by the carotenoid concentration of nutritional egg yolks. Thus, resonance Raman spectroscopy has been used to analyze the carotenoid concentration in the egg yolks of hens that were housed either in battery cages or on free-range grassland [23]. The egg yolks of the hens that had access to grassland contained approximately double the amount of carotenoid concentration of the egg yolks of hens housed in battery cages ($p < 0.001$). The kinetics of the carotenoid concentration in the egg yolks, depending on fodder, housing, and weather conditions, were also investigated.

Recent reports demonstrate that the oxidative status is related to various stress conditions in dairy cows, and carotenoids could serve as indicators of stress originating from the environment (e.g., heat stress or sun radiation) or from the animal itself (e.g., disease). Besides the invasive *in vitro* tests available, the optical noninvasive *in vivo* measurements of dermal carotenoids in cattle udder skin using a light-emitting diode (LED)-based portable spectroscopic system (miniaturized spectroscopic system [MSS]) for β-carotene analysis in the whole blood samples was applied to assess the oxidative status in cattle [24]. The system was calibrated using resonance Raman spectroscopy [25]. Correlations between the concentrations of dermal and blood carotenoids were calculated considering the nutritional status of the animals. A significant correlation ($R = 0.86$) was found for cattle with moderate to obese body conditions. Consequently, the blood and skin concentrations of β-carotene are comparable under stable stress conditions of the cattle. The other study aimed at investigating dermal carotenoid levels in cattle recovering from abomasal displacement [26].

In monkeys (similarly as in humans), lutein and zeaxanthin are found in significant amounts in the retina of the Japanese quail *Coturnix japonica* [27]. This makes the quail retina an excellent nonprimate small-animal model for studying the metabolic transformations of these important macular carotenoids. They are thought to play an integral role in protecting against light-induced oxidative damage, such as that found in age-related macular degeneration (AMD). The carotenoids present in the quail retina were identified by using C_{30} HPLC coupled with mass spectral and PDA detectors. Besides lutein (2.1%) and zeaxanthin (11.8%), other ocular carotenoids were identified: adonirubin (5.4%), 3′-oxolutein (3.8%), *meso*-zeaxanthin (3.0%), astaxanthin (28.2%), galloxanthin (12.2%), Σ,Σ-carotene (18.5%), and β-apo-2′-carotenol (9.5%). Moreover, deuterium-labeled lutein and zeaxanthin were used as dietary supplements to study the pharmacokinetics and metabolic transformations of these two ocular pigments in serum and ocular tissues. Using Raman spectroscopy (which supported HPLC coupled with mass spectrometry), the labeled carotenoids were detected and quantitated in the ocular tissue. It has been shown that dietary zeaxanthin is the precursor of 3′-oxolutein, β-apo-2′-carotenol, adonirubin, astaxanthin, galloxanthin, and Σ,Σ-carotene, whereas dietary lutein is the precursor for *meso*-zeaxanthin. These studies also revealed that the pharmacokinetic patterns of uptake, carotenoid absorption, and transport from serum into ocular tissues were similar to the results obtained in most human clinical studies.

Raman spectroscopy is a suitable method for the simultaneous, rapid, and nondestructive quantification of astaxanthin and cantaxanthin in salmon muscle tissue [28]. The spectra were collected with 785 nm excitation from 49 samples of ground muscle tissue of farmed Atlantic salmon (*Salmo salar* L.). The partial least-squares regression resulted in a root mean square error of prediction of 0.33 mg/kg (R^2=0.97) for carotenoids of the variable selected versions of all the preprocessed spectral data sets.

8.4 Humans

It has been shown (Chapter 1.2) that carotenoids are used as biomarkers to distinguish between the cancerous/malignant and healthy tissue or cells. Carotenoids in skin and their antioxidative role were broadly discussed in Chapter 1; thus, only a short report on *in situ* detection by using Raman spectroscopy is presented here. Moreover, the spectroscopic analysis of macula pigments that prevent damage that leads to AMD is discussed. There are also *in situ* studies on carotenoids at the level of a single human cell.

8.4.1 Skin

In many cases, determining the carotenoid content in human skin is related to the search for their antioxidant and protective activity against radicals. There are observations of change to the carotenoid content in human skin due to fruit, vegetable, or diet supplement

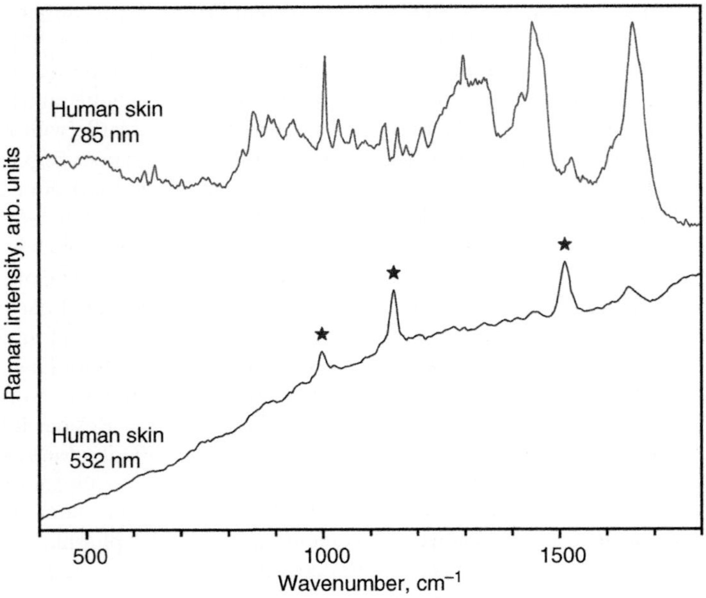

Figure 8.2 Raman spectra of human skin. Reprinted with permission from W. Werncke, I. Latka, S. Sassning, B. Dietzek, M. E. Darvin, M. C. Meinke, J. Popp, K. König, J. W. Fluhr, and J. Lademann, "Two-color Raman spectroscopy for the simultaneous detection of chemotherapeutics and antioxidative status of human skin," *Laser Phys. Lett.*, **8**, 895–900 (2011) [29]. Copyright (2011) IOP Publishing.

intake, as well as other factors (e.g., alcohol consumption, smoking, and radiation). The lifestyle impact on skin carotenoid content has also been examined.

The noninvasiveness of Raman spectroscopy is its most important advantage in determining carotenoids in human skin. The Raman spectrum of human skin depends on the incident laser wavelength. Using radiation around 500 nm, the carotenoid bands are selectively observed in the spectrum due to the resonance effect. With a laser of 785 nm yielding the pre-resonance Raman spectrum of carotenoids, the bands related to other skin structures are also observed (Figure 8.2) [29].

With multiline Ar^+ laser and excitations at 488 nm and 514.5 nm, it is possible to determine an absolute concentration of lycopene and β-carotene in human skin [30]. This method is based on lycopene and β-carotene's differing absorption spectra. The application of these two excitation lines results in different Raman-scattering efficiencies for both pigments. Lycopene and β-carotene represent 70% of all human skin carotenoids, and all of the carotenoids except lycopene have similar Raman spectra. This causes some errors in β-carotene determination in the human skin, mainly due to lutein content. But determining lycopene in human skin with an excitation of a 514.5 nm laser is not significantly influenced by other carotenoids, which are more pronounced when measured with a 488 nm line (Figure 8.3) [25, 30, 31]. Both excitations, 488 nm and 514 nm, were applied for the measurements of skin carotenoids as biomarkers of fruit and vegetable intake [32]. The total skin carotenoid level and lycopene skin level were determined in and correlated to the HPLC data. The single and multiple measurements of the cutaneous carotenoid level by using resonance Raman scatterng were compared, and a good agreement between them was found [33].

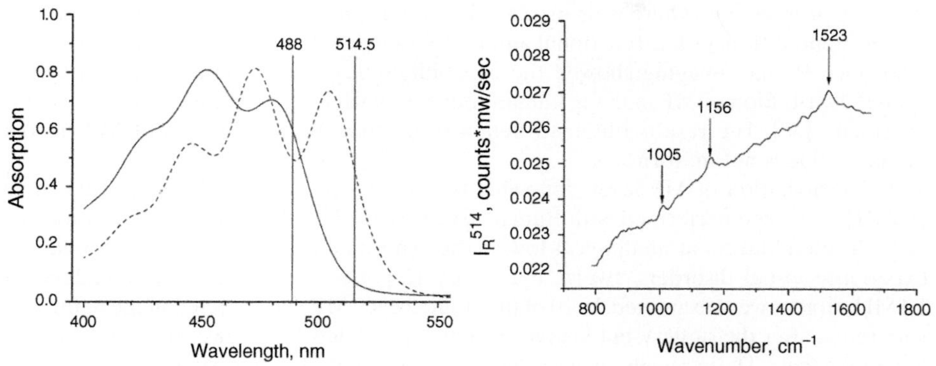

Figure 8.3 Left: Absorption spectra of β-carotene (solid line) and lycopene (dotted line) in ethanol solution. Right: Typical Raman spectra of β-carotene and lycopene in human skin measured *in situ* with 514.5 nm excitation. Reprinted with permission from M. E. Darvin, I. Gersonde, M. Meinke, W. Sterry, and J. Lademann, "Non-invasive in vivo determination of the carotenoids beta-carotene and lycopene concentrations in the human skin using the Raman spectroscopic method," *J. Phys. D-Appl. Phys.*, **38**, 2696–2700 (2005) [25]. Copyright (2005) IOP Publishing.

8.4.2 Macular pigment

Macular pigment (MP) is a name for the high concentration of lutein and zeaxanthin found in photoreceptor axons in the retina. Among carotenoids, these two are the only ones that cross the blood–retina barrier to form MP in the eye. MP plays an important role in protecting the macula, due to its antioxidative and spectroscopic activity. The absorption spectrum of MP shows a band maximum at 460 nm, so it absorbs blue light and protects the retina from photodamage. The higher the macular pigment optical density (MPOD), the greater the amount of blue light filtered. High MPOD could lower the risk of AMD, which is a disease that causes visual impairments. The relation between MOPD and AMD is one of the most popular topics in the study of macular pigment [34]. MPOD could be measured *in vivo* by means of many techniques, including resonance Raman spectroscopy [35].

The macular carotenoid level of age-related maculopathy (ARM) patients compared to that of healthy subjects has been investigated [36]. The decrease of carotenoid content in ARM patients and healthy older subjects was detected. Furthermore, for the patients with ARM in only one eye, the carotenoid level in the healthy eye was also lower, most likely due to ARM affecting the opposite eye as well. Whether the decreased carotenoid level in MP is one of ARM's causes or its effects remains uncertain, but it has been suggested that low macular carotenoid level could be one of the risk factors in the progression of this disease.

Secondary outcomes in a carotenoid clinical trial of early AMD have been collected by means of best-corrected visual acuity (BCVA), contrast sensitivity (CS), and Raman spectroscopy [37]. The randomized, double-masked, placebo-controlled clinical trial of carotenoids was developed together with other antioxidants. Raman spectroscopy was used for determining the carotenoid content in MP. Only persons with the highest risk for the progression of AMD were chosen for the survey. An increase of carotenoid content during the 36 months of the carotenoid trial was observed, whereas for the placebo group a small decrease in carotenoid content was detected. The observed decrease of MP in the placebo group is related to the loss of photoreceptors due to the disease's progression, whereas its increase in the treatment group shows the benefits of the carotenoid trial. Other functional and morphologic benefits were also found. *In vivo* resonance Raman imaging showed the capabilities of this method in determining the spatial distribution of MP in living human retina with very high resolution and molecular specificity [38]. The results obtained demonstrate that the distribution of MPs in the human retina is not uniform.

A determination of MP levels following the surgery of a full-thickness macular hole (FTMH) has been performed with Raman spectroscopy [39]. Patients with this syndrome lack all retinal layers at anatomical fovea. The syndrome also causes elderly patients to experience visual disorders. Twelve eyes from 12 patients who successfully underwent FTMH surgery were examined. In 10 of the studied eyes, MP was detected in the neurosensory retina after the surgery, but in nine of them, the MP level was lower than in the fellow healthy macula. These results suggest that the recovery of photoreceptors after surgery is very good.

The MP level in patients with malabsorption syndromes has also been studied [40]. The serum carotenoid level was examined using HPLC. The low uptake of carotenoids due to the malabsorption syndrome can cause an early-onset maculopathy. The results obtained show that normal subjects have higher levels of MP than malabsorption syndrome patients in any studied age (22–50 years for normal subjects and 17–57 years for malabsorption syndrome patients), although the carotenoid serum level is normal or even higher. Furthermore, lutein and zeaxanthin serum levels in both the healthy and the malabsorption syndrome patients increased, whereas MP levels decreased. This could be caused by the age-related breakdown of the biological processes of the transportation and absorption of carotenoids to the macula, which results from the decreased uptake of dietary carotenoids from the serum to the macula. In this case, even supplementing carotenoids could not raise the level of MP.

8.4.3 Carotenoids in single human cells

Carotenoids were detected not only in complex systems such as organs and tissues but also in singular human cells. Research in this area is mainly related to lymphocytes due to the protective role played by carotenoids in the human immune system [41–43]. The effects of the age [44] and health condition [45] of the organism has also been studied with Raman spectroscopy.

Leukocytes, the most diverse group of blood cells, can be divided into granulocytes (neutrophils, basophils, and eosinophils) and mononuclear cells (lymphocytes and monocytes) [41]. Different types of leukocytes can be distinguished microscopically due to the varying shapes of nuclei, sizes, and cellular components. However, Raman spectroscopy has often been used to determine the chemical composition of single blood cells and has shown its potential in the area of medical diagnostics [41–43].

Lymphocytes, monocytes, eosinophils, and neutrophils were measured with Raman imaging. From the spectra of nuclei and cytoplasm compartments of studied leukocytes (Figure 8.4, Color Supplement) [41], one can notice that only the cytoplasm of lymphocytes contains carotenoids. The identification of pigments was based on two marker bands observed in the Raman spectra at 1522 and 1158 cm^{-1}. However, no traces of carotenoids were observed for any other type of leukocytes [41].

Human lymphocytes are important to the adaptive part of the immune system. They are highly active cells that continuously generate reactive oxidative species (ROS) as part of their normal cellular activity. ROS are produced as part of the killing mechanism (e.g., to oxidize pollutants and viruses), but their overproduction can lead to tissue damage.

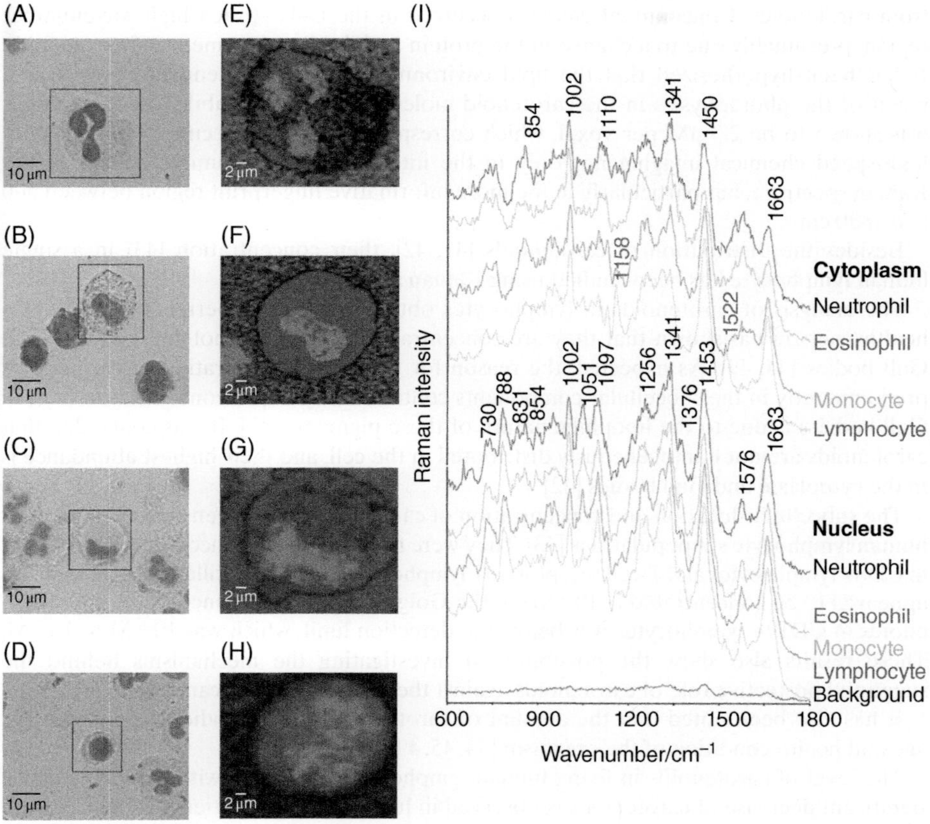

Figure 8.4 Morphological characteristics of the different leukocytes: neutrophil (A and E), eosinophil (B and F), monocyte (C and G), and lymphocyte (D and H). (A–D) White light images after Kimura staining; (E–H) false color Raman images of the same cell using the intensity at ~788 cm^{-1} to highlight the nucleus (pink) and the intensity of the CH stretching between 2800 and 3050 cm^{-1} to color code the overall cell area (blue). (I) Averaged Raman spectra of the cytoplasm, nucleus, and background region. Reprinted with permission from A. Ramoji, U. Neugebauer, T. Bocklitz, M. Foerster, M. Kiehntopf, M. Bauer, and J. Popp, "Toward a Spectroscopic Hemogram: Raman Spectroscopic Differentiation of the Two Most Abundant Leukocytes from Peripheral Blood," *Analytical Chemistry*, **84**, 5335–5342 (2012) [41]. Copyright (2012) American Chemical Society. (*See insert for color representation of the figure.*)

Therefore, the oxidant–antioxidant balance allowing normal cellular function and health needs to be maintained [46], and the role of antioxidants, including carotenoids (β-carotene or astaxanthin), is the protection of immune cells against oxidative stress and membrane damage [47, 48].

Time-lapse Raman imaging (TLRI) of living cells was a new approach in label-free chemical imaging through nonelectronic resonant, spontaneous Raman microspectroscopy [42]. Raman multiple images of an individual cell were obtained within a timespan of minutes. A full series of TLRI images typically resulted in more than 1.6 million data points per image. A fingerprint of molecular changes was observed before the cell was blebbing. The molecular fingerprint was related to a gradual disappearance of the Raman signal from carotenoids. Concomitant changes occurred in the C–H stretch high-wavenumber region, presumably due to a change in the protein and lipid environments of carotenoids. It has been hypothesized that the lipid environment of the carotenoids changes as a result of the photophysics in the carotenoid molecules. The detectability of carotenoids was shown to be 2.3 μM per voxel, which corresponds to 415 molecules. TLRI enables high-speed chemical imaging not only in the intense high-wavenumber region of the Raman spectrum, but particularly in the more informative fingerprint region between 500 and 1800 cm^{-1}.

Besides the distribution of carotenoids [41, 42], their concentration [43] in a single human lymphocyte has been studied using Raman spectroscopy.

The analysis of carotenoids in lymphocytes obtained from the peripheral blood of a healthy person has shown that they are concentrated (about 10^{-3} mol·dm^{-3}) in so-called Gall bodies [44, 49]. As expected, the reason for the high concentration of carotenoids predominantly in the subcellular components containing high lipid concentration (e.g., in Gall bodies) is due to the lipophilic nature of these pigments [43]. It was concluded that carotenoids are not homogeneously distributed in the cell, and their highest abundance is in the cytoplasm and Gall bodies [42].

The subcellular location and concentration of carotenoids have been studied in various human lymphocyte subpopulations [43]. They were found at a high concentration (~10^{-3} M) in CD8+ lymphocytes and T-cell receptor-γδ+ lymphocytes. In natural killer cells, carotenoids appeared to be concentrated (~10^{-4} M) in the Golgi complex. The concentration of carotenoids in CD19+ lymphocytes was below the detection limit, which was 10^{-6} M to 10^{-5} M. These results also show the possibility of investigating the mechanisms behind the suggested protective role of carotenoids against the development of cancers.

It has also been noted that the amount of carotenoids in Gall bodies depends on the age and health condition of the organism [44, 45, 49].

The level of carotenoids in living human lymphocytes decreases with age [49]. Also, a significant decrease of carotenoids is observed in lung carcinoma patients compared with healthy individuals, particularly in adenocarcinoma patients. Carotenoid supplementation raised the serum concentration in lung cancer patients up to normal levels, whereas intracellular content remained significantly lower [45].

8.5 Perspectives

This chapter presents the results of some selected published studies that describe various applications of Raman spectroscopy for an efficient measurement of carotenoids. This spectroscopic method has a potential to replace existing standard procedures used for biological sample analysis (mainly chromatographic techniques). A special advantage of vibrational spectroscopy is the possibility to perform *in situ* analysis of the intact cell or tissue without the necessity to perform any sample cleanup steps. Raman spectroscopy combined with microequipment and confocal microscopy can provide detailed molecular information with high spatial resolution at the cellular level. Imaging techniques have developed quickly over the last decade and, as a result, so has the potential application of vibrational methods in biological sample research. Usually, the sensitivity of these vibrational methods is lower compared to other analytical techniques. However, this is not the case for carotenoids, which can be analyzed at parts-per-million concentrations. Furthermore, some special Raman techniques, such as the SERS or TERS (tip-enhanced Raman scattering) methods, can increase the sensitivity of analysis. These methods enhance the signal by six or more orders of magnitude. In summary, the increased demand for solutions to the complex problems of plant and animal biochemistry requires a multidisciplinary approach in which Raman spectroscopy already plays a prominent role.

Acknowledgments

This project was supported by the National Science Centre (DEC-2012/07/B/ST5/00889).

References

1. H. Schulz, M. Baranska, and R. Baranski, "Potential of NIR-FT-Raman Spectroscopy in Natural Carotenoid Analysis," *Biopolymers*, **77**, 212–21 (2005).
2. H. Schulz, and M. Baranska, "Identification and quantification of valuable plant substances by IR and Raman spectroscopy," *Vib. Spectr.*, **43**, 13–25 (2007).
3. V. E. de Oliveira, H. V. Castro, H. G. M. Edwards, and L. F. C. de Oliveira, "Carotenes and carotenoids in natural biological samples: a Raman spectroscopic analysis," *J. Raman Spectrosc.*, **41**, 642–50 (2010).
4. C. Brackmann, A. Bengtsson, M. L. Alminger, U. Svanberg, and A. Enejder, "Visualization of β-carotene and starch granules in plant cells using CARS and SHG microscopy," *J. Raman Spectrosc.*, **42**, 586–92 (2011).
5. S. Gamsjaeger, M. Baranska, H. Schulz, P. Heiselmayer, and M. Musso, "Discrimination of carotenoid and flavonoid content in petals of pansy cultivars (*Viola x wittrockiana*) by FT-Raman spectroscopy," *J. Raman Spectrosc.*, **42**, 1240–7 (2011).
6. M. Baranska, R. Baranski, E. Grzebelus, and M. Roman, "*In situ* detection of a single carotenoid crystal in a plant cell using Raman microspectroscopy," *Vib. Spectr.*, **56**, 166–9 (2011).
7. M. Roman, K. M. Marzec, E. Grzebelus, P. W. Simon, M. Baranska, and R. Baranski, "Composition and (in)homogeneity of carotenoid crystals in carrot cells revealed by high resolution Raman imaging," *Spectrochim. Acta A*, **136**, 1395–400 (2015).
8. X. Qin, J. Zhu, W. Wang, X. Ding, K. Wang, Y. Fang, and T. Kuang, "A stable 'sandwich' system of surface-enhanced resonance Raman scattering for the analysis of β-carotenes in a photosynthetic pigment-protein complex," *J. Raman Spectrosc.*, **44**, 1111–9 (2013).
9. M. V. Cañamares, M. Leona, M. Bouchard, C. M. Grzywacz, J. Wouters, and K. Trentelman, "Evaluation of Raman and SERS analytical protocols in the analysis of Cape Jasmine dye (*Gardenia augusta* L.)," *J. Raman Spectrosc.*, **41**, 391–7 (2010).
10. A. Kaczor and M. Baranska, "*In situ* measurement of astaxanthin in biological material," *AIP Conf. Proc.*, **1267**, 338–9 (2010).
11. C. M. Thompson, E. W. North, S. N. White, and S. M. Gallager, "An analysis of bivalve larval shell pigments using micro-Raman spectroscopy," *J. Raman Spectrosc.*, **45**, 349–58 (2014).
12. J.C. Valmalette, A. Dombrovsky, P. Brat, C. Mertz, M. Capovilla, and A. Robichon, "Light-induced electron transfer and ATP synthesis in a carotene synthesizing insect," *Sci. Rep.*, **2**, 1–5 (2012).
13. A. Bonifacio, R. Guidetti, T. Altiero, V. Sergo, and L. Rebecchi, "Nature, source and function of pigments in tardigrades: *in vivo* Raman imaging of carotenoids in *Echiniscus blumi*," *PLoS One*, **7**, e50162 (2012).

14. L. N. de Oliveira, V. E. de Oliveira, S. D'ávila, H. G. M. Edwards, and L. F. de Oliveira, "Raman spectroscopy as a tool for polyunsaturated compound characterization in gastropod and limnic terrestrial shell specimens," *Spectrochim. Acta A*, **114**, 541–6 (2013).
15. G. Rusciano, G. Pesce, M. Salemme, L. Selvaggi, C. Vaccaro, A. Sasso, and R. Carotenuto, "Raman spectroscopy of *Xenopus laevis* oocytes," *Methods*, **51**, 27–36 (2010).
16. M. M. Mendes-Pinto, A. M. LaFountain, M. C. Stoddard, R. O. Prum, H. A. Frank, and B. Robert, "Variation in carotenoid-protein interaction in bird feathers produces novel plumage coloration," *J. Royal Soc. Interface.*, **9**, 3338–50 (2012).
17. C. J. Berg, A. M. LaFountain, R. O. Prum, H. O. Frank, and M. J. Tauber, "Vibrational and electronic spectroscopy of the retro-carotenoid rhodoxanthin in avian plumage, solid-state films, and solution," *Arch. Biochem. Biophys.*, **539**, 142–55 (2013).
18. T. A. Ilyina, A. B. Kerimov, M. V. Zagubizhenko, and G. V. Maksimov, "Seasonal dynamics of leaf-eating insects biomass and its influence on carotenoid content in feathers of Great Tit nestlings," *Russ. J. Ecol.*, **44**, 507–14 (2013).
19. D. B. Thomas, K.J. McGraw, H. F. James, and O. Madden, "Non-destructive descriptions of carotenoids in feathers using Raman spectroscopy," *Anal. Methods*, **6**, 1301–8 (2014).
20. D. B. Thomas, P. C. Nascimbene, C. J. Dove, D. A. Grimaldi, and H. F. James, "Seeking carotenoid pigments in amber-preserved fossil feathers," *Sci. Rep.*, **4**, 5226 (2014).
21. S. Tfaili, C. Gobinet, G. Josse, J.-F. Angiboust, M. Manfaita, and O. Piot, "Confocal Raman microspectroscopy for skin characterization: a comparative study between human skin and pig skin," *Analyst*, **137**, 3673 (2012).
22. C. Uragami, E. Yamashita, A. Gall, B. Robert, and H. Hashimoto, "Application of resonance Raman microscopy to in vivo carotenoid," *Acta Biochim. Polonica*, **59**, 53–56 (2012).
23. K. Hesterberg, S. Schanzer, A. Patzelt, W. Sterry, J. W. Fluhr, M. C. Meinke, J. Lademann, and M. E. Darvin, "Raman spectroscopic analysis of the carotenoid concentration in egg yolks depending on the feeding and housing conditions of the laying hens," *J. Biophotonics*, **5** (1), 33–9 (2012).
24. J. Klein, M. E. Darvin, M.C. Meinke, F. J. Schweigert, K. E. Müller, and J. J. Lademann, "Analyses of the correlation between dermal and blood carotenoids in female cattle by optical methods," *Biomed. Opt.*, **18**(6), 061219 (2013).
25. M. E. Darvin, I. Gersonde, M. Meinke, W. Sterry, and J. Lademann, "Non-invasive in vivo determination of the carotenoids beta-carotene and lycopene concentrations in the human skin using the Raman spectroscopic method," *J. Phys. D-Appl. Phys.*, **38**, 2696–700 (2005).
26. J. Klein, M. E. Darvin, K. E. Müller, and J. Lademann, "Serial non-invasive measurements of dermal carotenoid concentrations in dairy cows following recovery from abomasal displacement," *PLoS One*, **7**, 10, e47706 (2012).
27. P. Bhosale, B. Serban, D. Y. Zhao, and P. S. Bernstein, "Identification and metabolic transformations of carotenoids in ocular tissues of the Japanese quail *Coturnix japonica*," *Biochemistry*, **46**, 9050–7 (2007).
28. J. P. Wold, B. J. Marquardt, B. K. Dable, D. Robb, and B. Hatlen, "Rapid quantication of carotenoids and fat in Atlantic salmon (*Salmo salar* L.) by Raman spectroscopy and chemometrics," *Appl. Spectr.*, **58**(4), 395–403 (2004).
29. W. Werncke, I. Latka, S. Sassning, B. Dietzek, M. E. Darvin, M. C. Meinke, J. Popp, K. König, J. W. Fluhr, and J. Lademann, "Two-color Raman spectroscopy for the simultaneous detection of chemotherapeutics and antioxidative status of human skin," *Laser Phys. Lett.*, **8**, 895–900 (2011).

30. M. E. Darvin, I. Gersonde, H. Albrecht, S. A. Gonchukov, W. Sterry, and J. Lademann, "Determination of beta carotene and lycopene concentrations in human skin using resonance Raman spectroscopy," *Laser Physics*, **15**, 295–9 (2005).

31. M. E. Darvin, I. Gersonde, H. Albrecht, M. Meinke, W. Sterry, and J. Lademann, "Non-invasive in vivo detection of the carotenoid antioxidant substance lycopene in the human skin using the resonance Raman spectroscopy," *Laser Phys. Lett.*, **3**, 460–3 (2006).

32. S. T. Mayne, B. Cartmel, S. Scarmo, H. Lin, D. J. Leffell, E. Welch, I. Ermakov, P. Bhosale, P. S. Bernstein, and W. Gellermann, "Noninvasive assessment of dermal carotenoids as a biomarker of fruit and vegetable intake," *Am. J. Clin. Nutr.*, **92**, 794–800 (2010).

33. S. Scarmo, B. Cartmel, H. Lin, D. J. Leffell, I. V. Ermakov, W. Gellermann, P. S. Bernstein, and S. T. Mayne, "Single v. multiple measures of skin carotenoids by resonance Raman spectroscopy as a biomarker of usual carotenoid status," *Br. J. Nutr.*, **110**, 911–7 (2013).

34. O. Howells, F. Eperjesi and H. Bartlett, "Measuring macular pigment optical density in vivo: a review of techniques," *Graefes Arch. Clin. Exp. Ophthalmol.*, **249**, 315–47 (2011).

35. P. S. Bernstein, M. D. Yoshida, N. B. Katz, R. W. McClane, and W. Gellermann, "Raman detection of macular carotenoid pigments in intact human retina," *Invest. Ophthalmol. Vis. Sci.*, **39**, 2003–11 (1998).

36. A. Obana, T. Hiramitsu, Y. Gohto, A. Ohira, S. Mizuno, T. Hirano, P. S. Bernstein, H. Fujii, K. Iseki, M. Tanito, and Y. Hotta, "Macular carotenoid levels of normal subjects and age-related maculopathy patients in a Japanese population," *Ophthalmology*, **115**, 147–57 (2008).

37. S. Beatty, U. Chakravarthy, J. M. Nolan, K. A. Muldrew, J. V. Woodside, F. Denny, and M. R. Stevenson, "Secondary outcomes in a clinical trial of carotenoids with coantioxidants versus placebo in early age-related macular degeneration," *Ophthalmology*, **120**, 600–6 (2013).

38. M. Sharifzadeh, D. Y. Zhao, P. S. Bernstein, and W. Gellermann, "Resonance Raman imaging of macular pigment distributions in the human retina," *J. Opt. Soc. Am. A*, **25**, 947–57 (2008).

39. K. Neelam, N. O'Gorman, J. Nolan, O. O'Donovan, K. G. Au Eong, and S. Beatty, "Macular pigment levels following successful macular hole surgery," *Br. J. Ophthalmol.*, **89**, 1105–8 (2005).

40. M. S. Ward, D. Y. Zhao, and P. S. Bernstein, "Macular and serum carotenoid concentrations in patients with malabsorption syndromes," *J. Ocul. Biol. Dis. Inform.*, **1**, 12–18 (2008).

41. A. Ramoji, U. Neugebauer, T. Bocklitz, M. Foerster, M. Kiehntopf, M. Bauer, and J. Popp, "Toward a spectroscopic hemogram: Raman spectroscopic differentiation of the two most abundant leukocytes from peripheral blood," *Anal. Chem.*, **84**, 5335–42 (2012).

42. V. Pully, A. Lenferink, and C. Otto, "Time-lapse Raman imaging of single live lymphocytes," *J. Raman Spectrosc.*, **42**, 167–73 (2011).

43. G. Puppels, H. Garritsen, and J. Kummer, "Carotenoids located in human lymphocyte subpopulations and natural killer cells by Raman microspectroscopy," *Cytometry*, **14**, 251–6 (2005).

44. R. B. Ramanauskaite, I. Segers-Nolten, K. Grauw, N. M. Sijtsema, L. Van Der Maas, J. Greve, C. Otto, and C. G. Figdor, "Carotenoid levels in human lymphocytes, measured by Raman microspectroscopy," *Pure Appl. Chem.*, **69**, 2131–4 (1997).

45. T. C. Bakker Schut, G. J. Puppels, Y. M. Kraan, J. Greve, L. L. J. Van Der Maas, and C. G. Figdor, "Intracellular carotenoid levels measured by Raman microspectroscopy: Comparison of lymphocytes from lung cancer patients and healthy individuals," *Int. J. Canc. Prev.*, **74**, 20–5 (1997).

46. B. P. Chew, and J. S. Park, "Carotenoid action on the immune response," *J. Nutr.*, **134**, 257S–61S (2004).

47. A. P. Bolin, R. C. Macedo, D. P. Marin, M. P. Barros, and R. Otton, "Astaxanthin prevents in vitro auto-oxidative injury in human lymphocytes," *Cell Biol. Toxicol.*, **26**, 457–67 (2010).
48. H. Jyonouchi, R. J. Hill, Y. Tomita, and R. A. Good, "Studies of immunomodulating actions of carotenoids. 1. Effects of β-carotene and astaxanthin on murine lymphocyte functions and cell surface marker expression in vitro culture system," *Nutr. Cancer*, **16,** 93–105 (1991).
49. M. Stacewicz-Sapuntzakis, P. Bowen, J. Kikendall, and M. Burgess, "Simultaneous determination of serum retinol and various carotenoids: their distribution in middle-aged men and women," *J. Micronutr. Anal.*, **3**, 27–45 (1987).

9

Carotenoids in Pigment–Protein Complexes: Relation between Carotenoid Structure and Function

Wieslaw I. Gruszecki

Department of Biophysics, Institute of Physics, Maria Curie-Sklodowska University, Lublin, Poland

9.1 Biological functions of carotenoids

A conjugated double-bond system, which is a basic and typical structural element of a polyene, is responsible for both the photophysical and structural properties of carotenoids. On the one hand, a polyene chain is rigid, which, together with its length of circa 3 nm in the case of most abundant natural carotenoids [1, 2], provides unique opportunities to stabilize biomembranes and membrane-bound pigment–protein complexes [3–7]. On the other hand, a length of the conjugated double-bond system is responsible for absorption of light and therefore for the pigment properties of carotenoids. In the case of N values in the range of 7–11 (e.g., violaxanthin, N=9; lutein, N=10; or β-carotene, N=11; see Figure 9.1), the energies of the strongly allowed S0 to S2 electronic transition correspond to light energies from the blue-green spectral region (see Figure 9.2) [8].

Due to the same determinants, the energy of the first excited triplet state of the C_{40} carotenoids, with a sufficiently long conjugated double-bond system, is low enough to accept excitation energy from the triplet state of porphyrins, including chlorophylls, which are very effective photosensitizers able to generate singlet oxygen. Owing to the fact that the energy of both the triplet states of photosensitizers and the energy of singlet oxygen are higher than the triplet-state energy of the carotenoids listed above, they can play a photoprotective role via the energy quenching of photosensitizer triplet or oxygen singlet states.

Carotenoids: Nutrition, Analysis and Technology, First Edition. Edited by Agnieszka Kaczor and Malgorzata Baranska.

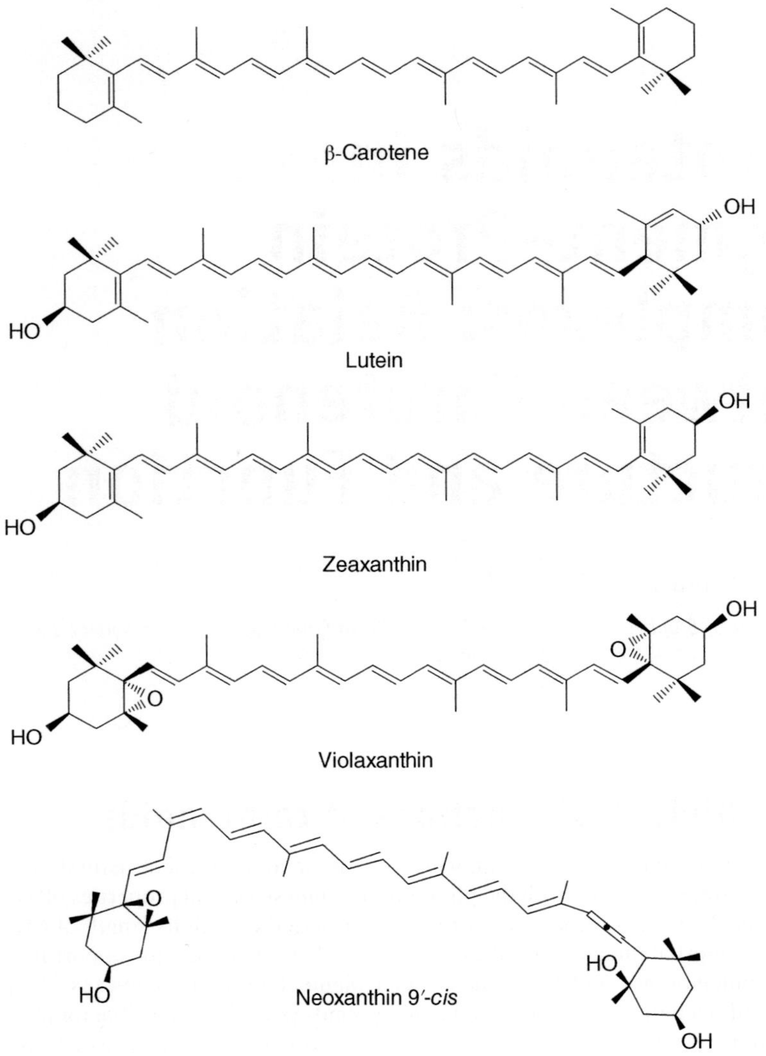

Figure 9.1 Chemical structures of the most abundant carotenoids, constituents of the pigment–protein complexes.

Carotenoids are assigned three major physiological functions in nature: photoprotection against oxidative damage [9, 10], structural stabilization of biomembranes and proteins, and light absorption (pigmentation and the photosynthetic light-harvesting function). As can be seen from the short discussion so far in this chapter, owing to the unique chemical structure of this class of molecules, carotenoids seem ideally suited to play important biological functions in living organisms.

There are two possible localizations of carotenoids in biomembranes; pigments can be directly present within the membrane lipid phase [3] and specifically bound to pigment–protein complexes. The distribution of carotenoids in the thylakoid membranes of the photosynthetic apparatus is a prominent example of such a localization. Almost an entire pool of the photosynthetically active carotenoids is protein bound, along with chlorophylls,

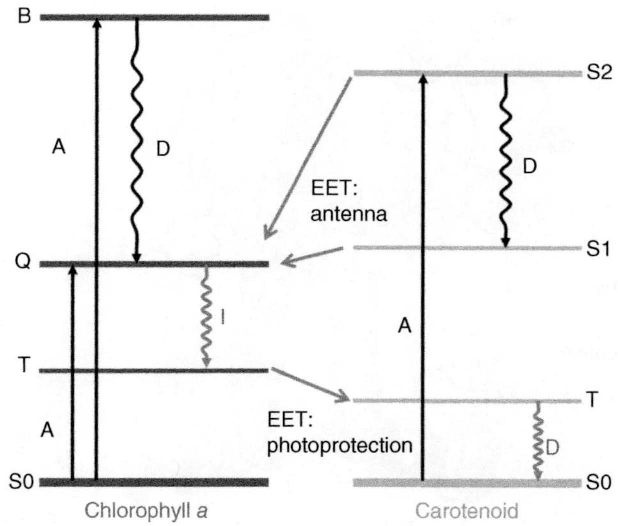

Figure 9.2 Scheme of energy levels of chlorophyll *a* and carotenoids with indicated selected electronic transitions. A stands for light absorption; D, thermal energy dissipation; I, intersystem crossing; EET, excitation energy transfer; S0 (ground), S1, and S2, the energy levels of a carotenoid; T, triplet states; Q, the Q_y state; and B, the B_x state of chlorophyll *a*.

and appears as functional pigment–protein complexes [11]. In addition to this, a certain poll of polar carotenoids, called xanthophylls, appears, at least transiently, directly in the lipid phase of the thylakoid membranes. Those xanthophylls are violaxanthin, antheraxanthin, and zeaxanthin, and such localization is associated with operation of the enzymatic interconversion between the pigments, referred to as the xanthophyll cycle [12]. The xanthophyll cycle pigments have one common structural feature, namely, the presence of two hydroxyl groups in the opposite ends of their molecules, at the C3 and C3′ positions. The distance between these polar groups (~3 nm) fits very well with the thickness of the hydrophobic core of the thylakoid membrane (~3 nm) [1, 7]. Owing to such compatibility, the xanthophylls can span the membrane and be anchored by their polar groups in the opposite hydrophilic zones of the membrane. Such pigment localization and orientation have been shown to influence considerably both the structural and dynamic properties of the membranes and, in consequence, protect the lipid phase against oxidative damage.

As mentioned in this chapter, most carotenoids are located *in vivo* in the functional pigment–protein complexes. A prominent example of such a complex is the plant photosynthetic antenna complex LHCII (light-harvesting pigment–protein complex of Photosystem II) [13, 14].

9.2 Carotenoids in pigment–protein complexes

LHCII (see Figure 9.3 in the Color Supplement) is a very abundant membrane protein in the biosphere, and it comprises virtually half of the chlorophyll molecules on Earth [15].

The main physiological function of this pigment–protein complex is capturing light quanta and transferring electronic excitations toward the reaction centers, to drive the photochemical reactions of photosynthesis.

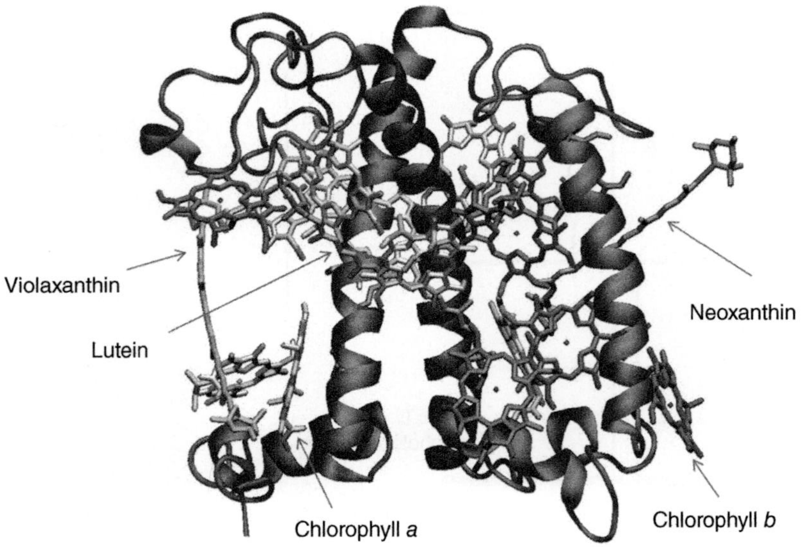

Figure 9.3 Model of the structure of the LHCII pigment–protein complex, based on the crystallographic data PDB: 2bhw. (*See insert for color representation of the figure.*)

A superficial analysis of the LHCII composition indicates enormously high pigment density per protein: eight molecules of chlorophyll *a*, six molecules of chlorophyll *b*, and four molecules of xanthophylls. The LHCII xanthophyll pool is constituted by two luteins, one neoxanthin, and one violaxanthin. Interestingly, the xanthophylls are not covalently bound to the complex but always occupy the same positions and bind to the complex at the same stoichiometry, both in the native LHCII and in the complex reconstituted *in vitro*, from the overexpressed lhcb apoprotein and pigment extract. This means that different xanthophylls play important and specific functions in the complex. LHCII is a photosynthetic antenna, and, therefore, it could be anticipated that the main physiological function of xanthophylls in the complex is to absorb light and direct their excitation energy toward chlorophylls [16]. In fact, such a nonradiative excitation energy transfer from xanthophylls to chlorophyll *a* can be very easily observed from the analysis of the chlorophyll fluorescence excitation spectra in which the contribution from carotenoid excitations can be noticed. Such energy transfer has to operate via the short-distance, energy-charge exchange mechanisms, referred to as Dexter-type energy transfers, due to the fact that carotenoids present a relatively low-fluorescence quantum yield, which is one of the determinants of the rate of the long-distance, Förster-type, nonradiative excitation energy transfer mechanism. A contribution of carotenoids to the antenna activity is very distinct in the case of the bacterial photosynthetic antenna complexes [17], but in the case of the plant LHCII complex, the xanthophyll absorption bands are almost overlapped by the combined Soret bands of chlorophyll *a* and chlorophyll *b*. This suggests that antenna activity of the LHCII-bound xanthophylls is not a vital biological function. Photosensitized generation of carotenoid triplet states in isolated LHCII, localized mostly on lutein, by time-resolved and pulse electron paramagnetic resonance (EPR) techniques [18] and also by Raman-scattering spectroscopy [19], shows that the antenna-bound xanthophylls act as photoprotectors via quenching of chlorophyll triplet states and preventing generation of singlet oxygen [20, 21]. Two molecules of lutein are located in the central part of the antenna protein, span the complex, and remain in close contact with numerous chlorophyll molecules. Such a localization provides favorable conditions for chlorophyll–lutein excitation energy transfer, including the chlorophyll triplet quenching by the xanthophyll, which is recognized as a basic photoprotective activity. It was suggested that circa 95% of chlorophyll triplet excitations in LHCII are effectively quenched by the protein-complexed molecules of lutein [20]. Moreover, the rigid xanthophyll molecules, located in the central, lutein-binding sites of LHCII (L1 and L2), play a fundamental physiological function in proper folding and stabilization of this pigment–protein complex [13, 14].

Most conclusions regarding the behavior of LHCII under light stress conditions, including those on xanthophyll-related photoprotection, are based on the model studies carried out with an isolated pigment–protein complex. Such observations are valuable from the physiological point of view due to the fact that isolated LHCII is not able to transfer excitation energy outward toward the reaction centers, and therefore it is a good model of this antenna complex under overexcitation conditions. Moreover, owing to the LHCII phosphorylation and the so-called State I–State II transition, the proteins migrate out of the membrane regions enriched with the reaction centers of Photosystem II [22–26]. Some antennae become energetically coupled to Photosystem I, but the majority remains energetically uncoupled from reaction centers in the thylakoid membranes. As mentioned in this chapter, chlorophylls are very efficient photosensitizers, basically due to the fact that the rate of intersystem crossing can reach ~60% in the case of chlorophyll *a*, and up to 88% in the case of chlorophyll *b*. Therefore, from the "strategic" standpoint, a better photoprotective activity, under overexcitation conditions, would be preventing the generation of chlorophyll triplets, rather than quenching them. A straightforward mechanism, acting according to such a rule, would be quenching of excessive chlorophyll singlet excitations. Chlorophyll *a* fluorescence quenching, observed at strong light conditions, is a manifestation of the operation of such a mechanism *in vivo*. Such observation is straightforward and technically very simple, contrary to explaining which exact mechanisms are directly responsible for that kind of excitation quenching. One of the popular concepts was directly based on the reversed antenna activity of the LHCII-bound xanthophylls, namely, on the singlet–singlet excitation energy transfer from chlorophyll to xanthophylls. The forward (from xanthophyll to chlorophyll) and the backward (from chlorophyll to xanthophyll) singlet–singlet excitation energy transfer was a core of the hypothesis, named the molecular gearshift mechanism [27]. The hypothesis has been put forward to explain the biological meaning of the xanthophyll cycle operating in the photosynthetic apparatus of higher plants. Within the xanthophyll cycle, violaxanthin, which is a xanthophyll present in the photosynthetic apparatus at physiological conditions, is enzymatically converted to zeaxanthin, under strong light conditions, via the two-step de-epoxidation (see Figure 9.4)

Owing to the fact that zeaxanthin is a xanthophyll with a longer conjugated double-bond system (N=11) than violaxanthin (N=9), corresponding energy levels in both xanthophylls will be different and located lower on the energy scale in the case of a longer polyene. Simply due to this fact, combined with the localization of the lowest singlet energy level of xanthophylls (S1, $1A^1_g$), which is comparable to the energy of the Q_y state of chlorophyll *a*, it could be anticipated that violaxanthin will be a xanthophyll predisposed to act as an antenna, contrary to zeaxanthin, which will be predisposed to act as a chlorophyll excitation quencher (see Figure 9.5).

Such a concept was originally presented as a hypothesis due to the fact that localization of the xanthophyll S1 level on the energy scale was uncertain, because direct S0→S1 electronic transition is forbidden for a single-photon absorption [28], due to the symmetry reasons. It appeared latter that the energy difference between the S1 states of violaxanthin and zeaxanthin was not as large as originally expected [29], which made the "molecular

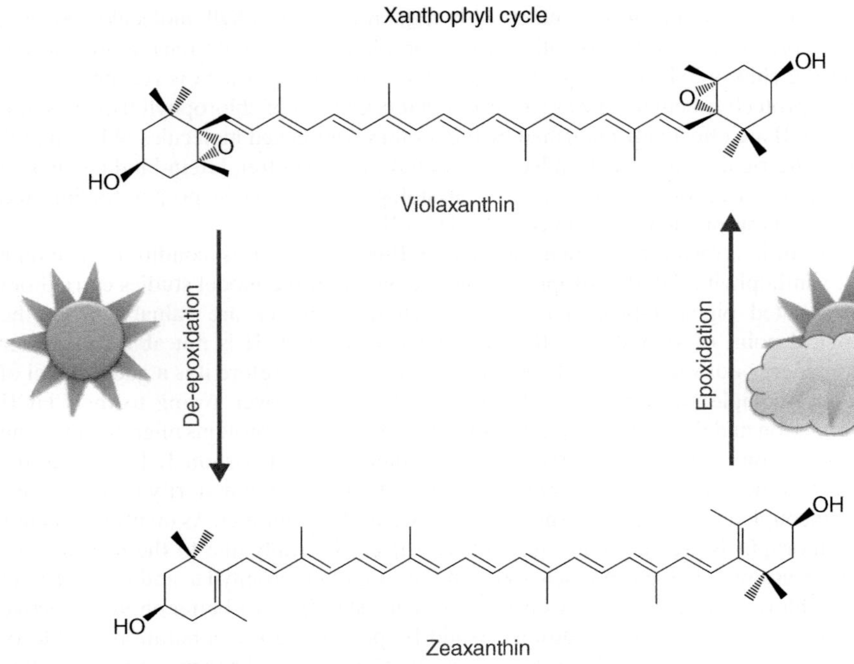

Figure 9.4 Schematic representation of the xanthophyll cycle operating in higher plants.

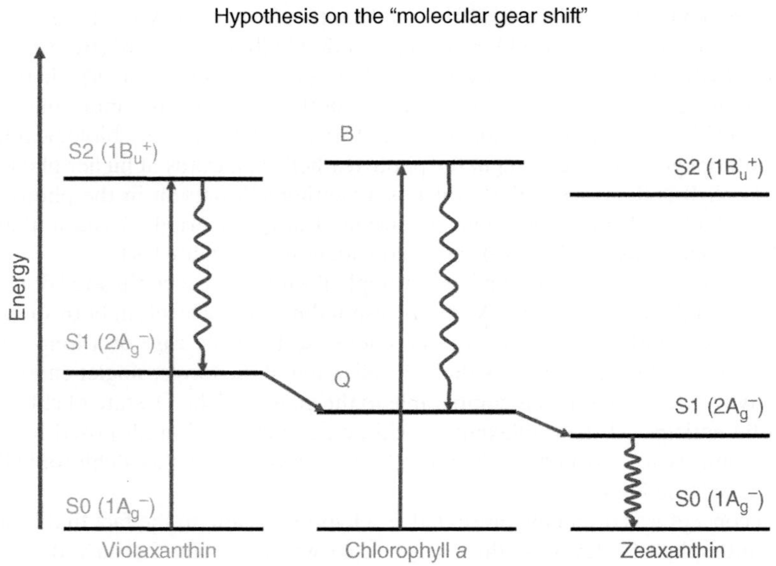

Figure 9.5 Comparison of the localization of the electronic energy levels of chlorophyll *a* and the xanthophyll cycle pigments, to discuss a direction of the excitation energy transfer.

gearshift model" less attractive. On the other hand, the vibronic bands of carotenoids are relatively broad and the S1 energy level could be almost isoenergetic relative to the Q_y state of chlorophylls; both the forward and the backward singlet–singlet excitation energy transfer between xanthophyll and chlorophyll molecules, embedded in the same pigment–protein complexes, is very probable, and it is also very likely that it plays a physiological function in regulation of the photosynthetic antenna function, under changing light intensity conditions [30].

As mentioned in this chapter, operation of the enzymatic reactions of the xanthophyll cycle requires violaxanthin, a xanthophyll bound to the protein environment (Figure 9.3), to be detached and transferred toward the lipid phase of the thylakoid membrane, in which the de-epoxidase enzyme dissolved in the luminal volume can act [12]. This process has been historically referred to as a light-dependent control of violaxanthin availability for enzymatic de-epoxidation. The resonance Raman study of xanthophylls in isolated LHCII has revealed that, under strong light conditions, violaxanthin is subjected to light-driven molecular configuration change, *in situ*, which makes the pigment binding to the protein less favorable for steric reasons. The localization site of violaxanthin in LHCII is at the border of monomers in the trimeric structure, which is a natural molecular organization form of this protein under physiological conditions. Owing to this fact, it has been hypothesized that the process of light-driven liberation of violaxanthin is associated with the light-induced LHCII trimer destabilization resulting in a monomer formation [31]. The process of light-induced trimer–monomer transition of LHCII was first observed by Garab and coworkers [32]. Such a LHCII transition was originally assigned as originating from a thermo-optical effect. It is very likely that violaxanthin undergoes a light-driven molecular configuration change not via a direct photoreaction but rather at the expense of thermal energy dissipated in the entire overexcited antenna system. In such a system, violaxanthin therefore can be recognized as a specific overexcitation sensor, triggering a cascade of processes leading to photoprotection via quenching of excessive excitations. One of the consequences of such a process is making violaxanthin available for the enzymatic de-epoxidation, which results in zeaxanthin accumulation. Another direct consequence is the presence of LHCII monomers instead of trimers in the photosynthetic membranes subjected to light stress. The possible physiological meaning of such a trimer–monomer conversion still remains an open question. The fact that the trimeric organization of LHCII has been conserved during biological evolution suggests that such a structure is optimized to assure efficient operation of the complex as a photosynthetic antenna. The fact that LHCII trimers disassemble into monomers, under light stress conditions, suggests a photoprotective meaning of this reorganization. Regarding accumulation of zeaxanthin, numerous observations has shown a correlation of zeaxanthin concentration and high-light-induced excitation quenching [33, 34]. However, the fact that a comparable extent of quenching could be observed in the zeaxanthin-less *Arabidopsis* mutants [35] raises a question on the causative character of the zeaxanthin level and excitation-quenching correlations. On the other hand, it can be hypothesized that, in the absence of zeaxanthin, other xanthophylls take over the role of excessive chlorophyll singlet excitation quenching [35]. In addition to the direct, photophysical effects of the xanthophyll cycle pigments on the pigment–protein complexes, indirect effects have been proposed, based on modulation of molecular organization of the antenna proteins (the formation of supramolecular structures) [14, 30, 36–38].

As emphasized here, each LHCII-bound xanthophyll represents a unique chemical structure and occupies a unique site in the protein. In contrast to lutein, which is tightly bound and hidden inside a protein core, or violaxanthin, which is relatively weakly bound and located at the periphery of the LHCII monomer (at the border of monomers in the trimeric structure), neoxanthin is anchored by one end in the protein, and half of its molecule protrudes out of the complex. Interestingly, in contrast to other LHCII-bound xanthophylls that remain in the all-*trans* molecular configuration, neoxanthin binds to the protein, adopting a 9′-*cis* molecular configuration. It seems that such a molecular configuration of the xanthophyll assures relatively tight protein binding, despite the fact that only half of the molecule is involved in interaction with the protein (a *hook effect*). Several light-controlled regulatory processes are assigned specifically to neoxanthin as a light-intensity-sensing photoreceptor. It has been demonstrated, based on the results of the resonance Raman analysis of the LHCII-bound xanthophylls, that neoxanthin undergoes light-driven molecular configuration changes, referred to as "twisting" [39]. Such a change has been proposed to alter the LHCII structure to a level that influences lutein–chlorophyll molecular distance and potentiates singlet–singlet excitation energy transfer to lutein (chlorophyll excitation quenching) [39]. Such a concept has been questioned for two reasons. In the first place, it is a relatively rigid protein core, which is, according to structural biologists, very unlikely to be subjected to reorganization [15]. Another line of criticism is associated with questioned chlorophyll excitation quenching by lutein [40]. Despite this dispute, the observation regarding light-driven twisting of neoxanthin is very important, certainly very interesting, and most likely physiologically relevant. It also has been demonstrated, with application of chromatographic analysis, that illumination of isolated LHCII, with relatively strong light, results in photo-isomerization of 9′-*cis* neoxanthin to other molecular configuration forms, in particular 9′,13′- and 9′,13-*dicis* [41]. It has been postulated that such a light-driven neoxanthin conversion facilities intertrimer LHCII interactions, leading to formation of the excitation-quenching molecular organization structures of LHCII. According to the authors, a close contact between the LHCII trimers in the membrane, which would result in the formation of excitation-quenching supramolecular structures of the complex, is blocked by neoxanthin protruding out of the protein but is potentiated after light-driven neoxanthin isomerization [42].

9.3 Final remarks

As can be concluded, based on the analysis of the molecular structure and physiological function of carotenoids bound to the pigment–protein complex LHCII, biological functions of pigments are potentiated by and specifically related to a chemical structure. Such a structure is responsible for both the structural and photophysical properties of carotenoids. Slightly altered xanthophyll composition of the other, minor photosynthetic pigment–protein antenna complexes (e.g., CP 24, CP 26, and CP 29) and, in particular, the presence of β-carotene in the photosynthetic reaction centers are believed to respond to the specific physiological functions of carotenoids in those pigment–protein complexes. This problem is still a subject of intensive research. Generally, both the structure-stabilizing and energy transfer functions are certainly basic ones assigned to carotenoids in the pigment–protein complexes. In the case of β-carotene, additionally, it has been hypothesized that a polyene chain may be directly involved in the electric charge transfer, for example in the cyclic electron transfer around Photosystem II [43]. A very interesting example of a pigment–protein complex that binds carotenoids is a water-soluble orange carotenoid protein called OCP [44, 45]. The OCP complex has been reported to act as a light intensity sensor in cyanobacteria, responsible for control of thermal energy dissipation under light stress conditions. The protein-embedded carotenoid (3′-hydroxyechinenone) remains in the all-*trans* configuration. A reversible phototransformation of OCP, from the "orange" form to the active "red" form, which takes place upon illumination with blue-green light, is associated with certain structural modifications of both the protein environment and the carotenoid cofactor, as demonstrated with application of the FTIR and resonance Raman techniques, respectively [45].

9.4 Perspectives

Despite the high activity of numerous research groups involved in studies on physiological functions of carotenoid pigments in the pigment–protein complexes, there are still many open questions that need clarification. One of these problems is associated with the potential involvement of a light-induced molecular configuration change of the LHCII-bound violaxanthin, in the process of light-driven trimer–monomer transition of the complex. A similar open question is related to the light-driven molecular configuration change of the LHCII-bound xanthophyll neoxanthin. It is possible that such a process influences (or maybe even potentiates?) supramolecular structure formation of LHCII, which is responsible for excessive excitation quenching in the photosynthetic apparatus of plants exposed to overexcitation conditions. These and similar open questions will be, most probably, addressed in the near future, and new findings will shed light on mechanistic aspects of unknown carotenoid functions in the pigment–protein complexes.

Acknowledgments

The research on carotenoids in pigment–protein complexes in the laboratory of the author is founded by the Foundation for Polish Science (program TEAM) within the project Molecular Spectroscopy for BioMedical Studies.

References

1. A. Milon, G. Wolff, G. Ourisson, and Y. Nakatani, "Organization of carotenoid-phospholipid bilayer systems. Incorporation of zeaxanthin, astaxanthin, and their C50 homologues into dimyristoylphosphatidylcholine vesicles," *Helvet. Chim. Acta,* **69**, 12–24 (1986).
2. T. Lazrak, A. Milon, G. Wolff, A. M. Albrecht, M. Miehe, G. Ourisson, and Y. Nakatani, "Comparison of the effects of inserted C40- and C50-terminally dihydroxylated carotenoids on the mechanical properties of various phospholipid vesicles," *Biochim. Biophys. Acta,* **903**, 132–41 (1987).
3. W. I. Gruszecki, "Carotenoids in membranes," in H. A. Frank, A. J. Young, G. Britton, and R. J. Cogdell (eds.), *The photochemistry of carotenoids*, Dordrecht: Kluwer Academic, 1999.
4. W. I. Gruszecki, "Carotenoid orientation: role in membrane stabilization," in N. I. Krinsky, S. T. Mayne, and H. Sies (eds.), *Carotenoids in health and disease*, New York: Marcel Dekker, 2004.
5. W. I. Gruszecki, "Carotenoids in lipid membranes," in J. T. Landrum (ed.), *Carotenoids: physical, chemical and biological functions and properties*, London: CRC Press, 2010.
6. W. I. Gruszecki and J. Sielewiesiuk, "Orientation of xanthophylls in phosphatidylcholine multibilayers," *Biochim. Biophys. Acta,* **1023**, 405–12 (1990).

7. W. I. Gruszecki and K. Strzalka, "Carotenoids as modulators of lipid membrane physical properties," *Biochim. Biophys. Acta,* **1740**, 108–15 (2005).
8. R. L. Christensen, "The electronic states of carotenoids," in H. A. Frank, A. J. Young, G. Britton, and R. J. Cogdell (eds.), *The photochemistry of carotenoids*, Dordrecht: Kluwer Academic, 1999.
9. N. I. Krinsky, "Carotenoid protection against oxidation," *Pure Appl. Chem.,* **51**, 649–60 (1979).
10. N. I. Krinsky, J. T. Landrum, and R. A. Bone, "Biologic mechanisms of the protective role of lutein and zeaxanthin in the eye," *Annu. Rev. Nutr.,* **23**, 171–201 (2003).
11. R. Croce and H. Van Amerongen, "Light-harvesting and structural organization of Photosystem II: from individual complexes to thylakoid membrane," *J. Photochem. Photobiol. B-Biol.,* **104**, 142–53 (2011).
12. R. Goss, M. Lohr, D. Latowski, J. Grzyb, A. Vieler, C. Wilhelm, and K. Strzalka, "Role of hexagonal structure-forming lipids in diadinoxanthin and violaxanthin solubilization and de-epoxidation," *Biochemistry,* **44**, 4028–36 (2005).
13. Z. Liu, H. Yan, K. Wang, T. Kuang, J. Zhang, L. Gui, X. An, and W. Chang, "Crystal structure of spinach major light-harvesting complex at 2.72 A resolution," *Nature,* **428**, 287–92 (2004).
14. R. Standfuss, A. C. T. Van Scheltinga, M. Lamborghini, and W. Kuhlbrandt, "Mechanisms of photoprotection and nonphotochemical quenching in pea light-harvesting complex at 2.5 A resolution," *EMBO J.,* **24**, 919–28 (2005).
15. T. Barros and W. Kuhlbrandt, "Crystallisation, structure and function of plant light-harvesting complex II," *Biochim. Biophys. Acta-Bioenerg.,* **1787**, 753–72 (2009).
16. M. Fuciman, M. M. Enriquez, T. Polivka, L. Dall'osto, R. Bassi, and H. A. Frank, "Role of xanthophylls in light harvesting in green plants: a spectroscopic investigation of mutant LHCII and Lhcb pigment-protein complexes," *J. Phys. Chem. B,* **116**, 3834–49 (2012).
17. J. Fiedor, M. Pilch, and L. Fiedor, "Tuning the thermodynamics of association of transmembrane helices," *J. Phys. Chem. B,* **113**, 12831–8 (2009).
18. M. Di Valentin, F. Biasibetti, S. Ceola, and D. Carbonera, "Identification of the sites of chlorophyll triplet quenching in relation to the structure of LHC-II from higher plants: evidence from EPR spectroscopy," *J. Phys. Chem. B,* **113**, 13071–8 (2009).
19. A. Gall, R. Berera, M. T. A. Alexandre, A. A. Pascal, L. Bordes, M. M. Mendes-Pinto, S. Andrianambinintsoa, K. V. Stoitchkova, A. Marin, L. Valkunas, P. Horton, J. T. M. Kennis, R. Van Grondelle, A. Ruban, and B. Robert, "Molecular adaptation of photoprotection: triplet states in light-harvesting proteins," *Biophys. J.*, **101**, 934–42 (2011).
20. M. Mozzo, L. Dall'osto, R. Hienerwadel, R. Bassi, and R. Croce, "Photoprotection in the antenna complexes of photosystem II: role of individual xanthophylls in chlorophyll triplet quenching," *J. Biol. Chem.,* **283**, 6184–92 (2008).
21. L. Dall'osto, C. Lico, J. Alric, G. Giuliano, M. Havaux, and R. Bassi, "Lutein is needed for efficient chlorophyll triplet quenching in the major LHCII antenna complex of higher plants and effective photoprotection in vivo under strong light," *BMC Plant Biology,* **6** (2006).
22. E. Janik, J. Bednarska, M. Zubik, M. Puzio, R. Luchowski, W. Grudzinski, R. Mazur, M. Garstka, W. Maksymiec, A. Kulik, G. Dietler, and W. I. Gruszecki, "Molecular architecture of plant thylakoids under physiological and light stress conditions: A study of lipid-light-harvesting complex II model membranes," *Plant Cell,* **25**, 2155–70 (2013).
23. H. Kirchhoff, "Architectural switches in plant thylakoid membranes," *Photosynth. Res.,* **116**, 481–7 (2013).

24. M. Tikkanen and E. M. Aro, "Thylakoid protein phosphorylation in dynamic regulation of photosystem II in higher plants," *Biochim. Biophys. Acta,* **1817**, 232–8 (2012).

25. M. Tikkanen, M. Grieco, and E. M. Aro, "Novel insights into plant light-harvesting complex II phosphorylation and 'state transitions'," *Trends Plant Sci.,* **16**, 126–31 (2011).

26. M. Tikkanen, M. Grieco, M. Nurmi, M. Rantala, M. Suorsa, and E. M. Aro, "Regulation of the photosynthetic apparatus under fluctuating growth light," *Phil. Trans. Royal Soc. B-Biol. Sci.,* **367**, 3486–93 (2012).

27. A. J. Young, D. Phillip, A. V. Ruban, P. Horton, and H. A. Frank, "The xanthophyll cycle and carotenoid-mediated dissipation of excess excitation energy in photosynthesis," *Pure Appl. Chem.*, **69**, 2125–30 (1997).

28. W. I. Gruszecki, H. Stiel, D. Niedzwiedzki, M. Beck, J. Milanowska, H. Lokstein, and D. Leupold, "Towards elucidating the energy of the first excited singlet state of xanthophyll cycle pigments by X-ray absorption spectroscopy," *Biochim. Biophys. Acta,* **1708**, 102–7 (2005).

29. T. Polivka, J. L. Herek, D. Zigmantas, H. E. Akerlund, and V. Sundstrom, "Direct observation of the (forbidden) S1 state in carotenoids," *Proc. Natl. Acad. Sci. USA,* **96**, 4914–7 (1999).

30. W. I. Gruszecki, M. Zubik, R. Luchowski, E. Janik, W. Grudzinski, M. Gospodarek, J. Goc, L. Fiedor, Z. Gryczynski, and I. Gryczynski, "Photoprotective role of the xanthophyll cycle studied by means of modeling of xanthophyll–LHCII interactions," *Chem. Phys.,* **373**, 122–8 (2010).

31. W. I. Gruszecki, M. Gospodarek, W. Grudzinski, R. Mazur, K. Gieczewska, and M. Garstka, "Light-induced change of configuration of the LHCII-bound xanthophyll (tentatively assigned to violaxanthin): a resonance Raman study," *J. Phys. Chem. B,* **113**, 2506–12 (2009).

32. G. Garab, Z. Cseh, L. Kovacs, S. Rajagopal, Z. Varkonyi, M. Wentworth, L. Mustardy, A. Der, A. V. Ruban, E. Papp, A. Holzenburg, and P. Horton, "Light-induced trimer to monomer transition in the main light-harvesting antenna complex of plants: thermo-optic mechanism," *Biochemistry,* **41**, 15121–9 (2002).

33. B. Demmig-Adams, "Survey of thermal energy dissipation and pigment composition in sun and shade leaves," *Plant and Cell Physiology,* **39**, 474–82 (1998).

34. B. Demmig-Adams and W. W. Adams, "Xanthophyll cycle and light stress in nature: uniform response to excess direct sunlight among higher plant species," *Planta,* **198**, 460–70 (1996).

35. M. P. Johnson, M. L. Perez-Bueno, A. Zia, P. Horton, and A. V. Ruban, "The zeaxanthin-independent and zeaxanthin-dependent qE components of nonphotochemical quenching involve common conformational changes within the photosystem II antenna in *Arabidopsis*," *Plant Physiol.*, **149**, 1061–75 (2009).

36. W. I. Gruszecki, W. Grudzinski, M. Gospodarek, M. Patyra, and W. Maksymiec, "Xanthophyll-induced aggregation of LHCII as a switch between light-harvesting and energy dissipation systems," *Biochim. Biophys. Acta,* **1757**, 1504–11 (2006).

37. L. Wilk, M. Grunwald, P. N. Liao, P. J. Walla, and W. Kuhlbrandt, "Direct interaction of the major light-harvesting complex II and PsbS in nonphotochemical quenching," *Proc. Natl. Acad. Sci. USA,* **110**, 5452–6 (2013).

38. A. V. Ruban, D. Phillip, A. J. Young, and P. Horton, "Carotenoid-dependent oligomerization of the major chlorophyll a/b light harvesting complex of photosystem II of plants," *Biochemistry,* **36**, 7855–59 (1997).

39. A. V. Ruban, R. Berera, C. Ilioaia, I. H. Van Stokkum, J. T. Kennis, A. A. Pascal, H. Van Amerongen, B. Robert, P. Horton, and R. Van Grondelle, "Identification of a mechanism of photoprotective energy dissipation in higher plants," *Nature,* **450**, 575–8 (2007).

40. M. G. Muller, P. Lambrev, M. Reus, E. Wientjes, R. Croce, and A. R. Holzwarth, "Singlet energy dissipation in the photosystem II light-harvesting complex does not Iinvolve energy transfer to carotenoids," *Chem. Phys. Chem.*, **11**, 1289–96 (2010).

41. M. Zubik, R. Luchowski, W. Grudzinski, M. Gospodarek, I. Gryczynski, Z. Gryczynski, J. W. Dobruckiand, and W. I. Gruszecki, "Light-induced isomerization of the LHCII-bound xanthophyll neoxanthin: possible implications for photoprotection in plants," *Biochim. Biophys. Acta,* **1807**, 1237–43 (2011).

42. M. Zubik, R. Luchowski, M. Puzio, E. Janik, J. Bednarska, and W. I. Gruszecki, "The negative feedback molecular mechanism which regulates excitation level in the plant photosynthetic complex LHCII: towards identification of the energy dissipative state," *Biochim. Biophys. Acta*, **1827**, 355–64 (2013).

43. W. I. Gruszecki, K. Strzalka, A. Radunz, and G. H. Schmid, "Cyclic electron flow around photosystem II as examined by photosynthetic oxygen evolution induced by short light flashes," *Zeitsch. Naturforsch. C-a J. Biosci.,* **52**, 175–9 (1997).

44. C. Boulay, L. Abasova, C. Six, I. Vass, and D. Kirilovsky, "Occurrence and function of the orange carotenoid protein in photoprotective mechanisms in various cyanobacteria," *Biochim. Biophys. Acta-Bioenerg.,* **1777**, 1344–54 (2008).

45. A. Wilson, C. Punginelli, A. Gall, C. Bonetti, M. Alexandre, J. M. Routaboul, C. A. Kerfeld, R. Van Grondelle, B. Robert, J. T. M. Kennis, and D. Kirilovsky, "A photoactive carotenoid protein acting as light intensity sensor," *Proc. Natl. Acad. Sci. USA* , **105**, 12075–80 (2008).

Part III

Technology

10

Carotenoid Biosynthesis and Regulation in Plants

Rafal Baranski[a] and Christopher I. Cazzonelli[b]

[a]*Institute of Plant Biology and Biotechnology, Faculty of Biotechnology and Horticulture, University of Agriculture in Krakow, Krakow, Poland*
[b]*Hawkesbury Institute for the Environment, University of Western Sydney, Hawkesbury Campus, Richmond, NSW, Australia*

10.1 Biosynthetic pathways

10.1.1 Occurrence in nature

Carotenoids are ubiquitous in living organisms where they play important functions, as shown in other chapters. They are found in organisms classified to all three domains of life (Bacteria, Archaea, and Eukaryota), including fungi, algae, higher plants, and animals [1, 2]. Most animals uptake carotenoids from food and accumulate or modify them through metabolic reactions, as they are not capable of carotenoid biosynthesis *de novo* due to the lack of essential enzymes. An exception to this rule was found in arthropods, specifically pea aphids (*Acyrthosiphon pisum*; class Insect, order Hemiptera), which accumulate their own carotenoids, carotenes, and torulene, responsible for color polymorphism between individuals [3]. Genetic analysis confirmed that the displayed color is inherited in the Mendelian fashion thus conferred by aphid genes. A unique bidirectionally transcribed arrangement of fused phytoene synthase and lycopene cyclase gene sequences, accompanied by the phytoene desaturase sequence, indicates that in the past an ancestor of pea aphids acquired a carotenoid gene cluster from zygomycete fungi via a horizontal transfer. Pigmentation observed in other aphid species, supported by their genomic analyses, extends the number of aphid species that may be able to perform carotenogenesis [4]. Recent phylogenetic analyses of other plant pests, spider mite (*Tetranychus urticae*; class Arachnida, order Trombidiformes) [5, 6] and gall midges (*Mayetiola destructor* and *Asteromyia carbonifer*; class Insect, order Diptera) [7], indicate analogous transfer of the same conserved gene cluster from fungal symbionts to arthropods with subsequent sequence duplications, rearrangements, and divergence.

Carotenoids: Nutrition, Analysis and Technology, First Edition. Edited by Agnieszka Kaczor and Malgorzata Baranska.

Identification of highly homologous sequences in three distinct taxonomic orders delivers molecular evidence for independent acquisition of carotenoid genes by those animals, although other scenarios cannot be neglected [8].

10.1.2 Cellular localization and compartmentalization

The evolutionary complexity of an organism determines how carotenoids are synthesized in cells. Archaea and bacteria lack internal organelles, so all steps of carotenoid biosynthesis must take place in the cytosol. The mevalonate pathway (MVA) is a multistep route leading to the synthesis of short, five-carbon (C_5) isoprenoid precursors of carotenoids in these organisms. For many years, the MVA pathway was considered as the only pathway of isoprenoid biosynthesis in eukaryotes. However, algae and higher plants have distinct cellular organelles surrounded by plasma membranes built of phospholipids and proteins that separate the biochemical environment from the rest of the cell. Such compartmentalization led to the separation of biosynthetic pathways in eukaryotes, with an alternative, nonmevalonate pathway formed in plastids (Figure 10.1).

In this pathway, the 2-C-methyl-D-erythritol 4-phosphate (MEP) pathway, the same C_5 isoprenoid precursors are synthesized as in the MVA pathway. It is now generally accepted that in eukaryotes, plastid C_5 isoprenoids are substrates for biosynthesis of carotenoids (tetraterpenes), chlorophylls, as well as mono- and diterpenes, while triterpenes and sesquiterpenes are generated from C_5 isoprenoids produced by the MVA pathway found in the cytosol [9, 10]. Metabolite exchange between plastids and cytosol occurs to some extent due to membrane permeability, but the MEP and MVA pathways cannot compensate for the absence of the other. Nevertheless, experiments with ^{13}C labeled glucose

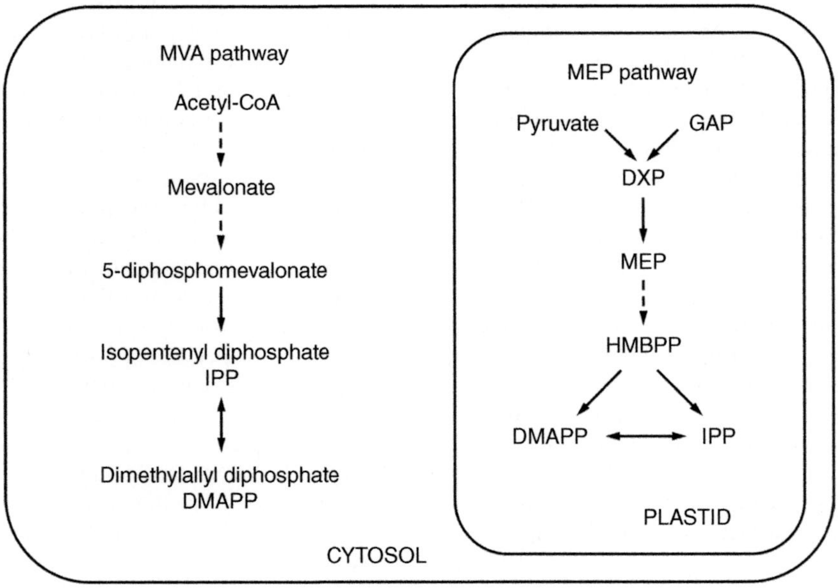

Figure 10.1 Cytosolic and plastidic pathways of C_5 isoprenoid biosynthesis in a plant cell. DXP, 1-deoxy-D-xylulose 5-phosphate; GAP, D-glyceraldehyde 3-phosphate; MEP, 2-C-methyl-D-erythritol 4-phosphate; HMBPP, (E)-1-hydroxy-2-methyl-2-butenyl diphosphate.

revealed that some microalgae like *Euglena gracilis* can synthesize carotenoids using precursors of both pathways [11]. In general, a consequence for the cellular compartmentalization is that carotenogenesis takes place in the plastids of plant cells.

10.1.3 Pathways to generate isoprenoid precursors for carotenoid biosynthesis

According to the International Union of Pure and Applied Chemistry (IUPAC) nomenclature, carotenoids are a class of hydrocarbons and their oxygenated derivatives that consist of eight C_5 isoprenoid units. Derivatives with more than 40 carbons in the chain can be also called carotenoids if they have more C_5 units joined in a manner similar to that of the C_{40} skeleton. Additionally, removal of one or both ends of the carotenoid molecule can result in shorter chain carotenoids, referred to as *apocarotenoids* [12]. Although shorter, C_{30} isoprenoids are not covered by the above definition; they are commonly classified as carotenoids. They are found in only a limited number of bacterial species (e.g., *Heliobacterium* sp., *Methylobacterium* sp. *Staphylococcus* sp., and *Streptococcus* sp.), which are able to condense two C_{15} isoprenoids [13, 14]. Thus, some organisms are capable of C_{30} and C_{40} carotenoid biosynthesis by making use of two divergent pathways; however, plants only use the C_{40} pathway [15].

Synthesis of a canonical 40-carbon carotenoid as well as other isoprenoids requires condensing C_5 units. Formation of these short isoprenoid precursors in the MEP pathway is processed by nuclear encoded enzymes that are targeted to plastids. Two substrates, pyruvate and D-glyceraldehyde 3-phosphate, are condensed by 1-deoxy-D-xylulose 5 phosphate (DXP) synthase (DXS), and then DXP is converted by DXP reductoisomerase (DXR) to MEP (Figure 10.1). As the outcome of the next multi-enzyme step, synthesis of (E)-1-hydroxy-2-methyl-2-butenyl diphosphate (HMBPP) and its subsequent reduction to two C_5 isoprenoid molecules, dimethylallyl diphosphate (DMAPP) and isopentenyl diphosphate (IPP), occur. DMAPP and IPP are isoprene isomers protonated at C_1 and C_3, respectively, and both have a five-carbon chain. Isoprene biosynthesis in the MVA pathway utilizes two units of acetyl-CoA that, after condensation, are converted to mevalonate undergoing phosphorylation. Decarboxylation of 5-diphosphomevalonate leads to IPP formation, which can then be isomerized to DMAPP [16–18].

Two mechanisms are involved in the elongation of the isoprene chain from five to 40 carbons. The carbon linear skeleton is elongated by five carbons each time when a C_5 unit is added. When two of the same isoprenoid molecules are condensed, the reaction results in duplication of the skeleton length. Thus, in a series of elongation reactions, DMAPP/IPP are converted to C_{10}, C_{15}, and C_{20} isoprenoid intermediates, and condensation of the latter gives the first C_{40} carotenoid (Figure 10.2). Bacteria, algae, and higher plants are capable of C_5–C_{20} and C_{40} isoprenoid biosynthesis in this manner. This pathway is extended to longer C_{45} and C_{50} carotenoids by a few selected bacteria such as *Flavobacterium dehydrogenans* [19], *Corynebacterium glutamicum* [20], *Dietzia* sp. [21], *Micrococcus luteus*, and halophilic archaea *Halobacterium* sp. and *Halococcus* sp. [22]. Biosynthesis of C_{45} and C_{50} carotenoids results from the condensation of their shorter C_{40} and C_{45} intermediates, respectively, by the addition of one C_5 unit.

Genetic engineering of *Escherichia coli* revealed that there are other functional routes for carotenoid biosynthesis. Depending on the combination of isoprenoid intermediates used in enzymatic reactions, carotenoids of various chain lengths can be synthesized (e.g., C_{35} carotenoids were synthesized after condensation of C_{15} and C_{20} intermediates) [23] (Figure 10.2). The engineering strategy revealed that biosynthesis of natural carotenoids

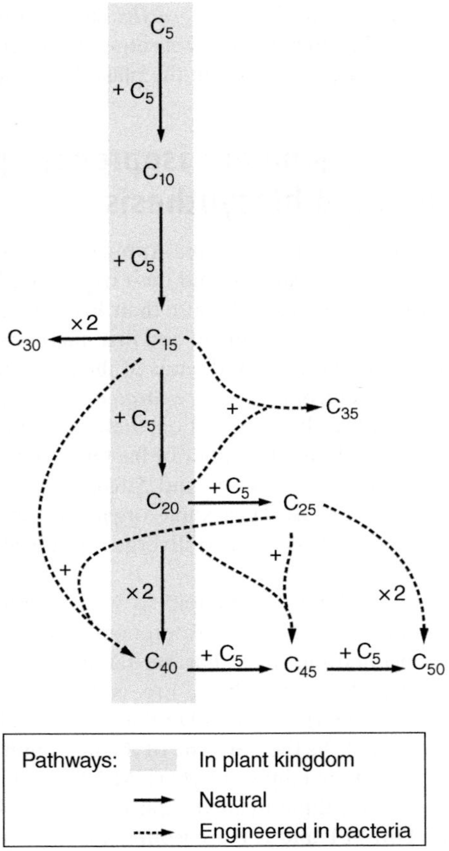

Figure 10.2 Isoprenoid chain elongation pathways known in living organisms, including plant kingdom, and engineered pathways in bacteria.

also can be achieved through alternative branches. For example, C_{40} carotenoids were obtained by fusion of C_{15} and C_{25} molecules instead of naturally occurring condensation of two C_{20} intermediates. Also the C_{45} carotenoid, naturally produced by condensation of a C_{40} molecule and C_5 unit, was synthesized in an engineered pathway by condensation of C_{20} and C_{25} intermediates, whereas the C_{50} carotenoid was produced by condensation of two C_{25} intermediates [14]. Clearly, there is some degree of flexibility in respect to engineering carotenoids in the bacterial world.

In plants, C_{40} carotenoids are synthesized after sequential, three-cycle condensation reactions (Figure 10.3 and Table 10.1). At first, geranylgeranyl diphosphate (GGPP) synthase catalyzes condensation of DMAPP and IPP and release of the allylic diphosphate group to form geranyl diphosphate (GPP) [18]. This C_{10} molecule with a doubled isoprene chain and one diphosphate end group binds to GGPP synthase, which repeats the condensation reaction with another IPP unit. The resulting farnesyl diphosphate (FPP) has a 15-carbon chain. In the third cycle, FPP and IPP condensation leads to formation of C_{20} GGPP. These three C_{10}, C_{15}, and C_{20} plastid isoprenoids are also precursors of many other classes of biologically active compounds, such as the mono- and diterpenes, phytol, chlorophylls, tocopherols, gibberelins, phylloquinone, ubiquinones, plastoquinones, and tocotrienol [16, 24].

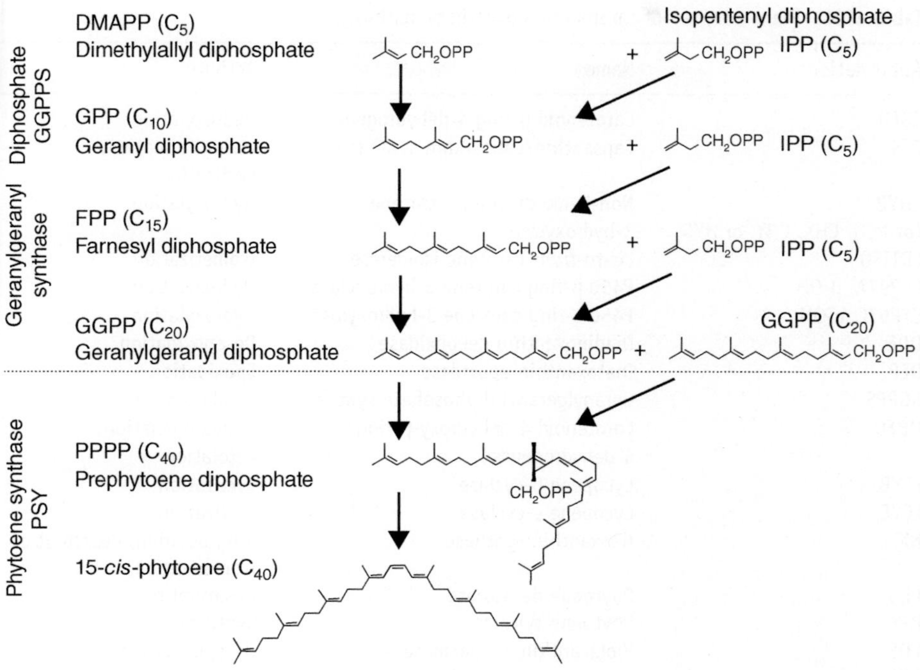

Figure 10.3 Biosynthesis of carotene precursors from C_5 units catalyzed by geranylgeranyl diphosphate synthase (GGPPS) and phytoene synthase (PSY).

10.1.4 The main pathway toward carotenoid biosynthesis

Plant carotenoids are hydrocarbons that may undergo various modifications through desaturation, isomerization, cyclization, oxygenation, hydroxylation, methylation, epoxidation, and esterification or their reversed reactions that lead to a diverse class of molecules of various structure and properties, and imply various biological functions of carotenoids (for comprehensive reviews, see [18, 25–31]). The carotenoid pathway can be arranged in a hierarchical manner with distinguished branches. The first carotenoids are subjected to desaturation and isomerization reactions that lead to formation of acyclic hydrocarbon molecules with an increased number of conjugated double bonds in the main chain (Figure 10.4). GGPP is the immediate precursor of plant carotenoids. Two GGPP molecules are condensed in a head-to-head orientation to form C_{40} prephytoene diphosphate (PPPP) with one diphosphate group at the central position. This reaction is catalyzed by phytoene synthase (PSY), the first enzyme of the carotenoid pathway in plants. Then the same enzyme converts PPPP to the first C_{40} carotenoid, 15-*cis*-phytoene, catalyzing a complex rearrangement at the site of diphosphate release.

Next, phytoene desaturase (PDS) catalyzes two-step desaturation of 15-*cis*-phytoene in which the number of conjugated double bonds increases from three to five in 15,9′-di-*cis*-phytofluene and then to seven in 9,15,9′-tri-*cis*-ζ-carotene. A desaturated fragment occupies the central bond and extends symmetrically toward both molecule ends. During these reactions, two *cis* bonds are also formed at 9 and 9′ positions.

Table 10.1 Plant enzymes of carotenoid biosynthetic pathway.

Abbreviation	Name	Activity
CBFD	Carotenoid β-ring 4-dehydrogenase	Hydroxylation
CCS	Capsanthin/capsorubin synthase	κ-ring formation, cyclization
CHYB (or BCH, CHX, CHY, or HYD)	Non-heme di-iron β-carotene 3-hydroxylase	Hydroxylation
CRTISO	*cis*-to-*trans* carotene isomerase	Isomerization
CYP97A, β-OH	P450 β-ring carotene 3-hydroxylase	Hydroxylation
CYP97C, ε-OH	P450 ε-ring carotene 3-hydroxylase	Hydroxylation
DDE	Diadinoxanthin deepoxidase	De-epoxidation
DEP	Diatoxanthin epoxidase	Epoxidation
GGPPS	Geranylgeranyl diphosphate synthase	Condensation
HBFD	Carotenoid 4-dehydroxy-β-ring 4-dehydrogenase	Dehydrogenation, ketolation
LCYB	Lycopene β-cyclase	Cyclization
LCYE	Lycopene ε-cyclase	Cyclization
NXS	Neoxanthin synthase	Ring opening, desaturation, isomerization
PDS	Phytoene desaturase	Desaturation
PSY	Phytoene synthase	Synthesis
VDE	Violaxanthin deepoxidese	De-epoxidation
ZDS	ζ-Carotene desaturase	Desaturation
ZEP	Zeinoxanthin epoxidase	Epoxidation
Z-ISO	15-*cis*-ζ-carotene isomerase	Isomerization

The enzyme 15-*cis*-ζ-carotene isomerase (Z-ISO) catalyzes isomerization of 9,15,9′-tri-*cis*-ζ-carotene at C_{15}, and 9,9′-di-*cis*-ζ-carotene is formed. This reaction can be light mediated, and therefore Z-ISO activity is not essential in light-exposed tissues. The second cycle of a two-step desaturation is carried out by ζ-carotene desaturase (ZDS). In these reactions, the length of the central unsaturated chain fragment increases to nine in 7,9,9′-tri-*cis*-neurosporene and then to 11 in 7,9,7′,9′-tetra-*cis*-lycopene (prolycopene). Similar to PDS, also ZDS generates two *cis* bonds at 7 and 7′ positions. The second isomerization catalyzed by *cis*-to-*trans* carotene isomerase (CRTISO) results in formation of all-*trans*-lycopene, also with 11 conjugated double bonds. The lack of CRTISO activity in light-exposed tissues does not prevent all-*trans*-lycopene formation; however, photoisomerization is less efficient [32–34]. The length of the desaturated chain fragment determines absorption properties of the polyene chromophore. A longer chromophore leads to a longer absorption wavelength, and thus phytoene is colorless, ζ-carotene (seven conjugated double bonds) is pale yellow, neurosporene (nine conjugated double bonds) is yellow, and lycopene (11 conjugated double bonds) is pinkish-red in color [35].

Cyclization of all-*trans*-lycopene forms asymmetric and then symmetric carotenes. Depending on the enzyme binding lycopene, the biosynthetic pathway bifurcates to produce β- or ε-carotenoids (Figure 10.5).

Lycopene β-cyclase (LCYB) is responsible for formation of the β-ionone ring, and lycopene ε-cyclase (LCYE) forms the ε-ionone ring. LCYB is capable of cyclization of both ends of linear lycopene. At first, cyclization leads to the formation of an asymmetric

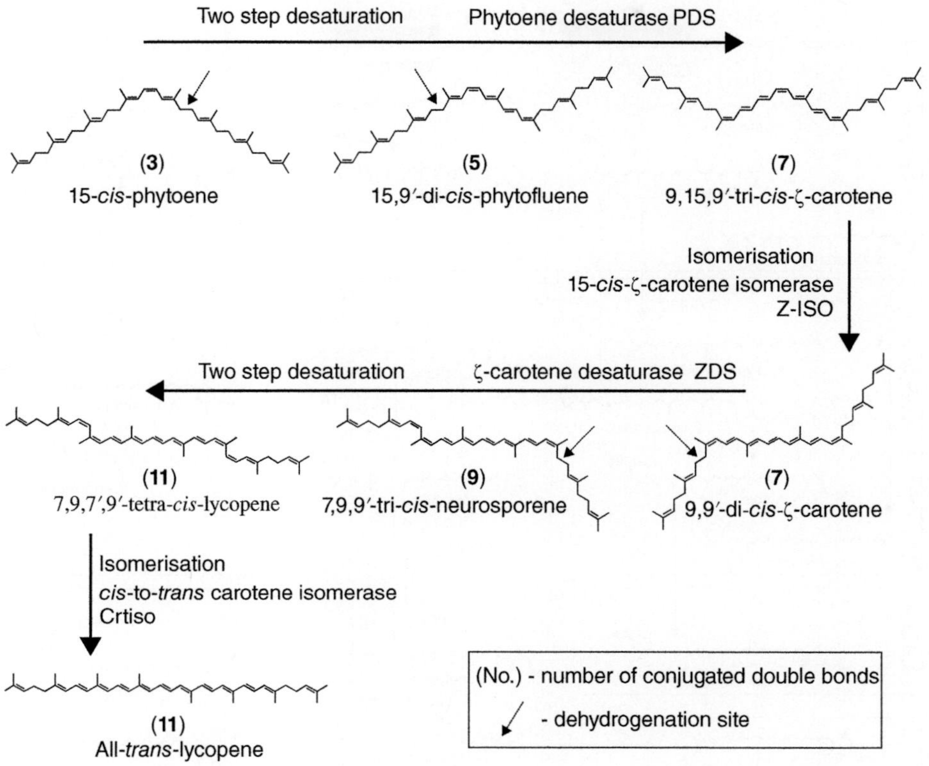

Figure 10.4 Desaturation and isomerization reactions of 15-*cis*-phytoene and intermediates in lycopene biosynthesis.

γ-carotene (β,ψ-carotene) with one β-ring and an acyclic second end. In the next reaction, the same enzyme completes cyclization of the acyclic end, forming the bicyclic β-carotene (β,β-carotene) with two β-rings. LCYE usually modifies one end of lycopene as it does not accept a monocyclic carotene as a substrate. LCYE converts one acyclic end of lycopene to the ε-ionone ring in δ-carotene (ε,ψ-carotene). The remaining acyclic end can be cyclized by LCYB, leading to formation of the bicyclic α-carotene (β,ε-carotene) with single β- and ε-ionone rings. Up till now, only one homolog of LCYE was found in lettuce that is capable of cyclization of both lycopene ends; thus, it forms the bicyclic ε,ε-carotene. Monocyclic carotenes are usually immediately converted to bicyclic carotenes, so both α- and β-carotene are much more common in plants, with the latter being predominant. Interestingly, the activity of LCYE to form the β-ring was also confirmed in the absence of LCYB. The ionone ring type determines the number of conjugated double bonds in a molecule. The β-ionone ring has a double bond in the the 5–6 position; thus, the bicyclic β-carotene has 11 conjugated double bonds determining an orange color of the compound. In the ε-ionone ring, a double bond is at the 4–5 position; thus, the chromophore of α-carotene (β,ε-carotene) is restricted to 10 conjugated double bonds and reflects a less intense orange color.

The next class of carotenoids to be formed from α- and β-carotene by hydroxylation are xanthophylls (Figure 10.5). Single hydroxylation of α- and β-carotene at the C_3 atom in the

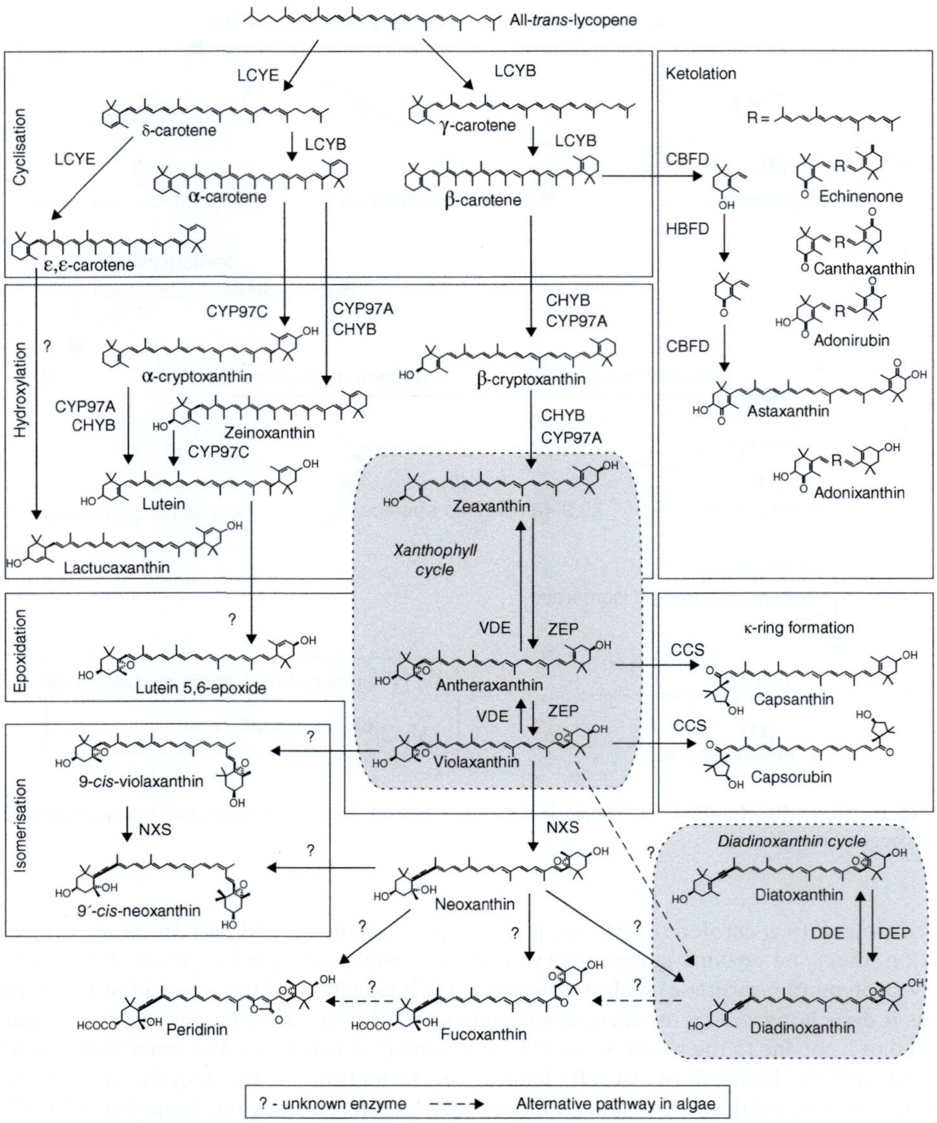

Figure 10.5 Plant carotenoid biosynthesis, enzymes, and reaction steps. Dashed line represents an alternative pathway in algae. Refer to Table 10.1 for enzyme abbreviations.

β-ring leads to zeinoxanthin and β-cryptoxanthin, respectively. Zeaxanthin is formed by the subsequent hydroxylation at C_3 of the second β-ring of β-cryptoxanthin, and lutein is produced by the hydroxylation of the ε ring of zeinoxanthin. Alternatively, α-carotene is hydroxylated at C_3 in the ε-ring, so the route to lutein goes through α-cryptoxanthin. Different enzymatic mechanisms are proposed to mediate α- and β-carotene hydroxylation, and they involve a ferrodoxin-dependent non-heme diiron monooxygenase (CHYB, alternatively abbreviated as HYD, β-OH, or BCH) and P450 heme cytochrome enzymes

CYP97A and CYP97C. Hydroxylation of β-carotene β-rings is mediated by a homodimer, β-carotene 3-hydroxylase (CHYB). CYP97A also exhibits some activity, but as it is not capable of homodimer formation, the reaction is less efficient. Hydroxylation of α-carotene requires interaction of CYP97A and CYP97C, which recognize β- and ε-rings, respectively. However, CYP97C and CHYB are also capable of β-ring hydroxylation although with lower efficiency than CYP97A [36]. As CYP97C prefers as a substrate a molecule with the β-ring already hydroxylated, zeinoxanthin is preferentially synthesized. There is also a *CYP97B3* gene in *Arabidopsis* with an unclear function [37]. CYP97B29 recently cloned from red algae has β-ring activity and probably also ε-ring activity, suggesting that the *CYP97A*, *B*, and *C* subfamily originated before the divergence of higher plants and green algae lineages [38, 39]. In addition, *CYP97B* subfamily members in genomes of probably all high plants are also reported [39]. A unique xanthophyll in the plant kingdom, lactucaxanthin (3,3′-ε,ε-carotene-diol), is formed after hydroxylation of both ε-rings of ε, ε-carotene, but its mechanism has not been fully elucidated yet [40].

Epoxidation reactions lead to formation of many carotenoids, of which the most common are those involved in the xanthophyll cycle. Two enzymes, zeinoxanthin epoxidase (ZEP) and violaxanthin deepoxidase (VDE), catalyze reversible reactions of epoxidation/de-epoxidation of three β,β-branch xanthophylls. Zeaxanthin is converted to antheraxanthin by epoxidation of its one β-ring, and then epoxidation of the second β-ring leads to formation of violaxanthin. Violaxanthin deepoxidase reverses these reactions in intense light. Epoxidation of α-branch xanthophyll lutein results in lutein 5,6-epoxide, which is found in small quantities in the leaves from plants. Neoxanthin synthase (NXS) opens one of the violaxanthin epoxy groups and desaturates the 6–7 bond in neoxanthin, which is isomerized to 9′-*cis*-neoxanthin. This xanthophyll also can be synthesized from the violaxanthin isomer 9-*cis*-violaxanthin. Both 9′-*cis*-neoxanthin and 9-*cis*-violaxanthin are the last β,β branch C_{40} carotenoids abundant in plants that are further metabolized by dioxygenases to xanthoxin, and ultimately produce abscisic acid (ABA).

10.1.5 Specialty branches of the pathway

In spite of the above-mentioned common pathway, some plant species synthesize specialty carotenoids. In the fruits of pepper (*Capsicum* spp.) [41, 42] and orange as well as the tepals of lily [43, 44], two dark red carotenoids, capsanthin and capsorubin, are present. They are converted from antheraxanthin and violaxanthin, respectively, by the same bifunctional enzyme capsanthin/capsorubin synthase (CCS) (Figure 10.5). The enzyme converts a six-carbon epoxy ring of antheraxanthin and violaxanthin to a κ-ring containing five carbons and one hydroxy group. CCS is highly homologous to LCYB, with 55% identity and 72% similarity. It also shows cyclization activity and is capable of lycopene conversion to β-carotene, although with much lower efficiency (estimated at 25% of that of *Capsicum* LCYB) [45–47].

Another unique carotenoid in higher plants is astaxanthin found in the petals of pheasant's eye (*Adonis* sp.) [48]. This carotenoid can be also found in many bacteria and algae (e.g., *Chlorella zofingiensis* and *Haematococcus pluvialis* [49, 50]), and it is responsible for a characteristic pink color of some animals (e.g., crustaceans and salmon) feeding on organisms capable of astaxanthin synthesis [51]. Two precursors of astaxanthin biosynthesis were proposed in higher plants, β-carotene and zeaxanthin. Recent findings revealed that β-carotene is converted in a three-step reaction involving hydroxylation and ketolation of β-rings [52] (Figure 10.5). At first, the β-ring of β-carotene is hydroxylated at C_4 by a carotenoid β-ring 4-dehydrogenase (CBFD). Then, the hydroxy group is dehydrogenated by a carotenoid 4-dehydroxy-β-ring 4-dehydrogenase (HBFD) to form a keton group. Next, a second hydroxylation reaction at C_3 by the same CBFD enzyme is carried out, and finally the β-ring has single keto and hydroxyl groups. Astaxanthin is a carotenoid with symmetric rearrangements in both end rings. Depending on the combination of end group moieties, various intermediates are synthesized. These include echinenone and canthaxanthin with one and two keto rings, respectively, and andonirubin with single keto and keto-hydroxyl rings. The exact order of intermediates in this keto-carotenoid branch of the biosynthetic pathway remains unrevealed. Presumably, astaxanthin can be converted to adonixanthin as the latter has a hydroxy group at the 3′ position and no keto group, so adonixathin may be synthesized by oxygen release from astaxanthin.

In algae, the C_{40} carotenoid biosynthesis is further extended [53] (Figure 10.5). Neoxanthin is proposed as the precursor of the diadinoxanthin cycle carotenoids, which is an alternative cycle to the xanthophyll cycle operating in land plants and plays a similar role in light-mediated photoprotection [54]. Diadinoxanthin has one epoxy ring and a hydroxylated β-ring at C_3 attached to the main polyene chain with a triple bond in the 7–8 position. The deepoxidation reaction catalyzed by diadinoxanthin deepoxidase (DDE) forms diatoxanthin with two hydroxylated end rings. The reaction is reversible by diatoxanthin epoxidase (DEP) in subsaturating light conditions. Several brown, red, and green algae also contain significant amounts of fucoxanthin [55, 56]. The high health-promoting properties of this carotenoid were given much attention recently [57], but the reactions leading to its formation remain unresolved, as biosynthesis of peridinin. The chemical structures of both carotenoids are similar to that of neoxanthin with the –OH group at C_3 substituted by $-OCOCH_3$. Modifications in the second ring are more complex and require multistep reactions. The role of neoxanthin as the precursor of diadinoxanthin, fucoxanthin, and peridinin has been questioned, as some algae, like small diatoms, do not have NXS converting violaxanthin to neoxanthin. In consequence, these organisms do not accumulate neoxanthin, and hence violaxanthin may be considered as the precursor of those specialty carotenoids. If this is true, fucoxanthin and peridinin might be products of diadinoxanthin conversion [58].

10.2 Regulation of carotenoid biosynthesis

The genes and biosynthetic enzymes controlling carotenogenesis have been extensively studied, and the next frontier is to discover what regulates carotenoid biosynthesis, accumulation, and storage. Carotenoid biosynthesis is under stringent control throughout the life of the plant, being finely tuned to developmental and environmental signals that control carotenoid gene expression, accumulation, and storage [1]. Carotenoids are important in photosynthesis, photoprotection, and the production of a range of hormones and signaling molecules [1]. They are also important in optimizing resource allocation, promoting color development in fruits and flowers, and altering the rates of catabolism. Carotenoid regulation and signaling are intriguing as the enzymes and pigments are localized in the plastid, whereas the genes are encoded in the nucleus. Therefore, some degree of communication between the plastid and the nucleus must occur in order to coordinate carotenoid biosynthesis as well as flux through the pathway to generate downstream phytohormones and apocarotenoid signaling metabolites. This section of this chapter will focus on regulatory aspects of carotenogenesis relating to (1) cross-talk between and within the carotenoid and MEP pathways, (2) environmental and developmental control, (3) epigenetic and posttranscriptional regulatory mechanisms, (4) plastid differentiation and communication, (5) enzyme localization and metabolon compartmentalization, and (6) carotenoid degradation and apocarotenoid signaling metabolites.

10.2.1 Cross-talk between and within the carotenoid and MEP pathways

Cross-talk or metabolic feedback signaling within and between the carotenoid, MEP, and ABA pathways is an enigmatic phenomenon. Cross-talk relies on the sensing of end product accumulation and the coordination of transcriptional and posttranscriptional regulatory mechanisms. Cross-talk modulates the entry of prenyl diphosphate precursors for carotenoid biosynthesis at different developmental stages and maintains flux through the carotenoid pathway to insure a sufficient supply of carotenoid derivatives for the downstream production of apocarotenoid signals [1]. Several genes encoding enzymes in isoprenoid and carotenoid biosynthesis are subject to negative and positive feedback regulatory processes, and several isoprenoid and/or carotenoid-derived molecules have been proposed to mediate these signaling processes [59–69]. Therefore, depending on the tissue and plastid type, a complex level of metabolic feedback coordination appears necessary to provide communication between pathways in order to deliver a balanced precursor supply for carotenogenesis and insure biosynthesis can be adjusted in response to environmental and developmental cues (reviewed in detail by Refs. [1, 30, 70, 71]).

10.2.2 Environmental and developmental control

There are reports describing environmental signals such as temperature, salt, CO_2, and water availability that can affect carotenoid composition, although the molecular mechanisms are awaiting a more detailed discovery [72–78]. Light is the most thoroughly studied environmental signal shown to elicit dramatic effects on carotenogenesis in a range of plant tissues during photomorphogenesis [79]. The light signal is transduced to a chemical signal by photoreceptors and chromeproteins that participate in the regulation of carotenoid pathway genes, particularly at the transcription level [80–82]. For example, when a seed positioned below the ground germinates, an etiolated (dark-grown) seedling develops, and photomorphogenesis is repressed in the absence of light. The cotyledons of etiolated seedlings contain etioplast plastid organelles instead of chloroplasts, and carotenoids become localized in prolemellar bodies (PLB), a lattice of tubular membranes that defines the etioplast [34, 61]. The exposure of light will cause the seedling to deetiolate, and etioplasts differentiate into chloroplasts concomitant with a burst in carotenoid biosynthesis that facilitates photomorphogenesis [34, 83, 84].

The expression of genes that encode rate-determining enzymes, PSY and DXS (1-deoxy-D-xylulose 5-phosphate synthase), becomes upregulated during seedling deetiolation [80, 85–88], whereas the transcription of *LCYB* in tomato and *Arabidopsis* increased when seedlings were transferred from low to high light [26]. The changes of carotenoid gene expression observed in correlation with light stimulation require different photoreceptors [89]. The transcription of maize *LCYB* and *VDE* was induced by red light illumination, revealing a dependence of carotenoid gene expression on phytochrome receptor types and their activities [89]. In maize, the upregulation of *PSY2* gene expression during deetiolation was shown to depend upon the PHY photoreceptors [73] and a family of Phytochrome Interacting Factors (PIF) proteins [87]. PIF proteins are transcription repressors that contain a basic helix–loop–helix motif and regulate *PSY* gene expression by coordinating carotenoid and chlorophyll biosynthesis during light-stimulated chloroplast differentiation [87, 90]. Although light is the best studied environmental signal controlling carotenoid biosynthesis, further studies are needed to unveil the molecular mechanisms by which light alters carotenogenesis and how this links to developmental programs.

Carotenoid biosynthesis is also dynamically regulated throughout the life cycle of a plant, from seed and root development to flowering and especially during fruit development, which will be a primary focus of this section (for detailed reviews, see [26, 71, 75, 76]). Tomato fruit ripening shows dramatic color changes reflective of carotenoid pigment changes. The carotenoid profile in green tomato fruits is rather similar to that of leaves, but during ripening the chlorophylls become degraded and a dramatic accumulation of carotenoids, in particular lycopene, is produced at the branch in the pathway to β- and ε-carotenoids [91]. During the ripening process, chloroplasts differentiate into chromoplast organelles, which sequester large amounts of carotenoids [92].

Fruit ripening is associated with transcriptional upregulation of the MEP pathway gene *DXS*, followed by *PSY* and *PDS* as well as other carotenogenic genes encoding desaturases and isomerases that facilitate a burst in carotenoid biosynthesis [91, 93–96]. The carotenoid content in marigold petals, resulting in light-yellow to dark-orange colored flowers, also correlates positively with the expression of *PSY* and *DXS* transcripts [97]. In contrast, the expression of the cyclase genes, *LCYB* and *LCYE*, at the branch in the pathway diminishes during fruit ripening [98] and clearly correlates with an enhanced flux through the initial stages of the pathway as well as a restriction to carotenoid end products, which leads to a massive accumulation of lycopene and a reduction in xanthophylls [99–101]. In contrast, an unknown mutation in the tomato *delta* mutant caused an increase in *LCYE* gene expression and accumulation of δ-carotene in fruit tissues, whereas upregulation of *LCYB2* transcript abundance in the *beta* mutant led to accumulation of β-carotene [98]. The tomato *LCYB2* promoter contains RAP2.2 and ERE (ethylene responsive element) *cis*-acting DNA motifs, which can bind transcription factors and trigger regulation of carotenoid accumulation in fruits and flowers [102]. Although there are other relevant examples in the literature, these few pieces of evidence highlight how regulation of carotenogenesis is finely tuned to developmental changes. The evidence for carotenoids to mediate developmental programs is emerging fast, and perhaps their roles in controlling organelle biogenesis, differentiation, signaling, and communication are the ripest areas for discovery.

10.2.3 Regulation by epigenetic and posttranscriptional mechanisms

A paradigm shift for secondary metabolism was the discovery of an epigenetic regulatory mechanism that controls carotenogenesis and links the production of secondary metabolites to memory-forming processes in *Arabidopsis* [103]. The carotenoid biosynthetic pathway bifurcates after lycopene to produce lutein or β-carotenes, and their derivatives. Using *Arabidopsis* as a model, it was shown how the branch point was regulated by a chromatin-modifying histone methyltransferase, Set Domain Group 8 (SDG8), which targets the carotenoid isomerase (CRTISO) [104]. CRTISO is a key rate-limiting enzyme in carotenogenesis that controls composition of the downstream xanthophyll pigments and accumulation of the upstream *cis*-carotenes [34]. SDG8 alters the histone-3-lysine-4 trimethylation surrounding the *CRTISO* gene, thereby facilitating permissive *CRTISO* gene expression and lutein biosynthesis [105].

The *sdg8* and *crtiso* mutants have reduced lutein in leaves, but tend to also accumulate *cis*-carotenoids in etiolated seedlings, which results from the reduction in *CRTISO* transcript abundance. The changed carotenoid profile in these mutants was proposed to cause an increase in shoot branching, presumably by perturbing strigolactone biosynthesis [71, 104]. Further characterization of the *CRTISO* and *SDG8* promoters revealed overlapping tissue-specific expression in tissues important in epigenetic programming (shoot meristem) and reprogramming (anthers) events, which link the control of carotenogenesis to plant development [106]. Together, these two enzymes control carotenoid flux through the branch from prolycopene to the synthesis of α- and β-carotenes. Investigations have indicated that both *crtiso* and *sdg8* mutants have an inhibitory effect on *LCYE* transcript levels, revealing that metabolic feedback may partially explain the reduced lutein levels [61, 104].

Another intriguing example of an epigenetic regulatory mechanism involving microRNA (miRNA) control of carotenogenesis opens a new frontier to control carotenogenesis. Overexpression of the *Arabidopsis AtmiR156b* gene in *Brassica napus* enhanced the levels of lutein and β-carotene in seeds as well as increased reproductive shoot branching [107, 108]. The *AtmiR156* gene regulates 11 members of the squamosa promoter binding protein-like (SPL) family, and each SPL gene further regulates numerous other genes through a complex gene regulation network [108]. It is very interesting to note that microarray analysis showed that SDG8 controls the expression of certain miRNA genes in *Arabidopsis*, in particular *AtmiRNA156*, which regulates SPL-15 [109]. *AtmiRNA156* was shown to be upregulated by 24-epibrassinolide (a highly active brassinosteroid), highlighting a new link between SDG8 regulation of brassinosteroid-regulated miRNA gene expression, shoot branching, and carotenogenesis [110]. Given that SDG8 controls specific developmental and stress-responsive pathways in plants [111–113], and the fact that miRNA targeted gene silencing and chromatin modification perturb carotenogenesis, the future is bright to uncover how the regulation of carotenoid-derived phytohormones and apocarotenoid signaling metabolites is linked to developmental programs. The collective evidence is getting stronger to continue the speculation that carotenoids may play a significant role in the epigenetic programming of developmental events in response to environmental stimuli.

10.2.4 Carotenoids in plastid biogenesis, differentiation, and control

A major form of carotenoid sink regulation involves the sequestration and storage of carotenoids, which are determined in part by the type of plastid organelle and specific plastidial structures that promote sequestration. The biogenesis and differentiation of plastid operations have a major effect upon carotenoid composition and storage. For example, overexpression of *PSY* in *Arabidopsis* did not affect the carotenoid levels in chloroplasts of photosynthetic tissues; however, in proplastids of seed-derived calli, carotenoid levels increased by over 100-fold, being deposited in crystals, similar to crystalline-type chromoplasts of nongreen tissues present in several other taxa [114]. Carotenoids are usually localized in photosynthetic membranes of chloroplasts, whereas in chromoplasts the storage of esterfied carotenoids is associated with fibrillins, which are lipoprotein structures in plastoglobuli [115]. The cauliflower (*Brassica oleracea* var. *botrytis*) *or* mutant displays an arrest in plastid division that causes chromoplast-like plastids that contain membranous compartments to form instead of leucoplasts [116, 117]. The *or* mutant accumulates high carotenoid levels, in particularly β-carotene, which causes an orange color in edible tissues that are normally white [117]. The *OR* gene encodes a DnaJ-like protein with a conserved Cys-rich domain that chaperones target substrates to DnaK/Hsp70 for the correct folding and assembly [92, 116, 117]. Similarly, the Hsp21 protein chaperone from tomato was also found to promote chloroplast-to-chromoplast transition, in turn resulting in the accumulation of carotenoids [118]. Clearly, changes to plastid division can have profound outcomes for creating a new carotenoid sink.

The size and replication (number) of plastids can also affect carotenoid sequestration. The tomato *high-pigment* mutants *hp1* and *hp2* accumulate carotenoids, and it was concluded that this was likely due to elevated plastid biogenesis [119–122]. The *DDB1* gene that is mutated in *hp1* [122] and the *DET1* gene that is mutated in *hp2* [120] are both involved in light-mediated regulation of carotenogenesis and plastid biogenesis. Again, there were no changes in carotenoid gene expression observed in tomato lines with suppressed *DET1* expression; instead, the size and/or number of plastids was elevated [121]. Similarly, the tomato *hp3* mutant has a defective *ZEP* gene involved in the xanthophyll cycle and enhances carotenoid accumulation by increasing both plastid numbers and the size of the plastid compartment [123]. A deeper insight into the molecular mechanisms that control plastid size and number is needed to shed light on how the storage of carotenoids can be further manipulated for biofortication projects.

Plastid organelles communicate with each other and the nucleus by a process known as retrograde signaling (reviewed by Ref. [124]). This can involve two processes: (1) operational control—signals produced in mature organelles in response to environmental cues to maintain the "optimal" running of metabolic processes; and (2) biogenic control—signals produced in developing organelles required for the production and correct assembly of structures and complexes. *Cis*-carotene metabolites are produced only in the upper part of the pathway, and their function remains unknown. Searching for novel *cis*-carotene-derived signals has proved difficult due to the fact that mutations in early stages of carotenoid biosynthesis are lethal and prevent the production of carotenoids important in photosynthesis. However, very recently there appears to be an exciting hunt for novel *cis*-carotenoid-derived signaling molecules [66, 67, 125]. These metabolites are hypothesized to mediate chloroplast to nuclear communication by controlling nuclear gene expression [125]. In summary, plastids are dynamic organelles, and developmental and environmental signals can alter their biogenesis, number, structure, and metabolism to have intriguing effects upon carotenoid storage and regulation.

10.2.5 Enzyme localization and metabolon compartmentalization

Perhaps the reassembly and relocalization of carotenoid metabolic complexes referred to as metabolons represent the next wave of the carotenoid regulatory world. Carotenoid biosynthesis is localized in plastid membranes, whereby a metabolon that links multiple coordinating enzymes by noncovalent interactions channels the intermediary products through an enzyme complex(es) along a biosynthetic route [126, 127]. Enzyme complexes with high molecular weights containing carotenoid biosynthesis enzymes have been identified in plastids [25, 128–130], although the intermediates in the carotenoid pathway are largely absent. In principal, the formation of metabolon could result in interactions between enzymes and is likely to affect enzyme activity and protein localization.

The shape, size, and polarity of carotenoid metabolites can ultimately affect the molecular interactions between proteins and membrane localization within the plastid organelle. Carotenoids can have different geometric *cis*-isomers formed due to rotations at any of their conjugated double bonds, and therefore affect their ability to align within subcellular structures and reduce the stability of metabolon complexes by altering the rigidity of the lipid membranes and limiting oxygen penetration to the hydrophobic core of the membrane [131, 132]. For example, the altered shape of *cis*-carotenoids can reduce how they crystallize and aggregate when compared with their counterpart all-*trans* isomers, and this was indeed the case in chromoplasts from tomato and watermelon fruits where all-*trans*-lycopene crystallized and aggregated [133, 134]. PSY is likely to represent the head of an enzyme metabolon. In *Arabidopsis* and rice, different PSY isoforms localize to plastoglobuli and attach to the chloroplast thylakoids [127, 135]. The physical localization of the Maize PSY1 isoforms can change depending on the allelic variant, and it was hypothesized that different types of plastoglobuli, being fibrillar or globular, in combination with different PSY1 isoforms might direct carotenogenesis to different plastid compartments [135]. Carotenoid enzymes are usually thought to be localized to the chloroplast envelope, and in chromoplasts the plastid sequesters carotenoids as plastoglobuli. However, it could be possible that chromoplast carotenoids are synthesized and sequestered in plastoglobuli. Indeed, this is an insightful view recently proposed to explain carotenogenic regulation and availability for biosynthesis [127].

10.2.6 Carotenoid degradation and production of signaling metabolites

Carotenoids are rather stable compounds, and their rate of biosynthesis, capacity for storage, and degradation are key processes controlling carotenoid homeostatic steady-state levels. It was long thought that the rate of carotenoid degradation was slow, but new evidence using $^{14}CO_2$ pulse-chase labeling demonstrated that degradation rates in *Arabidopsis* are much higher than expected [136]. Carotenoids are large nonpolar molecules, and their cleavage is required to allow movement out of the hydrophobic chloroplast membrane and into a more hydrophilic environment where they can perhaps act as signaling metabolites mediating cellular and nuclear processes. Non-enzymatic photooxidation and enzymatic cleavage of carotenoids are two well-studied processes that can degrade carotenoids to apocarotenoid signaling molecules.

Singlet oxygen ($^1O_2$), the main reactive oxygen species (ROS) in photosynthetic organisms, can non-enzymatically attack β-carotene or xanthophylls by oxidization [137]. Similarly, lipoxygenases and peroxidases can also unspecifically break down carotenoids by oxidative degradation [138]. Carotenoids help to quench the $^1O_2$ reactive oxygen stress signal in the photosystem reaction centers, and in the process a variety of β-apocarotenoids, including β-carotene endoperoxide, geranylacetone, pseudoionone β-cyclocitral, β-carotene-5,6-epoxide, and β-ionone, are produced [139–142]. These β-apocarotenoids appear to have different functions, although many are involved in high-light stress responses in plants by repressing genes through the chloroplast to nucleus signal transduction pathways that function to moderate development, growth, and biogenesis of cellular components [142].

A few carotenoid-derived signaling molecules are produced via the oxidative cleavage catalyzed by carotenoid cleavage dioxygenases (CCDs) in plants, and they affect the synthesis of color, apocarotenoid flavor, and developmental processes. The CCD gene family consists of nine members, four CCDs and five NCEDs (9-*cis*-epoxycarotenoid dioxygenases), whose enzymes have emerged as exciting areas of discovery [29, 143–145]. Members of the CCD family have different substrate preferences, and they contribute to the turnover of carotenoids with a high degree of enzymatic cleavage specificity in non-photosynthetic tissues of plants [146, 147]. Interestingly, the expression profile of CCD family enzymes shows a stronger correlation with apocarotenoid biosynthesis than with the degradation of carotenoids [29].

The synthesis, catabolism, and transport of the phytohormone ABA are controlled by physiological (sugar sensing, and stomatal guard cell transpiration), developmental (seed germination and dormancy, cell division, and elongation), and environmental stress (drought, salinity, cold, pathogen, and UV stress responses) processes in plants [148]. *In vitro* biochemical assays have shown that ABA is a cleavage product of 9-*cis*-violaxanthin and/or 9′-*cis*-neoxanthin by the NCED. These enzymes catalyze the 11,12-cleavage of 9-*cis*-epoxy carotenoids to produce C_{25} apocarotenoids and the rate-limiting ABA precursor, xanthoxin. The path from xanthoxin to absicisic acid requires cytosolic oxidation and has been extensively reviewed elsewhere [148–150]. Factors that regulate the expression or activity of upstream carotenoid enzymes can affect the levels of xanthophylls and hence ABA synthesis. For example, the β-carotene hydroxylase from rice can alter the levels of xanthophylls, thereby affecting tolerance to the oxidative stress associated with drought [151]. Drought stress can induce PSY levels in rice and maize, thereby enhancing carotenogensis and ABA production [63, 64]. Conversely, *zds* and *crtiso* mutants have been associated with reduced ABA levels [152]. Collectively, these few pieces of evidence show how important upstream regulatory steps are in modulating downstream carotenoid-derived products such as ABA.

The strigolactone class of carotenoid-derived terpenoids functions to (1) inhibit shoot branching in *Arabidopsis*, pea, petunia, and rice by presumably inhibiting bud outgrowth and maintaining apical dominance [153, 154]; (2) influence mycorrhizal hyphal branching in order to stimulate a symbiotic relationship in the root rhizosphere [155]; and (3) encourage germination of parasitic plant seeds such as striga [156]. β-carotene has been shown to be the substrate for strigolactone biosynthesis [157], and it has yet to be determined if changes in β-carotene levels can actually perturb strigolactone production. D27 is a β-carotene isomerase that converts all-*trans*-β-carotene into 9-*cis*-β-carotene, which is needed for subsequent CCD7 cleavage and strigolactone synthesis [158]. Next CCD7 catalyzes the 9′,10′-cleavage of 9-*cis*-β-carotene to give 9-*cis*-β-apo-10’-carotenal, and CCD8 catalyzes the oxidative cleavage and intramolecular cyclization of 9-*cis*-apo-10’-carotenal to produce carlactone [158]. Recent evidence shows that two rice members of CYP711 enzymes homologous to the *Arabidopsis* More Axillary Growth 1 (MAX1; encodes a cytochrome P450) act as carlactone oxidases to stereoselectively convert carlactone into ent-2′-epi-5-deoxystrigol and to the orobanchol revealing structural diversification step in the production of strigolactones. The biological relevance of different strigolactones remains to be discovered [159]. Given that CCD8 was originally shown to cleave *trans*-apo-10’-carotenal to apo-13-carotenone, a precursor to strigolactone, other strigolactone-like molecules are likely to exist, and this highlights that the biosynthesis of carlactone to striglactone is awaiting further exciting discovery.

CCD enzymes are also required for the production of several biologically and commercially important apocarotenoids. *In planta*, CCD1 seems responsible for producing fragrance and flavor apocarotenoids; 9,10-cleavage of β-carotene yields an aromatic volatile β-ionone [139, 160, 161]. In maturing *Arabidopsis* seeds, a loss of function of

CCD1 activity leads to higher carotenoid levels and may have a role in synthesis of apocarotenoid flavor and aroma volatiles [162]. The tomato LeCCD1 enzyme contributes to the formation of the flavor volatiles β-ionone, pseudoionone, and geranylacetone [139]. In Satsuma mandarin (*Citrus unshiu*), the CCD4 enzyme cleaves β-cryptoxanthin and zeaxanthin asymmetrically at the 7,8 or 7′,8′ positions to yield β-citraurin and apo-8′-β-carotenal [163]. *Arabidopsis* CCD4 was also identified as a negative regulator of carotenoid content by two independent approaches: identification of quantitative trait loci and fine mapping, and a genome-wide association study that showed that CCD4 plays a major role in the degradation of β-carotene during seed desiccation and dark-induced leaf senescence [164]. Furthermore, CCD4 was recently shown to be involved in leaf development [125]. The *Arabidopsis clb5/zds* (chloroplast biogenesis-5 and ζ-carotene desaturase) mutants accumulate one or more *cis*-carotenoids, and their accumulation was associated with an abnormal needle-like leaf abnormality and the repression of several nuclear encoded genes involved in early chloroplast development, photosynthetic activity, and carotenoid biosynthesis. Through use of the fluridone carontenoid inhibitor (targets PDS) and the *ccd4 clb5* double mutant, the authors rescued *clb5* mutant phenotypes [125]. Given that proteomic analysis has shown that CCD4 is localized to plastoglobules, where carotenoids accumulate in high concentration, the functions of CCD4 are beginning to emerge [165].

There are other apocarotenoid signaling molecules such as C_{13} cyclohexenone derivatives (e.g., blumenol) and $C_{13/14}$ apocarotenoids (e.g., mycorradicin) that appear to function in controlling beneficial arbuscular mycorrhizal fungi symbiosis and/or triggering hyphal branching in the rhizosphere [155, 166–168]. There is evidence for other novel mobile carotenoid-derived signaling metabolites required for normal root and shoot development. These include an unknown *Arabidopsis* graft transmissible signal produced in the roots of *bps1* (*bypass1*) mutants that can move and arrest shoot development [169]. The mobile signal does not require the activity of any single carotenoid cleavage dioxygenases, and it is related to neither ABA nor strigolactone [170]. Periodic lateral root (LR) branching in *Arabidopsis* has been reported to require biosynthesis of an uncharacterized apocarotenoid that is directly involved in LR formation [171]. Genetic analysis ruled out ABA and strigolactone as candidates, and by use of CCD inhibitor D15 [172], it was concluded that an apocarotenoid derived from β-carotene or β,β-xanthophylls by oxidative cleavage acted in conjunction with an oscillatory LR-clock. Interestingly, application of D15 treatment resulted in higher overall carotenoid content in roots [171]. Finally, signals derived from the *cis*-carotenoids tetra-*cis*-lycopene and tri-*cis*-neurosporene were proposed to produce apocarotenoids signals in tomato that regulate metabolic feedback of *PSY1* transcription and link organellar metabolic status to overall plant development [66].

The time is ripe for more discoveries to elucidate the novel chemical structures of apocarotenoid signaling molecules regulated by BPS1, controlling a lateral root clock, leaf development, or retrograde gene expression that controls metabolic feedback in tomato fruit ripening. A deeper understanding of the control processes and apocarotenoid signaling pathways will facilitate the fine-tuning of plant responses to environmental and developmental cues. Carotenoids play essential roles during photosynthesis, and they serve as precursor substrates for the production of a variety of hormones and signaling metabolites that link secondary metabolism to fundamental processes such as growth, development, and reproduction. Unraveling the regulation of biosynthesis, storage, and degradation of carotenoid-derived signaling molecules will undoubtedly provide fascinating new insights into the roles that carotenoids have in nature.

10.3 Biofortification and health perspectives

The carotenoid biosynthetic pathway in plants is complex and tightly regulated, as discussed in this chapter. The biochemical steps in the pathway have been discovered, and the discovery of complex mechanisms regulating carotenoid gene expression, protein activity, and localization are at the forefront of active research combining information from different higher plant species and genomic approaches. By enhancing our knowledge of the regulation of biosynthetic processes and flux through the pathway, undoubtedly new possibilities will emerge to enhance plant biofortification as a convenient resource to produce valuable micronutrient compounds. Special interest in carotenoid biosynthesis in plants is attributed to the highly beneficial chemical properties of carotenoid compounds that are well recognized in promoting human health, for example due to their antioxidant properties and provitamin A activity. They are also valuable ingredients used commercially in animal food and the aquaculture feed industry. Several drawbacks can be identified when considering plants as a sink for carotenoid storage: (1) the level of carotenoid accumulation in various plant organs can be low or absent, (2) biosynthesis can be tissue and organ dependent, (3) environmental factors can alter carotenoid accumulation, and (4) some carotenoids are only synthesized by specific species.

High homology between carotenoid genes among different plant species as well as some microorganisms makes genetic engineering a powerful tool to enhance carotenoid content in plant organs or redirect pathway flux to produce different carotenoid species. This can be accomplished by (1) the overexpression of carotenoid genes to elevate total carotenoids or individual compounds, (2) the silencing of carotenoid gene expression to perturb the pathway at specific steps and elevate the levels of specific carotenoid metabolites, and (3) transfer a single or stack of carotenoid genes from one organism to another in order to enhance biosynthesis or perhaps introduce new pathway branches to produce new carotenoids [10]. Several attempts to modify the carotenoid pathway have commenced and successfully enhanced biofortification [28, 173], with Golden Rice being the most recognized. Golden Rice produces provitamin A carotenoids, mainly β-carotene, in grains due to the expression of the *Pantoea ananatis* phytoene desaturase (*CrtI*) gene and plant *PSY* gene from *Narcissus pseudonarcissus,* later replaced by maize *PSY* in the second-generation Golden Rice (GR2). This modification allowed β-carotene to accumulate up to 31 μg/g grain tissue, which is a sufficient dietary intake for combating vitamin A deficiency in people relying exclusively on a diet of rice [174]. Release of GR2 to farmers and further production may be a turning point in commercial adoption of plants with engineered biosynthetic pathways. The approach of pathway modification may be of particular interest to develop varieties of commercial significance for industrial purposes in future ventures. An interesting example has already been presented by Jayaraj *et al.* [175], who produced carrots that accumulate several keto-carotenoids in the root, mainly astaxanthin, adonirubin, and canthaxanthin, which are rare in plants but essential for feed use in the aquaculture industry.

Natural biosynthetic pathways in algae are less understood, although the major steps have been identified. Most intriguing is that algae can synthesize many carotenoids not present in higher land plants. For example, considerable attention has been directed to the synthesis of fucoxanthin due to its health-beneficial properties [56, 58]. A deeper discovery of the enzymes responsible for algae carotenoid biosynthesis and mechanisms regulating accumulation, storage, and degradation will ultimately benefit carotenoid biofortification of land plants and the screening for new varieties that are rich in carotenoids species important for human health.

Acknowledgments

The support of the National Science Centre, Poland is acknowledged (decision No. DEC-2013/09/B/NZ9/02379).

References

1. C. I. Cazzonelli, "Carotenoids in nature: insights from plants and beyond," *Funct. Plant Biol.,* **38**, 833–47 (2011).
2. S. Takaichi, "Carotenoids in algae: distributions, biosyntheses and functions," *Marine Drugs,* **9**, 1101–18 (2011).
3. N. A. Moran and T. Javik, "Lateral transfer of genes from fungi underlies carotenoid production in aphids. *Science,* **328**, 624–7 (2010).
4. E. Novakova and N. A. Moran, "Diversification of genes for carotenoid biosynthesis in aphids following an ancient transfer from a fungus," *Mol. Biol. Evol.,* **29**, 313–23 (2012).
5. M. Grbić, T. Van Leeuwen, R. M. Clark, S. Rombauts, P. Rouze, V. Grbić, *et al.*, "The genome of *Tetranychus urticae* reveals herbivorous pest adaptations," *Nature,* **479**, 487–92 (2011).
6. B. Altincicek, J. L. Kovacs, and N. M. Gerardo, "Horizonatally transferred fungal carotenoid genes in the two-spotted spider mite *Tetranychus urticae*," *Biol. Lett.*, **8**, 253–7 (2012).
7. C. Cobbs, J. Heath, J. O. Stireman III, and P. Abbot, "Carotenoids in unexpected places: Gall midges, lateral gene transfer, and carotenoid biosynthesis in animals," *Mol. Phylogen. Evol.*, **68**, 221–8 (2013).
8. L. Boto, "Horizontal gene transfer in the acquisition of novel traits by metazoans," *Proc. Royal Soc. London B*, **281**, 2013–450 (2014).
9. K. Wang and S.-I. Ohnuma, "Chain-length determination mechanism of isoprenyl diphosphate synthases and implications for molecular evolution," *Trends Biochem. Sci.,* **24**, 445–51 (1999).
10. V. M. Ye and S. K. Bhatia, "Metabolic engineering strategies for the production of beneficial carotenoids in plants," *Food Sci. Biotech.*, **21**, 1511–7 (2012).
11. D. Kim, M. R. Filtz, and P. J. Proteau, "The methylerythritol phosphate pathway contributes to carotenoid but not phytol biosynthesis in *Euglena gracilis*," *J. Nat. Products*, **67**, 1067–9 (2004).
12. IUPAC-IUB, "Nomenclature of carotenoids," 1974, http://www.chem.qmul.ac.uk/iupac/carot/ (last accessed July 2, 2015).
13. S. Takaichi, K. Inoue, M. Akaike, M. Kobayashi, H. Oh-oka, and M. T. Madigan, "The major carotenoid in all known species of heliobacteria is the C30 carotenoid 4,4'-diaponeurosporene, not neurosporene," *Arch. Microbiol.*, **168**, 277–81 (1997).
14. F. Wang, J. G. Jiang, and Q. Chen, "Progress on molecular breeding and metabolic engineering of biosynthesis pathways of C_{30}, C_{35}, C_{40}, C_{45}, C_{50} carotenoids," *Biotechnol. Adv.*, **25**, 211–22 (2007).
15. D. Umeno, A. V. Tobias, and F. H. Arnold, "Diversifying carotenoid biosynthetic pathways by directed evolution," *Microbiol. Mol. Biol. Rev.*, **69**, 51–78 (2005).
16. P. M. Dewick, "The biosynthesis of C_5–C_{25} terpenoid compounds," *Nat. Prod. Rep.*, **19**, 181–222 (2002).
17. M. Rodríguez-Concepción and A. Boronat, "Elucidation of the methylerythritol phosphate pathway for isoprenoid biosynthesis in bacteria and plastids. A metabolic milestone achieved through genomics," *Plant Physiol.*, **130**, 1079–89 (2002).

18. A. R. Moise, S. Al-Babili, and E. T. Wurtzel, "Mechanistic aspects of carotenoid biosynthesis," *Chem. Rev.*, **114**, 164–93 (2014).
19. O. B. Weeks, A. G. Andrewes, B. O. Brown, *et al.*, "Occurrence of C40 and C45 carotenoids in the C50 carotenoid system of *Flavobacterium dehydrogenans*," *Nature*, **224**, 879–82 (1969).
20. P. Krubasik, M. Kobayashi, and G. Sandmann, "Expression and functional analysis of gene cluster involved in the synthesis of decaprenoxanthin reveals the mechanisms for C_{50} carotenoid formation," *Euro. J. Biochem.*, **268**, 3702–8 (2001).
21. L. Tao, H. Yao, and Q. Cheng, "Genes from a *Dietzia* sp. for synthesis of C40 and C50 beta-cyclic carotenoids," *Gene*, **386**, 90–7 (2007).
22. R. Netzer, M. H. Stafsnes, T. Andreassen, A. Goksøyr, P. Bruheim, and T. Brautaset, "Biosynthetic pathway for γ-cyclic sarcinaxanthin in *Micrococcus luteus*: heterologous expression and evidence for diverse and multiple catalytic functions of C(50) carotenoid cyclases," *J. Bacteriol.*, **192**, 5688–99 (2010).
23. D. Umeno and F. H. Arnold, "A C_{35} carotenoid biosynthetic pathway," *Appl. Environ. Microbiol.*, **69**, 3573–9 (2003).
24. V. S. Dubey, R. Bhalla, and R. Luthra, "An overview of the non-mevalonate pathway for terpenoid biosynthesis in plants," *J. Biosci.*, **28**, 637–46 (2003).
25. F. J. Cunningham and E. Gantt, "Genes and enzymes of carotenoid biosynthesis in plants," *Ann. Rev. Plant Physiol. Plant Mol. Biol.*, **49**, 557–83 (1998).
26. J. Hirschberg, "Carotenoid biosynthesis in flowering plants," *Curr. Opin. Plant Biol.*, **4**, 210–18 (2001).
27. P. D. Fraser and P. M. Bramley, "The biosynthesis and nutritional uses of carotenoids," *Prog. Lipid Res.*, **43**, 228–65 (2004).
28. C. Rosati, G. Diretto, and G. Giuliano, "Biosynthesis and engineering of carotenoids and apocarotenoids in plants: state of the art and future prospects," *Biotech. Gen. Engin. Rev.*, **26**, 151–74 (2009).
29. M. H. Walter and D. Strack, "Carotenoids and their cleavage products: Biosynthesis and functions," *Nat. Products Rep.*, **28**, 663–92 (2011).
30. M. A. Ruiz-Sola and M. Rodriguez-Concepcion, "Carotenoid biosynthesis in *Arabidopsis*: a colorful pathway," *Arabidopsis Book*, **10**, e0158 (2012).
31. G. Giuliano, "Plant carotenoids: genomics meets multi-gene engineering," *Curr. Opin. Plant Biol.*, **19**, 111–7 (2014).
32. G. Giuliano, L. Giliberto, and C. Rosati, "Carotenoid isomerase: a tale of light and isomers," *Trends Plant Sci.*, **7**, 427–9 (2002).
33. T. Isaacson, G. Ronen, D. Zamir, and J. Hirschberg, "Cloning of tangerine from tomato reveals a carotenoid isomerase essential for the production of beta-carotene and xanthophylls in plants," *Plant Cell*, **14**, 333–42 (2002).
34. H. Park, S. S. Kreunen, A. J. Cuttriss, D. DellaPenna, and B. J. Pogson, "Identification of the carotenoid isomerase provides insight into carotenoid biosynthesis, prolamellar body formation, and photomorphogenesis," *Plant Cell*, **14**, 321–32 (2002).
35. D. B. Rodriguez-Amaya, *A guide to carotenoid analysis in foods*, Washington, DC: ILSI (International Life Sciences Institute) Press, 2001.
36. R. F. Quinlan, M. Shumskaya, L. M. T. Bradbury, J. Beltrán, C. Ma, E. J. Kennelly, and E. T. Wurtzel, "Synergistic interactions between carotene ring hydroxylases drive lutein formation in plant carotenoid biosynthesis," *Plant Physiol.*, **160**, 204–14 (2012).

37. J. E. Kim, K. M. Cheng, N. E. Craft, B. Hamberger, and C. J. Douglas, "Overexpression of *Arabidopsis thaliana* carotenoid hydroxylases individually and in combination with a β-carotene ketolase provides insight into in vivo functions," *Phytochemistry,* **71**, 168–78 (2010).
38. S. Bak, F. Beisson, G. Bishop, B. Hamberger, R. Höfer, S. Paquette, and D. Werck-Reichhart, "Cytochromes P450," *Arabidopsis Book*, **9**, e0144 (2011).
39. L.-E. Yang, X.-Q. Huang, Y. Hang, Y.-Y. Deng, Q.-Q. Lu, and S. Lu, "The P_{450}-type carotene hydroxylase $PuCHY_1$ from *Porphyra* suggests the evolution of carotenoid metabolism in red algae," *J. Integr. Plant Biol.*, **56**, 902–15 (2014).
40. D. Siefermann-Harms, S. Hertzberg, G. Borch, and S. Liaaen-Jensen, "Lactucaxanthin, an ε,ε-carotene-3,3′-diol from *Lactuca sativa*," *Phytochemistry,* **20**, 85–8 (1981).
41. J. Deli, P. Molnar, Z. Matus, and G. Toth, "Carotenoid composition in the fruits of red paprika (*Capsicum annuum* var. *lycopersiciforme rubrum*) during ripening; biosynthesis of carotenoids in red paprika," *J. Agric. Food Chem.*, **49**, 1517–23 (2001).
42. I. Guzman, S. Hamby, J. Romero, P. W. Bosland, and M. A. O'Connell, "Variability of carotenoid biosynthesis in orange colored *Capsicum* spp.," *Plant Sci.,* **179**, 49–59 (2010).
43. M. Yamagishi, S. Kishimoto, and M. Nakayama, "Carotenoid composition and changes in expression of carotenoid biosynthetic genes in tepals of Asiatic hybrid lily," *Plant Breeding,* **129**, 100–7 (2010).
44. M. R. Gómez-García and N. Ochoa-Alejo, "Biochemistry and molecular biology of carotenoid biosynthesis in chili peppers (*Capsicum* spp.)," *Intl. J. Mol. Sci.,* **14**, 19025–53 (2013).
45. P. Hugueney, A. Badillo, H. Chen, A. Klein, J. Hirschberg, B. Camara, and M. Kuntz, "Metabolism of cyclic carotenoids: a model for the alteration of this biosynthetic pathway in *Capsicum annuum* chromoplasts," *Plant J.,* **8**, 417–24 (1995).
46. Z. Jeknić, J. T. Morré, S. Jeknić, S. Javremović, A. Subotić, and T. H. H. Chen "Cloning and functional characterization of a gene for capsanthin/capsorubin synthase from tiger lily (*Lilium lancifolium* Thunb 'Splendens')," *Plant Cell Physiol.*, **53**, 1899–912 (2012).
47. M. Yamagishi, "How genes paint lily flowers: Regulation of colouration and pigmentation patterning," *Scienta Horticulturae*, **163**, 27–36 (2013).
48. T. Maoka, T. Etoh, S. Kishimoto, and S. Sakata, "Carotenoids and their fatty acid esters in the petals of *Adonis aestivalis*," *J. Oleo Sci.*, **60**, 47–52 (2011).
49. Y. Wang and T. Chen, "The biosynthetic pathway of carotenoids in the astaxanthin-producing green alga *Chlorella zofingiensis*," *World J. Microbiol Biotech.,* **24**, 2927–32 (2008).
50. D. Han, Y. Li, and Q. Hu, "Astaxanthin in microalgae: pathways, functions and biotechnological implications," *Algae*, **28**, 131–47 (2013).
51. T. Matsuno, "Aquatic animal carotenoids," *Fisheries Sci.*, **67**, 771–83 (2001).
52. F. X. Cunningham and E. Gantt, "Elucidation of the pathway to astaxanthin in the flowers of *Adonis aestivalis*," *Plant Cell*, **23**, 3055–69 (2011).
53. M. Bertrand, "Carotenoid biosynthesis in diatoms," *Phytosynthesis Res.*, **106**, 89–102 (2010).
54. M. Dambek, U. Eilers, J. Breitenbach, S. Steiger, C. Büchel, and G. Sandmann, "Biosynthesis of fucoxanthin and diadinoxanthin and function of initial pathway genes in *Phaeodactylum tricornutum*," *J. Exper. Botany,* **63**, 5607–12 (2012).
55. P. Heydarizadeh, I. Poirer, D. Loizeau, L. Ulmann, V. Mimouni, B. Schoefs, and M. Bertrand, "Plastids of marine phytoplankton produce bioactive pigments and lipids," *Marine Drugs,* **11**, 3425–71 (2013).

56. S. R. Kumar, M. Hosokawa, and K. Miyashita, "Fucoxanthin: a marine carotenoid exerting anti-cancer effects by affecting multiple mechanisms," *Marine Drugs,* **11**, 5130–47 (2013).

57. E. Christaki, E. Bonos, I. Giannenas, and P. Flotou-Paneri, "Functional properties of carotenoids originating from algae," *J. Sci. Food Agric.,* **93**, 5–11 (2013).

58. K. Mikami and M. Hosokawa, "Biosynthetic pathway and health benefits of fucoxanthin, an algae-specific xanthophyll in brown seaweeds," *Int. J. Mol. Sci.*, **14**, 13763–81 (2013).

59. S. Römer, P. D. Fraser, J. W. Kiano, C. A. Shipton, N. Misawa, W. Schuch, and P. M. Bramley, "Elevation of the provitamin A content of transgenic tomato plants," *Nature Biotechnol.,* **18**, 666–9 (2000).

60. P. Beyer, S. Al-Babili, X. Ye, P. Lucca, P. Schaub, R. Welsch, and I. Potrykus, "Golden Rice: introducing the beta-carotene biosynthesis pathway into rice endosperm by genetic engineering to defeat vitamin A deficiency," *J. Nutr.,* **132**, 506S–10S (2002).

61. A. J. Cuttriss, A. Chubb, A. Alawady, B. Grimm, and B. Pogson, "Regulation of lutein biosynthesis and prolamellar body formation in *Arabidopsis*," *Funct. Plant Biol.,* **34**, 663–72 (2007).

62. G. Qin, H. Gu, L. Ma, Y. Peng, X. W. Deng, Z. Chen, and L. J. Qu, "Disruption of phytoene desaturase gene results in albino and dwarf phenotypes in Arabidopsis by impairing chlorophyll, carotenoid, and gibberellin biosynthesis," *Cell Res.*, **17**, 471–82 (2007).

63. F. Li, R. Vallabhaneni, and E. T. Wurtzel, "*PSY3*, a new member of the phytoene synthase gene family conserved in the Poaceae and regulator of abiotic stress-induced root carotenogenesis," *Plant Physiol.,* **146**, 1333–45 (2008a).

64. R. Welsch, F. Wust, C. Bar, S. Al-Babili, and P. Beyer, "A third phytoene synthase is devoted to abiotic stress-induced abscisic acid formation in rice and defines functional diversification of phytoene synthase genes," *Plant Physiol.,* **147**, 367–80 (2008).

65. L. Bai, E. H. Kim, D. DellaPenna, and T. P. Brutnell, "Novel lycopene epsilon cyclase activities in maize revealed through perturbation of carotenoid biosynthesis," *Plant J.,* **59**, 588–99 (2009).

66. D. E. Kachanovsky, S. Filler, T. Isaacson, and J. Hirschberg, "Epistasis in tomato color mutations involves regulation of phytoene synthase 1 expression by *cis*-carotenoids," *Proc. Natl. Acad. Sci. USA*, **109**, 19021–6 (2012).

67. E. Fantini, G. Falcone, S. Frusciante, L. Giliberto, and G. Giuliano, "Dissection of tomato lycopene biosynthesis through virus-induced gene silencing," *Plant Physiol.*, **163**, 986–98 (2013).

68. J. Arango, M. Jourdan, E. Geoffriau, P. Beyer, and R. Welsch, "Carotene hydroxylase activity determines the levels of both alpha-carotene and total carotenoids in orange carrots," *Plant Cell,* **26**, 2223–33 (2014).

69. L. P. Wright, J. M. Rohwer, A. Ghirardo, A. Hammerbacher, M. Ortiz-Alcaide, B. Raguschke, J. P. Schnitzler, J. Gershenzon, and M. A. Phillips, "Deoxyxylulose 5-phosphate synthase controls flux through the methylerythritol 4-phosphate pathway in Arabidopsis," *Plant Physiol.,* **165**, 1488–504 (2014).

70. A. Rodriguez-Villalon, E. Gas, and M. Rodriguez-Concepcion, "Colors in the dark: a model for the regulation of carotenoid biosynthesis in etioplasts," *Plant Sign. Behav.,* **4**, 965–7 (2009a).

71. C. I. Cazzonelli and B. J. Pogson, "Source to sink: regulation of carotenoid biosynthesis in plants," *Trends Plant Sci.,* **15**, 266–74 (2010).

72. A. J. Thompson, B. J. Mulholland, A. C. Jackson, J. M. McKee, H. W. Hilton, R. C. Symonds, T. Sonneveld, A. Burbidge, P. Stevenson, and I. B. Taylor, "Regulation and manipulation of ABA biosynthesis in roots," *Plant Cell Environ.,* **30**, 67–78 (2007).

73. F. Li, R. Vallabhaneni, J. Yu, T. Rocheford, and E. T. Wurtzel, "The maize phytoene synthase gene family: overlapping roles for carotenogenesis in endosperm, photomorphogenesis, and thermal stress tolerance," *Plant Physiol.,* **147**, 1334–46 (2008b).

74. M. L. Perez-Bueno and P. Horton, "The role of lutein in the acclimation of higher plant chloroplast membranes to suboptimal conditions," *Physiol. Plant.,* **134**, 227–36 (2008).

75. A. L. Fanciullino, L. P. Bidel, and L. Urban, "Carotenoid responses to environmental stimuli: integrating redox and carbon controls into a fruit model," *Plant Cell Environ.,* **37**, 273–89 (2014).

76. L. Liu, Z. Shao, M. Zhang, and Q. Wang, "Regulation of carotenoid metabolism in tomato," *Mol. Plant* (2014), DOI: 10.1093/mp/ssu121.

77. M. A. Ruiz-Sola, V. Arbona, A. Gomez-Cadenas, M. Rodriguez-Concepcion, and A. Rodriguez-Villalon, "A root specific induction of carotenoid biosynthesis contributes to ABA production upon salt stress in arabidopsis," *PLoS ONE*, **9**, e90765 (2014).

78. Z. Zhang, L. Liu, M. Zhang, Zhang Y., and Q. Wang, "Effect of carbon dioxide enrichment on health-promoting compounds and organoleptic properties of tomato fruits grown in greenhouse," *Food Chem.*, **153**, 157–63 (2014b).

79. C. A. Howitt and B. J. Pogson, "Carotenoid accumulation and function in seeds and non-green tissues," *Plant Cell Environ.*, **29**, 435–45 (2006).

80. M. Ghassemian, J. Lutes, J. M. Tepperman, H. S. Chang, T. Zhu, X. Wang, P. H. Quail, and B. M. Lange, "Integrative analysis of transcript and metabolite profiling data sets to evaluate the regulation of biochemical pathways during photomorphogenesis," *Arch. Biochem. Biophys.,* **448**, 45–59 (2006).

81. A. Castillon, H. Shen, and E. Huq, "Phytochrome Interacting Factors: central players in phytochrome-mediated light signaling networks," *Trends Plant Sci.,* **12**, 514–21 (2007).

82. C. Stange and C. Flores, "Carotenoids and photosynthesis: regulation of carotenoid biosyntesis by photoreceptors," in M. Najafpour (ed.), *Advances in photosynthesis: fundamental aspects*, Zagreb, Croatia: InTech, 2012.

83. S. Römer and P. D. Fraser, Recent advances in carotenoid biosynthesis, regulation and manipulation," *Planta,* **221**, 305–8 (2005).

84. A. Rodriguez-Villalon, E. Gas, and M. Rodriguez-Concepcion, "Phytoene synthase activity controls the biosynthesis of carotenoids and the supply of their metabolic precursors in dark-grown Arabidopsis seedlings," *Plant J.,* **60**, 424–35 (2009b).

85. J. von Lintig, R. Welsch, M. Bonk, G. Giuliano, A. Batschauer, and H. Kleinig, "Light-dependent regulation of carotenoid biosynthesis occurs at the level of phytoene synthase expression and is mediated by phytochrome in *Sinapis alba* and *Arabidopsis thaliana* seedlings," *Plant J.,* **12**, 625–34 (1997).

86. P. Botella-Pavia, O. Besumbes, M. A. Phillips, L. Carretero-Paulet, A. Boronat, and M. Rodriguez-Concepcion, "Regulation of carotenoid biosynthesis in plants: evidence for a key role of hydroxymethylbutenyl diphosphate reductase in controlling the supply of plastidial isoprenoid precursors," *Plant J.,* **40**, 188–99 (2004).

87. G. Toledo-Ortiz, E. Huq, and M. Rodriguez-Concepcion, "Direct regulation of phytoene synthase gene expression and carotenoid biosynthesis by phytochrome-interacting factors," *Proc. Natl. Acad. Sci. USA*, **107**, 11626–31 (2010).

88. S. Meier, O. Tzfadia, R. Vallabhaneni, C. Gehring, and E. T. Wurtzel, "A transcriptional analysis of carotenoid, chlorophyll and plastidial isoprenoid biosynthesis genes during development and osmotic stress responses in *Arabidopsis thaliana*," *BMC Systems Biol.*, **5**, 77 (2011).

89. S. Woitsch and S. Romer, "Expression of xanthophyll biosynthetic genes during light-dependent chloroplast differentiation," *Plant Physiol.,* **132**, 1508–17 (2003).
90. P. Leivar and P. H. Quail, "PIFs: pivotal components in a cellular signaling hub," *Trends Plant Sci.,* **16**, 19–28 (2011).
91. P. M. Bramley, "Regulation of carotenoid formation during tomato fruit ripening and development," *J. Exper. Botany,* **53**, 2107–13 (2002).
92. G. Giuliano and G. Diretto, "Of chromoplasts and chaperones," *Trends Plant Sci.,* **12**, 529–31 (2007).
93. I. Pecker, D. Chamovitz, H. Linden, G. Sandmann, and J. Hirschberg, "A single polypeptide catalyzing the conversion of phytoene to zeta-carotene is transcriptionally regulated during tomato fruit ripening," *Proc. Natl. Acad. Sci. USA*, **89**, 4962–6 (1992).
94. V. Corona, B. Aracri, G. Kosturkova, G. E. Bartley, L. Pitto, L. Giorgetti, P. A. Scolnik, and G. Giuliano, "Regulation of a carotenoid biosynthesis gene promoter during plant development," *Plant J.,* **9**, 505–12 (1996).
95. L. M. Lois, M. Rodriguez-Concepcion, F. Gallego, N. Campos, and A. Boronat, "Carotenoid biosynthesis during tomato fruit development: regulatory role of 1-deoxy-D-xylulose 5-phosphate synthase," *Plant J.,* **22**, 503–13 (2000).
96. J. Giovannoni, "Molecular biology of fruit maturation and ripening," *Ann. Rev. Plant Physiol. Plant Mol. Biol.,* **52**, 725–49 (2001).
97. C. P. Moehs, L. Tian, K. W. Osteryoung, and D. DellaPenna, "Analysis of carotenoid biosynthetic gene expression during marigold petal development," *Plant Mol. Biol.*, **45**, 281–93 (2001).
98. G. Ronen, M. Cohen, D. Zamir, and J. Hirschberg, "Regulation of carotenoid biosynthesis during tomato fruit development: expression of the gene for lycopene epsilon-cyclase is down-regulated during ripening and is elevated in the mutant Delta," *Plant J.,* **17**, 341–51 (1999).
99. G. Giuliano, G. E. Bartley, and P. A. Scolnik, "Regulation of carotenoid biosynthesis during tomato development," *Plant Cell,* **5**, 379–87 (1993).
100. P. D. Fraser, M. R. Truesdale, C. R. Bird, W. Schuch, and P. M. Bramley, "Carotenoid biosynthesis during tomato fruit development (evidence for tissue-specific gene expression)," *Plant Physiol.,* **105**, 405–13 (1994).
101. I. Pecker, R. Gabbay, F. X. Cunningham, and J. Hirschberg, "Cloning and characterization of the cDNA for lycopene β-cyclase from tomato reveals decrease in its expression during fruit ripening," *Plant Mol. Biol.*, **30**, 807–19 (1996).
102. M. Dalal, V. Chinnusamy, and K. C. Bansal, "Isolation and functional characterization of lycopene beta-cyclase (CYC-B) promoter from *Solanum habrochaites*," *BMC Plant Biol.*, **10**, 61 (2010).
103. C. I. Cazzonelli, K. Yin, and B. J. Pogson, "Potential implications for epigenetic regulation of carotenoid biosynthesis during root and shoot development," *Plant Signal Behav.*, **4**, 339–41 (2009a).
104. C. I. Cazzonelli, A. J. Cuttriss, S. B. Cossetto, W. Pye, P. Crisp, J. Whelan, E. J. Finnegan, C. Turnbull, and B. J. Pogson, "Regulation of carotenoid composition and shoot branching in *Arabidopsis* by a chromatin modifying histone methyltransferase, SDG8," *Plant Cell,* **21**, 39–53 (2009b).
105. C. I. Cazzonelli, T. Millar, E. J. Finnegan, and B. J. Pogson, "Promoting gene expression in plants by permissive histone lysine methylation," *Plant Signal Behav.*, **4**, 484–8 (2009c).

106. C. I. Cazzonelli, A. C. Roberts, M. E. Carmody, and B. J. Pogson, "Transcriptional control of set domain group8 and carotenoid isomerase during *Arabidopsis* development," *Molecular Plant*, **3**, 174–91 (2010).

107. S. Wei, B. Yu, M. Y. Gruber, G. G. Khachatourians, D. D. Hegedus, and A. Hannoufa, "Enhanced seed carotenoid levels and branching in transgenic Brassica napus expressing the *Arabidopsis* miR156b gene," *J. Agric. Food Chem.*, **58**, 9572–8 (2010).

108. S. Wei, M. Y. Gruber, B. Yu, M. J. Gao, G. G. Khachatourians, D. D. Hegedus, I. A. Parkin, and A. Hannoufa, "*Arabidopsis* mutant sk156 reveals complex regulation of SPL15 in a miR156-controlled gene network," *BMC Plant Biol.*, **12**, 169 (2012).

109. G. Dong and J. Li, "MicroRNAs profiling reveals a potential link between the SDG8 methyltransferase and brassinosteroid-regulated gene expression in *Arabidopsis*," *Data Mining Genom. Proteom.*, **4**, e110 (2013).

110. L. L. Lin, C. C. Wu, H. C. Huang, H. J. Chen, Hsieh H. L., and H. F. Juan, "(2013) Identification of MicroRNA 395a in 24-epibrassinolide-regulated root growth of *Arabidopsis thaliana* using MicroRNA arrays," *Intl. J. Mol. Sci.*, **14**, 14270–86 (2013).

111. A. Berr, E. J. McCallum, A. Alioua, D. Heintz, T. Heitz, and W. H. Shen, "*Arabidopsis* histone methyltransferase Set Domain Group8 mediates induction of the jasmonate/ethylene pathway genes in plant defense response to necrotrophic fungi," *Plant Physiol.*, **154**, 1403–14 (2010).

112. C. I. Cazzonelli, N. Nisar, A. C. Roberts, K. D. Murray, J. O. Borevitz, and B. J. Pogson, "A chromatin modifying enzyme, SDG8, is involved in morphological, gene expression, and epigenetic responses to mechanical stimulation," *Frontiers Plant Sci.*, **5**, 533 (2014).

113. X. Wang, J. Chen, Z. Xie, S. Liu, T. Nolan, H. Ye, M. Zhang, H. Guo, P. S. Schnable, Z. Li, and Y. Yin, "Histone lysine methyltransferase SDG8 is involved in brassinosteroid-regulated gene expression in *Arabidopsis thaliana*," *Molecular Plant*, **7**, 1303–15 (2014).

114. D. Maass, J. Arango, F. Wust, P. Beyer, and R. Welsch, "Carotenoid crystal formation in Arabidopsis and carrot roots caused by increased phytoene synthase protein levels," *PLoS ONE*, **4**, e6373 (2009).

115. M. Vishnevetsky, M. Ovadis, and A. Vainstein, "Carotenoid sequestration in plants: the role of carotenoid-associated proteins," *Trends Plant Sci.*, **4**, 232–5 (1999).

116. D. J. Paolillo, Jr., D. F. Garvin, and M. V. Parthasarathy, "The chromoplasts of *Or* mutants of cauliflower (*Brassica oleracea* L. var. botrytis)," *Protoplasma*, **224**, 245–53 (2004).

117. S. Lu, J. V. Van Eck, X. Zhou, A. B. Lopez, D. M. O'Halloran, K. M. Cosman, B. J. Conlin, D. J. Paolillo, D. F. Garvin, J. Vrebalov, L. V. Kochian, H. Küpper, E. D. Earle, J. Cao, and L. Li, "The cauliflower Or gene encodes a DnaJ cysteine-rich domain-containing protein that mediates high levels of β-carotene accumulation," *Plant Cell*, **18**, 3594–605 (2006).

118. I. Neta-Sharir, T. Isaacson, S. Lurie, and D. Weiss, "Dual role for tomato heat shock protein 21: protecting photosystem II from oxidative stress and promoting color changes during fruit maturation," *Plant Cell*, **17**, 1829–38 (2005).

119. Y. S. Liu, S. Roof, Z. B. Ye, C. Barry, A. van Tuinen, J. Vrebalov, C. Bowler, and J. Giovannoni, "Manipulation of light signal transduction as a means of modifying fruit nutritional quality in tomato," *Proc. Natl. Acad. Sci. USA*, **101**, 9897–902 (2004).

120. G. R. Davuluri, van A. Tuinen, P. D. Fraser, A. Manfredonia, R. Newman, D. Burgess, D. A. Brummell, S. R. King, J. Palys, J. Uhlig, P. M. Bramley, H. M. Pennings, and C. Bowler, "Fruit-specific RNAi-mediated suppression of DET1 enhances carotenoid and flavonoid content in tomatoes," *Nature Biotechnol.*, **23**, 890–5 (2005).

121. I. Kolotilin, H. Koltai, Y. Tadmor, C. Bar-Or, M. Reuveni, A. Meir, S. Nahon, H. Shlomo, L. Chen, and I. Levin, "Transcriptional profiling of high pigment-2dg tomato mutant links early fruit plastid biogenesis with its overproduction of phytonutrients," *Plant Physiol.,* **145**, 389–401 (2007).

122. R. Azari, M. Reuveni, D. Evenor, S. Nahon, H. Shlomo, L. Chen, and I. Levin, "Overexpression of UV-Damaged DNA Binding Protein 1 links plant development and phytonutrient accumulation in high pigment-1 tomato," *J. Exper. Botany,* **61**, 3627–37 (2010).

123. N. Galpaz, Q. Wang, N. Menda, D. Zamir, and J. Hirschberg, "Abscisic acid deficiency in the tomato mutant high-pigment 3 leading to increased plastid number and higher fruit lycopene content," *Plant J.,* **53**, 717–30 (2008).

124. B. J. Pogson, N. S. Woo, B. Forster, and I. D. Small, "Plastid signalling to the nucleus and beyond," *Trends Plant Sci.,* **13**, 602–9 (2008).

125. A. O. Avendano-Vazquez, E. Cordoba, E. Llamas, C. San Roman, N. Nisar, S. De la Torre, M. Ramos-Vega, M. D. Gutierrez-Nava, C. I. Cazzonelli, B. J. Pogson, and P. Leon, "An uncharacterized apocarotenoid-derived signal generated in zeta-carotene desaturase mutants regulates leaf development and the expression of chloroplast and nuclear genes in *Arabidopsis*," *Plant Cell,* **26**, 2524–37 (2014).

126. K. Jorgensen, A. V. Rasmussen, M. Morant, A. H. Nielsen, N. Bjarnholt, M. Zagrobelny, S. Bak, and B. L. Moller, "Metabolon formation and metabolic channeling in the biosynthesis of plant natural products," *Curr. Opin. Plant Biol.*, **8**, 280–91 (2005).

127. M. Shumskaya and E. T. Wurtzel, "The carotenoid biosynthetic pathway: thinking in all dimensions," *Plant Sci.*, **208**, 58–63 (2013).

128. S. Al-Babili, J. von Lintig, H. Haubruck, and P. Beyer, "A novel, soluble form of phytoene desaturase from Narcissus pseudonarcissus chromoplasts is Hsp70-complexed and competent for flavinylation, membrane association and enzymatic activation," *Plant J.*, **9**, 601–12 (1996).

129. M. Bonk, B. Hoffmann, J. Von Lintig, M. Schledz, S. Al-Babili, E. Hobeika, H. Kleinig, and P. Beyer, "Chloroplast import of four carotenoid biosynthetic enzymes in vitro reveals differential fates prior to membrane binding and oligomeric assembly," *Euro. J. Biochem.,* **247**, 942–50 (1997).

130. A. B. Lopez, Y. Yang, T. W. Thannhauser, and L. Li, "Phytoene desaturase is present in a large protein complex in the plastid membrane," *Physiol. Plant.,* **133**, 190–8 (2008).

131. A. Kostecka-Gugała, D. Latowski, and K. Strzałka, "Thermotropic phase behaviour of α-dipalmitoylphosphatidylcholine multibilayers is influenced to various extents by carotenoids containing different structural features: evidence from differential scanning calorimetry," *Biochim. Biophys. Acta Biomemb.*, **1609**, 193–202 (2003).

132. W. I. Gruszecki and K. Strzalka, "Carotenoids as modulators of lipid membrane physical properties," *Biochim Biophys Acta,* **1740**, 108–15 (2005).

133. G. Britton, "Structure and properties of carotenoids in relation to function," *FASEB J.*, **9**, 1551–8 (1995).

134. W. W. Fish, "Interaction of sodium dodecyl sulfate with watermelon chromoplasts and examination of the organization of lycopene within the chromoplasts," *J. Agric. Food Chem.,* **54**, 8294–300 (2006).

135. M. Shumskaya, L. M. Bradbury, R. R. Monaco, and E. T. Wurtzel, "Plastid localization of the key carotenoid enzyme phytoene synthase is altered by isozyme, allelic variation, and activity," *Plant Cell,* **24**, 3725–41 (2012).

136. K. G. Beisel, S. Jahnke, D. Hofmann, S. Koppchen, U. Schurr, and S. Matsubara, "Continuous turnover of carotenes and chlorophyll a in mature leaves of Arabidopsis revealed by 14CO2 pulse-chase labeling," *Plant Physiol.,* **152**, 2188–99 (2010).

137. S. Gonzalez-Perez, J. Gutierrez, F. Garcia-Garcia, D. Osuna, J. Dopazo, O. Lorenzo, J. L. Revuelta, and J. B. Arellano, "Early transcriptional defense responses in *Arabidopsis* cell suspension culture under high-light conditions," *Plant Physiol.,* **156**, 1439–56 (2011).

138. F. Leenhardt, B. Lyan, E. Rock, A. Boussard, J. Potus, E. Chanliaud, and C. Remesy, "Genetic variability of carotenoid concentration, and lipoxygenase and peroxidase activities among cultivated wheat species and bread wheat varieties," *Euro. J. Agron.*, **25**, 170–6 (2006).

139. A. J. Simkin, S. H. Schwartz, M. Auldridge, M. G. Taylor, and H. J. Klee, "The tomato carotenoid cleavage dioxygenase 1 genes contribute to the formation of the flavor volatiles beta-ionone, pseudoionone, and geranylacetone," *Plant J.*, **40**, 882–92 (2004).

140. L. M. Bradbury, M. Shumskaya, O. Tzfadia, S. B. Wu, E. J. Kennelly, and E. T. Wurtzel, "Lycopene cyclase paralog CruP protects against reactive oxygen species in oxygenic photosynthetic organisms," *Proc. Natl. Acad. Sci. USA*, **109**, E1888–97 (2012).

141. F. Ramel, S. Birtic, C. Ginies, L. Soubigou-Taconnat, C. Triantaphylides, and M. Havaux, "Carotenoid oxidation products are stress signals that mediate gene responses to singlet oxygen in plants," *Proc. Natl. Acad. Sci. USA*, **109**, 5535–40 (2012).

142. M. Havaux, "Carotenoid oxidation products as stress signals in plants," *Plant J.,* **79**, 597–606 (2014).

143. F. Bouvier, J. C. Isner, O. Dogbo, and B. Camara, "Oxidative tailoring of carotenoids: a prospect towards novel functions in plants," *Trends Plant Sci.,* **10**, 187–94 (2005).

144. E. Lewinsohn, Y. Sitrit, E. Bar, Y. Azulay, M. Ibdah, A. Meir, E. Yosef, D. Zamir, and Y. Tadmor, "Not just colors: carotenoid degradation as a link between pigmentation and aroma in tomato and watermelon fruit," *Trends Food Sci. Tech.*, **16**, 407–15 (2005).

145. P. J. Harrison and T. D. H. Bugg, "Enzymology of the carotenoid cleavage dioxygenases: reaction mechanisms, inhibition and biochemical roles," *Arch. Biochem. Biophys.*, **544**, 105–11 (2014).

146. R. Campbell, L. J. Ducreux, W. L. Morris, J. A. Morris, J. C. Suttle, G. Ramsay, G. J. Bryan, P. E. Hedley, and M. A. Taylor, "The metabolic and developmental roles of carotenoid cleavage dioxygenase4 from potato," *Plant Physiol.,* **154**, 656–64 (2010).

147. R. Vallabhaneni, L. M. Bradbury, and E. T. Wurtzel, "The carotenoid dioxygenase gene family in maize, sorghum, and rice," *Arch. Biochem. Biophys.,* **504**, 104–11 (2010).

148. R. Finkelstein, "Abscisic acid synthesis and response," *Arabidopsis Book,* **11**, e0166 (2013).

149. M. Seo and T. Koshiba, "Complex regulation of ABA biosynthesis in plants," *Trends Plant Sci.,* **7**, 41–48 (2002).

150. E. Nambara and A. Marion-Poll, "Abscisic acid biosynthesis and catabolism," *Ann. Rev. Plant Biol.*, **56**, 165–85 (2005).

151. H. Du, N. Wang, F. Cui, X. Li, J. Xiao, and L. Xiong, "Characterization of the beta-carotene hydroxylase gene *DSM2* conferring drought and oxidative stress resistance by increasing xanthophylls and abscisic acid synthesis in rice," *Plant Physiol.,* **154**, 1304–18 (2010).

152. J. Fang, C. Chai, Q. Qian, *et al.*, "Mutations of genes in synthesis of the carotenoid precursors of ABA lead to pre-harvest sprouting and photo-oxidation in rice," *Plant J.,* **54**, 177–89 (2008).

153. V. Gomez-Roldan, S. Fermas, P. B. Brewer, *et al.*, "Strigolactone inhibition of shoot branching," *Nature,* **455**, 189–94 (2008).

154. M. Umehara, A. Hanada, S. Yoshida, *et al.*, "Inhibition of shoot branching by new terpenoid plant hormones," *Nature,* **455**, 195–200 (2008).

155. K. Akiyama, K. Matsuzaki, and H. Hayashi, "Plant sesquiterpenes induce hyphal branching in arbuscular mycorrhizal fungi," *Nature*, **435**, 824–7 (2005).

156. R. Matusova, K. Rani, F. W. Verstappen, M. C. Franssen, M. H. Beale, and H. J. Bouwmeester"The strigolactone germination stimulants of the plant-parasitic *Striga* and *Orobanche* spp. are derived from the carotenoid pathway," *Plant Physiol.,* **139**, 920–34 (2005).

157. S. H. Schwartz, X. Qin, and M. C. Loewen, "The biochemical characterization of two carotenoid cleavage enzymes from Arabidopsis indicates that a carotenoid-derived compound inhibits lateral branching," *J. Biol. Chem.*, **279**, 46940–5 (2004).

158. A. Alder, M. Jamil, M. Marzorati, M. Bruno, M. Vermathen, P. Bigler, S. Ghisla, H. Bouwmeester, P. Beyer, and S. Al-Babili, "The path from beta-carotene to carlactone, a strigolactone-like plant hormone," *Science,* **335**, 1348–51 (2012).

159. Y. Zhang, A. D. van Dijk, A. Scaffidi, *et al.*, "Rice cytochrome P450 MAX1 homologs catalyze distinct steps in strigolactone biosynthesis," *Nature Chem. Biol.*, **10**, 1028–33 (2014a).

160. M. Ibdah, Y. Azulay, V. Portnoy, *et al.* "Functional characterization of CmCCD1, a carotenoid cleavage dioxygenase from melon," *Phytochemistry,* **67**, 1579–89 (2006).

161. F. C. Huang, G. Horvath, P. Molnar, E. Turcsi, J. Deli, J. Schrader, G. Sandmann, H. Schmidt, and W. Schwab, "Substrate promiscuity of RdCCD1, a carotenoid cleavage oxygenase from Rosa damascena," *Phytochemistry,* **70**, 457–64 (2009).

162. M. E. Auldridge, D. R. McCarty, and H. J. Klee, "Plant carotenoid cleavage oxygenases and their apocarotenoid products," *Curr. Opin. Plant Biol.,* **9**, 315–21 (2006).

163. G. Ma, L. Zhang, A. Matsuta, K. Matsutani, K. Yamawaki, M. Yahata, A. Wahyudi, R. Motohashi, and M. Kato, "Enzymatic formation of beta-citraurin from beta-cryptoxanthin and zeaxanthin by carotenoid cleavage dioxygenase4 in the flavedo of citrus fruit," *Plant Physiol.,* **163**, 682–95 (2013).

164. S. Gonzalez-Jorge, S. H. Ha, M. Magallanes-Lundback, L. U. Gilliland, A. Zhou, A. E. Lipka, Y. N. Nguyen, R. Angelovici, H. Lin, J. Cepela, H. Little, C. R. Buell, M. A. Gore, and D. Dellapenna, "Carotenoid cleavage dioxygenase4 is a negative regulator of beta-carotene content in *Arabidopsis* seeds," *Plant Cell,* **25**, 4812–26 (2013).

165. P. K. Lundquist, A. Poliakov, N. H. Bhuiyan, B. Zybailov, Q. Sun, and K. J. van Wijk, "The functional network of the *Arabidopsis* plastoglobule proteome based on quantitative proteomics and genome-wide coexpression analysis," *Plant Physiol.,* **158**, 1172–92 (2012).

166. G. Giuliano, S. Al-Babili, and J. von Lintig, "Carotenoid oxygenases: cleave it or leave it," *Trends Plant Sci.*, **8**, 145–9 (2003).

167. D. S. Floss, W. Schliemann, J. Schmidt, D. Strack, and M. H. Walter, "RNA interference-mediated repression of MtCCD1 in mycorrhizal roots of *Medicago truncatula* causes accumulation of C27 apocarotenoids, shedding light on the functional role of CCD1," *Plant Physiol.,* **148**, 1267–82 (2008).

168. M. H. Walter, D. S. Floss, and D. Strack, "Apocarotenoids: hormones, mycorrhizal metabolites and aroma volatiles," *Planta,* **232**, 1–17 (2010).

169. J. M. Van Norman, R. L. Frederick, and L. E. Sieburth, "*BYPASS1* negatively regulates a root-derived signal that controls plant architecture," *Curr. Biol.*, **14**, 1739–46 (2004).

170. J. M. Van Norman and L. E. Sieburth, "Dissecting the biosynthetic pathway for the *bypass1* root-derived signal," *Plant J.*, **49**, 619–28 (2007).

171. J. M. Van Norman, J. Zhang, C. I. Cazzonelli, B. J. Pogson, P. J. Harrison, T. D. Bugg, K. X. Chan, A. J. Thompson, and P. N. Benfey, "Periodic root branching in Arabidopsis requires synthesis of an uncharacterized carotenoid derivative," *Proc. Natl. Acad. Sci. USA*, **111**, E1300–9 (2014).

172. M. J. Sergeant, J. J. Li, C. Fox, N. Brookbank, D. Rea, T. D. Bugg, and A. J. Thompson, "Selective inhibition of carotenoid cleavage dioxygenases: phenotypic effects on shoot branching," *J. Biol. Chem.*, **284**, 5257–64 (2009).

173. G. Farré, G. Sanahuja, S. Naqvi, C. Bai, T. Capell, C. Zhu, and P. Christou, "Travel advice on the road to carotenoids in plants," *Plant Sci.*, **179**, 28–48 (2010).

174. J. A. Paine, C. A. Shipton, S. Chaggar, R. M. Howells, M. J. Kennedy, G. Vernon, S. Y. Wright, E. Hinchliffe, J. L. Adams, A. L. Silverstone, and R. Drake, "Improving the nutritional value of Golden Rice through increased pro-vitamin A content," *Nature Biotechnol.*, **23**, 482–7 (2005).

175. Y. Jayaraj, R. Devlin, and Z. Punja, "Metabolic engineering of novel ketocarotenoid production in carrot plants," *Transgenic Res.*, **17**, 489–501 (2008).

11

Carotenoid Bioavailability from the Food Matrix: Toward Efficient Extraction Procedures

Hartwig Schulz

Julius Kühn Institute (JKI), Federal Research Centre for Cultivated Plants, Institute for Ecological Chemistry, Plant Analysis and Stored Product Protection, Berlin, Germany

11.1 Introduction

The colors of fruits and vegetables are composed mainly by the individual amounts of different carotenoids, anthocyanins, flavonoids, and chlorophylls. The most important function of these pigments is to attract animals (e.g., mammals and birds), which are responsible for distributing the seeds and thus guaranteeing the reproductive success of the individual plant species [1]. In a process of co-evolution, carotenoids possess various biological functions for humans, predominantly provitamin A activity, antioxidative properties, and enhancement of the immune system.

Carotenoids occur in all plants and are therefore among the most important nutrients in food materials. They are fat-soluble microconstituents that have beneficial effects to human health, including protection against cancer, various cardiovascular diseases, and macular degeneration. Today, approximately 700 carotenoids have been detected in nature, and they are divided into different carotenes (e.g., α-carotene, β-carotene, and lycopene) and xanthophylls, which represent the oxygenated carotenoid fraction (lutein, zeaxanthin, canthaxanthin, and astaxanthin). The chemical structures of the most frequently occurring carotenoids are presented in Figure 11.1.

In plants, carotenoids play a crucial role in protecting chlorophyll with antioxidant activity, and these properties are one of the many reasons that carotenoids are of interest to humans. All carotenoids exist in plants in the *trans*-geometric form; however, thermal

Carotenoids: Nutrition, Analysis and Technology, First Edition. Edited by Agnieszka Kaczor and Malgorzata Baranska.

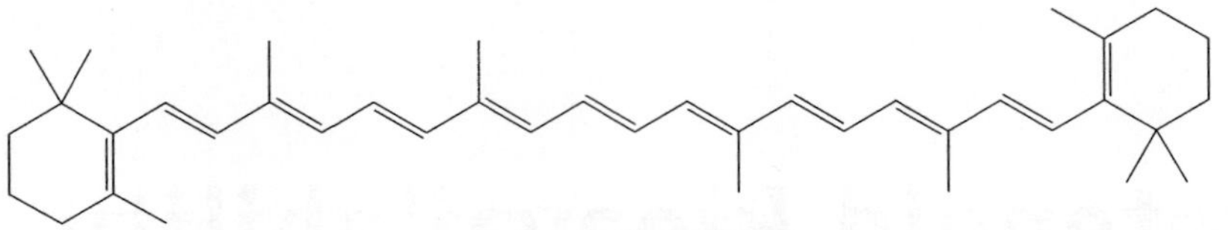

β-carotene

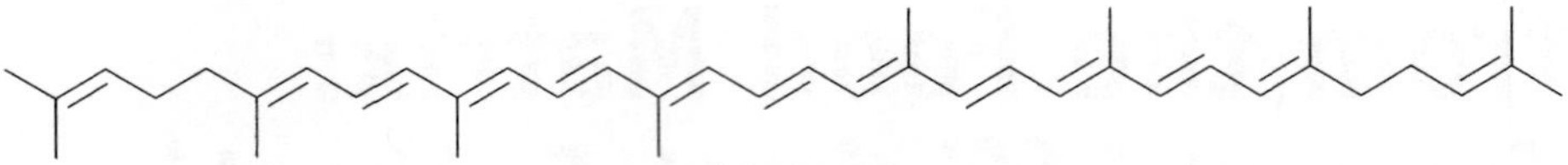

Lycopene

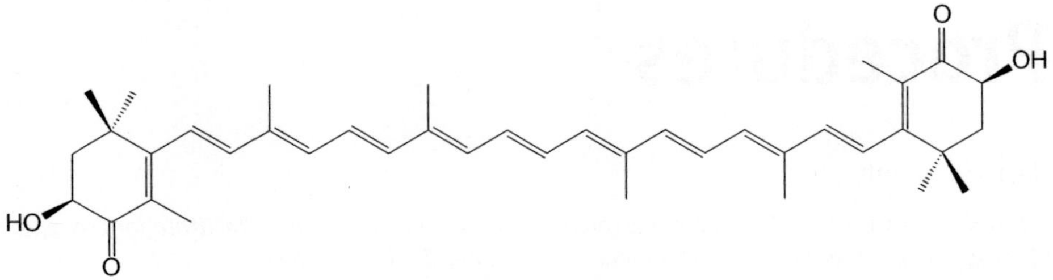

Astaxanthin

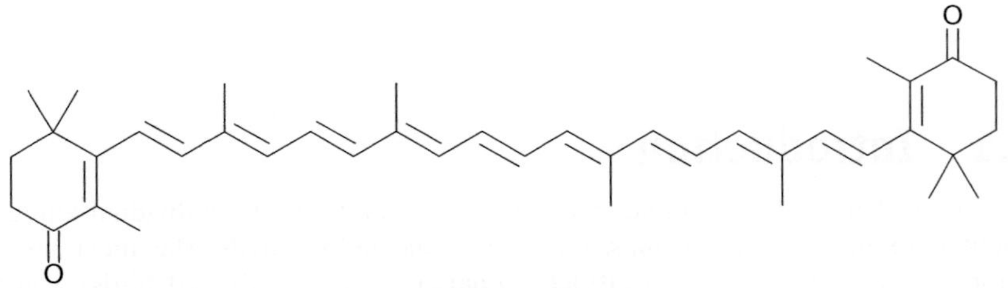

Canthaxanthin

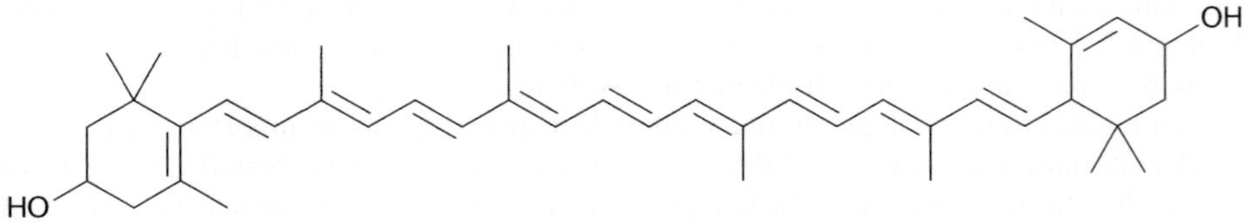

Zeaxanthin

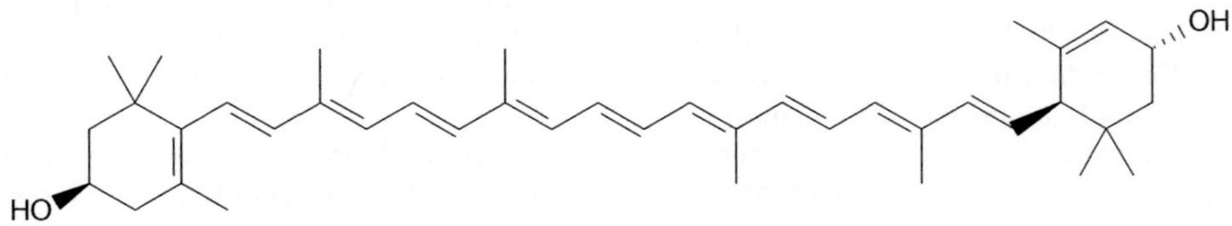

Lutein

Figure 11.1 Chemical structures of those carotenoids most frequently found in fruits and vegetables.

processing can induce *trans*-to-*cis* carotenoid isomerization. The content of carotenoids in plants is influenced by different factors related to the genetic background, the environment, and cultivation strategies used to manage the crop during its growth. In particular, cultivation strategies can result in an increase in the concentration of carotenoids. However, postharvest processes also may induce some changes concerning the chemistry of carotenoids, hence their individual bioavailability.

11.2 Occurrence of carotenoids in food materials

In higher plants, carotenoids are mainly detected in leaves, flowers, and fruits. But recent studies confirm that large amounts of carotenoids also occur in numerous macro- and microalgae [2, 3]. Furthermore, photosynthetic bacteria and fungi also are able to produce various carotenoids, such as canthaxanthin. Contrary to that, animals are unable to biosynthesize carotenoids *de novo* and are therefore dependent on the carotenoid supply from their diet. It is well known that several yellow- or red-colored birds, some fish species such as salmon, and numerous marine invertebrates accumulate various carotenoids (mainly astaxanthin) from nature. In human blood plasma, usually the following six carotenoids are detected: α- and β-carotene, lycopene, zeaxanthin, lutein, and β-cryptoxanthin [4]. With respect to provitamin A activity, the most prominent substances are α- and β-carotene, several xantophylls including β-cryptoxanthin, and some apocarotenoids [5]. However, the enzymatic processes involved in the conversion of these precursors with provitamin A activity are influenced by different factors, such as the consistency of the food matrix, vitamin A, and the health status of the individual [6]. Among the group of carotenoids that are converted to retinol, their individual provitamin A activity was determined several years ago [7]. As can be seen from Table 11.1, β-carotene has the highest provitamin A activity because every molecule produces two of retinal, which is subsequently reduced to retinol. Today, it is well known that only those carotenoids can be converted into vitamin A that possess at least one β-type ring, no oxygenated functional groups, and a polyene chain containing at least 11 carbon atoms.

Table 11.1 Carotenoids with provitamin A acitivity. The individual provitamin A value is relative to ß-carotene according to Bauernfeind [7].

Carotenoid	Percent Vitamin A Activity
trans-β-Carotene	100
9-*cis*-β-Carotene	38
13-*cis*-β-Carotene	53
trans-α-Carotene	53
9-*cis*-α-Carotene	13
13-*cis*-α-Carotene	16
trans-β-Crypthoxanthin	57
9-*cis*-β-Crypthoxanthin	27
15-*cis*-β-Crypthoxanthin	42
β-Carotene-5,6-epoxide	21
γ-Carotene	42–50
β-Zeacarotene	20–40

During fruit development, several metabolic changes influence their chemical composition and structural characteristics, especially at the end of the process during fruit ripening. Fruit development covers a maturation phase consisting of initial cell division, followed by a period of cell growth and an increase in the size of laticiferous canals and intercellular spaces, until a maximum organ expansion is reached [8]. Vasquez-Caicedo *et al.* [9] analyzed the morphological changes of the structures with the aim to understand where the plant pigments are exactly deposited during maturation of mango (*Mangifera indica*). They also got a deeper insight into the nature and availability of carotenoids during postharvest ripening and described the nutritional and sensory quality of mango fruits. In capsicum (*Capsicum annuum*) fruits, early ripening stages were characterized by the presence of chloroplasts [10], where carotenoids are part of the pigment–protein complex of Photosystems I and II in the stroma- and grana-thylakoids. The authors were able to prove that during fruit ripening, chloroplasts differentiate into chromoplasts by disintegration of the thylakoid membranes and by the development of new pigment-bearing structures.

11.3 Bioavailability and bioefficiency of carotenoids

It has been reported that humans consume around 60 different carotenoids with their intake of vegetables and fruits. Small amounts of carotenoid uptake are related to the consumption of eggs, fish, and poultry for which plant and algal materials (e.g., zeaxanthin from maize) are very often ingredients of the animal feed [11]. Numerous epidemiological studies also have been performed to understand more precisely the beneficial effect of various carotenoids on human health. In this context especially, lycopene and β-carotene have been found to act as important protectors against cancer and cardiovascular diseases [11–14]. Therefore, today growing interest exists in getting reliable information regarding the bioavailability of carotenoids, with respect to both carotenoids per se and the vitamin A value of provitamin A carotenoids in foods or supplement preparations [15]. Such data are needed for dietary recommendations, supplement formulation, and design of intervention strategies involving carotenoids. At present, scarce quantitative information is available, which is related to the lack of adequate methods to measure carotenoid bioavailability. Reported ranges of carotenoid bioavailability (% dose absorbed) range from 1 to 99, and variability is generally high both within and between treatments. Currently available methods allow one to determine relative bioavailability, but in most cases these approaches are not applicable to assess data for absolute bioavailability. The most commonly applied methods include measuring the increase in plasma carotenoid concentration following chronic intervention, and use of postprandial chylomicron (PPC) carotenoid or retinyl ester response following a single dose of carotenoid [15]. Based on the currently available data, it can be suggested that oil solutions of carotenoids are more bioavailable than those from food matrices. Furthermore, it has been recognized that heating can improve the bioavailability of carotenoids from some selected food products.

Generally, the bioactivity of carotenoids requires their preceding release from the food matrix and subsequent absorption. However, today the bioavailability of carotenoids still is not yet fully understood because numerous factors influence this diverse process, which has been reviewed in detail previously [6, 16, 17]. According to several studies, it has been presented that the chemical structure of an individual carotenoid has a high impact on its bioavailability. In this context, van het Hof *et al.* [18] registered a fivefold higher bioavailability of lutein compared to β-carotene from a mixed-vegetable diet. Similar results were obtained by Kostic *et al.* [19], who administered equimolar doses of lutein and β-carotene dissolved in oil to their study participants. Furthermore, the effects of interactions between different carotenoids and the total amount of carotenoid on bioavailability have been studied intensively, and it was discovered that different carotenoids compete for their absorption [20]. However, the chemical environment of the carotenoids in the plant tissue also plays an important role regarding their release and subsequent absorption. Today, it is well known that in plants, carotenoids are deposited in different types of plastids, such as chloroplasts and chromoplasts. The low bioavailability of carotenoids from raw green vegetables is related to the fact that the pigment is bound in various complexes with protein that are located in the chloroplasts. If food material is heated, carotenoids are released from these complexes and thus will enhance their bioavailability [21]. It is assumed that the morphology of chromoplasts in yellow, orange, and red fruits and vegetables has a significant impact on the bioavailability of carotenoids. Thus, it has been reported that carrot root cells contain comparatively large, crystalline aggregations of β-carotene, whereas nanoscale substructures of lipid-dissolved and liquid-crystalline β-carotene can be found in papaya fruits [22, 23]. At the same time, crystalloid accumulations of lycopene have been identified in both papayas and tomatoes.

A series of in vitro digestion experiments have been carried out in which an enhanced release of lycopene and β-carotene from papayas has been detected, whereas the release from carrots and tomatoes was significant lower [24]. Because all three mentioned fruits contain β-carotene, the authors developed a three-way cross-over clinical trial to evaluate the bioavailability of the vitamin A precursor. Furthermore, they also determined the bioavailability of β-cryptoxanthin from papaya fruits, which are known to contain high amounts of this provitamin A carotenoid. A total of 16 participants were recruited for the randomized cross-over study. Test meals containing raw carrots, tomatoes, and papayas were adjusted to provide an equal amount of β-carotene and lycopene. For the evaluation of bioavailability, lipoprotein fractions containing newly absorbed carotenoids were analyzed over 9.5 hours after test meal consumption. The bioavailability of β-carotene from papayas was found to be approximately three times higher than that from carrots and tomatoes, whereas differences in the bioavailability of β-carotene from carrots and tomatoes were insignificant. Retinyl esters appeared in the lipoprotein fractions at a significantly higher concentration after the consumption of the papaya test meal. The authors mention that lycopene was approximately 2.6 times more bioavailable from papayas than from tomatoes. Furthermore, the bioavailability of β-cryptoxanthin from papayas was shown to be 2.9 and 2.3 times higher than that of the other papaya carotenoids β-carotene and lycopene, respectively. It is assumed that the morphology of chromoplasts and the physical deposition form of carotenoids play major roles in the context of their individual bioavailability from the foods investigated. Particularly, the liquid-crystalline deposition of β-carotene and the storage of lycopene in very small crystalloids in papayas were found to be associated with their high bioavailability. In conclusion, papaya was shown to provide highly bioavailable β-carotene, β-cryptoxanthin, and lycopene and is therefore recommended as a readily available dietary source of provitamin A for reducing the incidence of vitamin A deficiencies in many subtropical and tropical developing countries [23]. Based on liquid chromatography–mass spectroscopy (LC-MS) data (Figure 11.2, Color Supplement), it has been found that yellow fruits contain only trace amounts of lycopene, whereas this substance occurs as the main carotenoid in red papaya (51% of total carotenoids).

In addition, the developmental pathway of red papaya chromoplasts was investigated during fruit ripening and carotenogenesis. The authors found that carotenoids from papaya

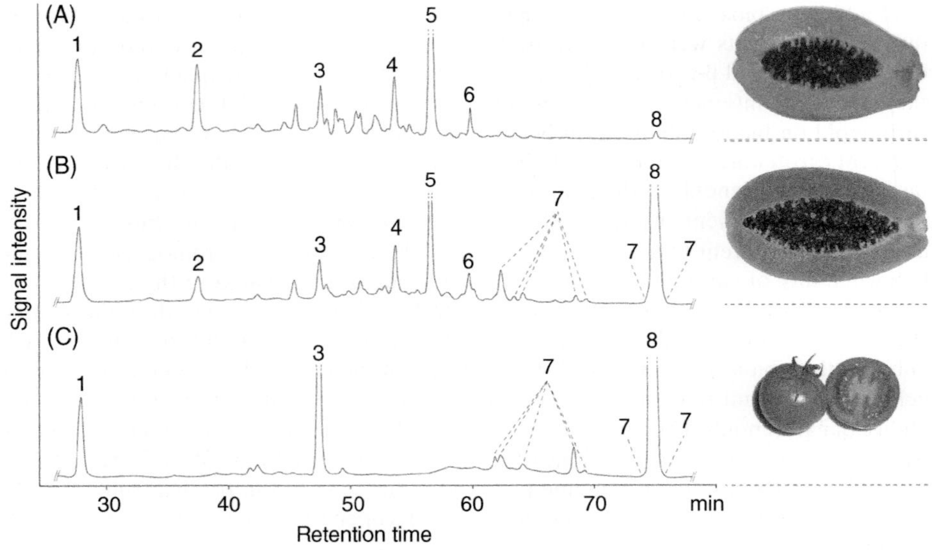

Figure 11.2 Separation of carotenoids and carotenoid esters from (A) yellow papaya, (B) red papaya, and (C) tomato fruit by high-performance liquid chromatography (HPLC) monitored at 450 nm. 1: β-Apo-8-carotenal (added as internal standard); 2: β-cryptoxanthin; 3: β-carotene; 4: β-cryptoxanthin caprate; 5: β-cryptoxanthin laurate; 6: β-cryptoxanthin myristate; 7: *Z*-lycopene isomers; and 8: all-*E*-lycopene. (Reproduced with permission from Schweiggert *et al.*, 2011 [22]. © Springer.) (*See insert for color representation of the figure.*)

and mango were accumulated in globular and tubular structures, where they are present in a lipid-dissolved or liquid-crystalline form [22]. Contrary to that, the studies prove that chromoplasts obtained from carrots and tomatoes show large crystalloid β-carotene and lycopene aggregates, respectively (Figure 11.3, Color Supplement).

The same authors recognized for the first time that fruits collected from papaya and tomato plants accumulate a crystalline form of lycopene, whereas in papaya fruits a much smaller size of lycopene crystalloids was deposited [22, 24].

In 1967, the World Health Organization (WHO) defined the term *bioefficiency* as "the fraction of ingested carotenoids with provitamin A activity that is absorbed and converted to its active form retinol." Estimating that the bioefficacy of carotenoids from a diet is one-third of that of retinol and recognizing that the equivalence between β-carotene and retinol is 2:1, a ratio value of 6 was introduced to calculate the efficacy for β-carotene and 12 for other carotenoids. The term *bioavailability* has been formed by a fusion of the two words *biological* and *availability* [25]. Generally, it is defined as the amount of a nutrient that is released from a food during the digestion process. In contrast to the term *bioaccessibility*, which is usually described as the sum of digestibility and assimilation, bioavailability covers metabolism, transport and tissue distribution, and bioactivity of a certain active substance [26]. Numerous fruits and vegetables contain various carotenoids that possess high bioactivity with regard to human health. In particular, β-carotene as the precursor of vitamin A represents an important nutritional issue in many developing countries due to its role in immune function and growth [27]. But also other carotenoids that are not converted to vitamin A, such as lycopene, are well known for their health-promoting properties [28].

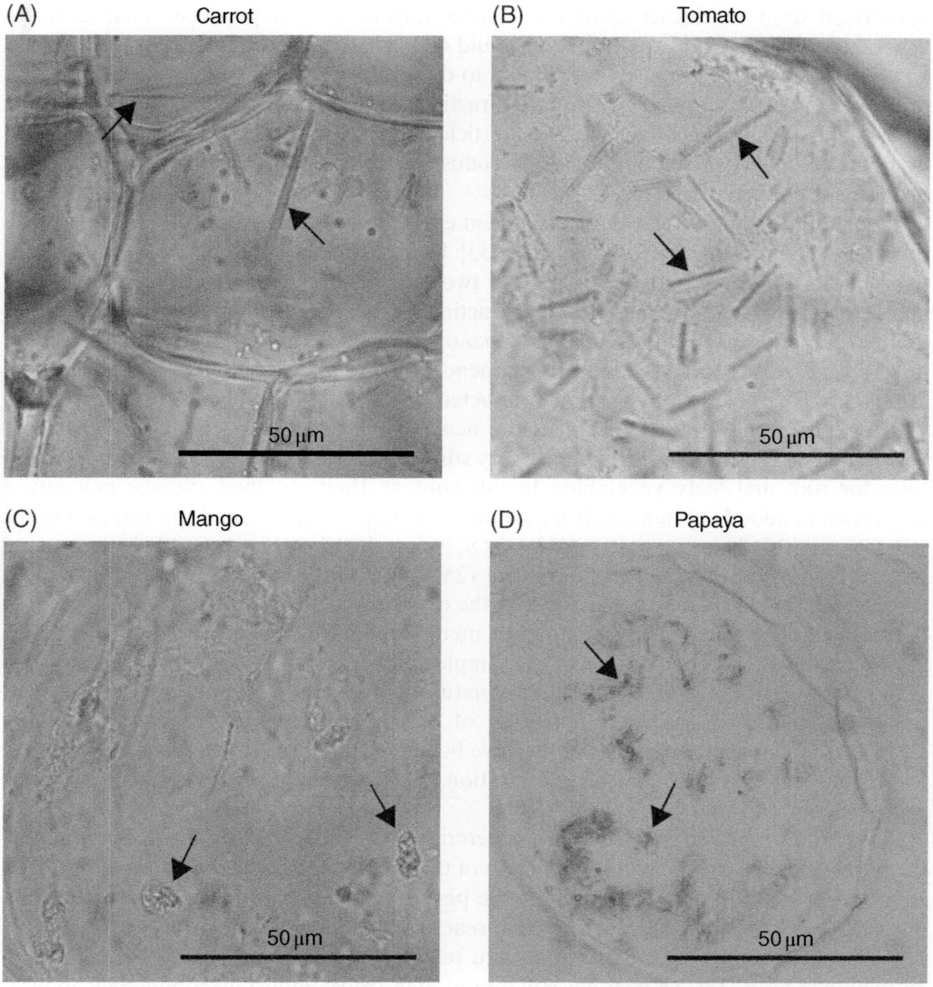

Figure 11.3 Light micrographs of carrot root and mango, papaya, and tomato fruits. The chromoplasts are marked with arrows. (Reproduced with permission from Schweiggert *et al.*, 2012 [24]. © Elsevier.) (*See insert for color representation of the figure.*)

11.4 Extraction of carotenoids from various food matrices

Several extraction and purification studies have been performed to obtain carotenoids from natural sources, including solvent extraction, supercritical fluid extraction (SFE), distillation, membrane separation, chromatography, and crystallization. Furthermore, biotechnological methods have been applied to produce carotenoids in bioreactors with appropriate microorganisms. Nevertheless, also today solvent extraction is mainly used to isolate natural carotenoids in industrial-scale amounts [29, 30]. In the past, different organic solvents such as acetone, tetrahydrofuran, n-hexane, pentane, methanol, and chloroform have been used to extract carotenoids from various natural products, such as fruits, vegetables, and seafood [31–33]. Today, liquid CO_2 is becoming increasingly important as an extraction solvent because of its ability to diffuse into natural tissues and its nontoxic properties. In order to purify the isolated fractions, carotenoids are usually crystallized or co-crystallized [34]. In literature, most articles related to various extraction methods describe analytical procedures, whereas industrial applications are scarce and in most instances explained in patents.

Taungbodhitham *et al.* developed a solvent extraction method suitable for a wide range of sample matrices in carotenoid analysis [33]. Using canned tomato juice as a representative sample, they were able to present that two solvents of low biological hazard, ethanol and hexane, are the most suitable for extracting carotenoids from the matrix. The use of double extraction, each with 35 ml of an ethanol–hexane mixture (4:3, by volume), resulted in good recoveries of carotenoids (lycopene 96%, α-carotene 102%, and β-carotene 93–100%). Coefficients of variation conducted on different days were for lycopene 5% and for β-carotene 7%. They applied the new established method to various fruit and vegetable matrices, and performed recovery studies with carrot and spinach as representatives for root and leafy vegetables. In this context, they obtained average percentage recoveries of added carotenoids from canned tomato juice, carrot, and spinach as follows: 101, 99.8, and 101% for α-carotene (12.4, 24.8, 49.6, and 99.2 μg/10 ml of added α-carotene); and 98.1, 99.7, and 96.1% for β-carotene (25.5, 50.9, 101, and 201 μg/10 ml of added β-carotene). These similar recoveries over the explored concentration ranges confirm that the application of the developed extraction method seems to be more or less unaffected by differences in matrix composition of the samples.

In recent years, the growing demand for natural products in foods, pharmaceuticals, and cosmetics caused a significant reduction of organic solvents in extraction processes. Following this trend, numerous patents have been registered related to the use of physical techniques such as precipitation, distillation, filtration and centrifugation, enzymatic processes, and SFE.

Extraction of natural products with supercritical CO_2 has received much attention for the past several years. The main advantages of this technique are that no extraction solvent residues remain and the extractions can be performed at low to moderate temperatures, insuring that less destruction or chemical reactions will occur during the extraction process. The first uses of CO_2 extraction were related to decaffeination of coffee [35] and extraction of hops [36], which today still represent the most important commercial applications in this field. In addition, it prevents the oxidation of carotenoids during the extraction process. In recent years, the growing interest in nutraceuticals has led to increased efforts to find potential carotenoid sources in several products and by-products obtained from the agricultural and fishing industries [37–39].

Table 11.2 summarizes some of the most important approaches to isolate carotenoids from various natural materials. Nevertheless, it has to be stressed here that even today organic solvents are still widely used, and many patents involve the use of ethanol and ethyl acetate but also describe the advantages of so-called green solvents such as ethyl lactate [40].

Roots of carrot (*Daucus carota* L. var. Caro Pride) were successfully extracted with supercritical fluid CO_2 under various combinations of pressures and solvent modifiers at 40 °C, and the resulting ratio of α- and β-carotene content was determined by high-performance LC (HPLC). The supercritical fluid CO_2 extraction at 40 °C and 60.6 MPa with 5% chloroform as modifier afforded 111.16 and 148.32 mg of α- and β-carotene per gram of dried carrot, respectively. Compared to solvent extraction using chloroform as the extraction solvent, the new method extracted only 92.70% of the total carotenoid fraction [41]. The effects of thermal treatments during blanching, pasteurization, and sterilization

Table 11.2 Recent patents related to the extraction of carotenoids (according to Riggi [77]).

Title	Patent Number	Method	Raw Materials	References
Solventless extraction	CA2397655	Broth cells; thermal lysing (>50 °C), centrifuge cell mixture, light layer enriched, non-emulsified enriched components	Algae, fungi, bacteria	Engelhardt *et al.*, 2001 [78]
Pigment extraction system and method	US2003091704	Raw materials; homogenization, washing, centrifugation, pigment recovery	Citrus fruits, mainly grapefruit	Lee Hyoung & Coates, 2003 [79]
Natural color concentrates and antimicrobial nutraceutical from plants	CA2303352	Raw materials + food-grade polyvinyl pyrollidone Mixing, removing the juice Substrate enriched in carotenoids	Flower, fruit (mainly cranberry and blueberry) and vegetable juice or homogenate	Hoffman *et al.*, 2004 [80]
Processes for extracting carotenoids and for preparing feed materials	CA2395319	Raw materials + solvent, Mixing, separating water layer Carotenoid solution in an edible oil	Shellfish, krill, algae, fungi, vegetables, tomatoes	Kagan & Braun, 2001 [81]
Isolation of carotenoid crystals	CA2396167	Oily suspension from disrupted microbial cells + alkali (pH 9–12), kept at 50–75 °C, separated and washed Crystalline suspension with a salty aqueous solution	Microbial sources (bacteria, fungi, algae, yeast)	Wolf *et al.*, 2001 [82]
Carotenoid extraction process	US2003044499	Diluted raw materials (Brix <10°), crushing, decantation, centrifugation, extraction with organic solvents, carotenoid-containing plant oleoresin	Tomato paste, carrots, dried carrots, wolfberry fruit (*Lycium barbarum*), corn, *Dunaliella* biomass	Zelkha & Sedlov, 2003 [83]
Method for producing carotenoid concentrate from green mass of plant material	UA73556	Raw materials–oil (0.5 to 2:1) Filtration or thermal pressing and milling, carotenoid-enriched substrate	Green mass of plant material	Postoienko *et al.*, 2004 [84]

(*continued*)

Table 11.2 (*Continued*)

Title	Patent Number	Method	Raw Materials	References
Process for extracting carotenoids from fruit- and vegetable-processing waste	AU2003287701	Macerated source–alcohol–surfactant, slurry + carbon disulfide, decantation, centrifugation, liquid fraction + solid fraction, separating liquid fraction, concentrating, carotenoid crystals precipitated	Fruit- or vegetable-processing waste	Rusnack & Allen, 2004 [85]
Method for production of fat-soluble carotenoid complex from hydrobios and waste	RU2004100513	Raw materials: heated fat (<40 °C), agitation, centrifugation, carotenoid-enriched substrate	Fish industry by-products	Mukhin *et al.*, 2006 [86]
Production of lycopene enriched antioxidants	ES2241503	Raw materials–lipid, high-speed stirring (<120 °C), carotenoid-enriched substrate	Any plant product (tomatoes, watermelons, wild berries, flowers, etc.)	Rey, 2005 [87]
Isolation and purification of carotenoids from marigold flowers	AU2005331246	Marigold flower petals Ensilaging, dehydration, dried meal pelletizing, pellet + hexane solvent extraction, marigold oleoresin, homogenizing in alcohol, hydrolysis with alkali, carotenoid esters precipitation using water and alcohol (50/50) Mixture, washing with hot water, filtration of carotenoid crystals, centrifugation, filtration, drying, carotenoid crystals	Marigold flower petals	Madavalappil & Swaminathan, 2006 [53]
Process for production of carotenoids	JP2007319015	Microorganism culture + alcohols heated (>80 °C), mixing, alcohol solution, concentration and mixing with water, carotenoid-enriched precipitate, washing and filtration	Microorganism cultures	Ishikawa *et al.*, 2007 [88]

Extraction of carotenoids from plant material	US20097572468	Dried and milled raw materials–ethyl lactate/ethanol (93/7, v/v), filtration, centrifugation and membrane separation, carotenoid-enriched solution, evaporation	Tomato, watermelon, papaya, guava, mango, grapefruit, olive, carrots, parsley, spinach	Ishida *et al.*, 2009 [89]
Separation of carotenoids from fruits and vegetables	CA2305091	Mechanically crushed, cooked, homogenized, and freeze-dried raw materials Mixing the powder with an edible oil SFE (45 to 50 °C / 35 to 38 mpa / 120 to 180 min.	Fruits and vegetables, especially tomatoes	Shi, 2001 [90]
Method for extracting chlorophyll and carotenoid pigments from seaweeds, crustacean, and echinodermata	KR20020000660	CO_2 + alcohol entrainer 80 °C / 5 to 50 mpa	Seaweeds, crustaceans, echinoderms	Chun & Hong, 2002 [91]
Method for producing organic solvent-free lycopene concentrate	AU2369002	Drying (moisture < 10%) and milling, optionally adding virgin olive oil and oligoresin, SFE: <80 °C, 30–70 mpa, depressurisation 10–20 mpa, 40–60 °C	Industrial wastes from the tomato-processing industry	Rey *et al.*, 2002 [92]
Improvements in or relating to separation technology	CA2483191	Lipophilic compound and urea solution, near-critical fluid (35–80 °C / 15–50 mpa), depressurizing, lipophilic compound	By-product of transesterification processes	Mackenzie *et al.*, 2003 [93]
Method for extracting lutein from green plant materials	US20046737552	Two-step supercritical fluid extraction First pressure: 10–40 mpa Second pressure: 41–80 mpa Entrainer (ethanol 1 to 5% (v/v) of the supercritical fluid)	Alfalfa, wheat, barley, kale, broccoli, spinach, cabbage beans, soybean, mustard greens, collards, turnip greens	Crombie, 2004 [94]
Process and apparatus for modifying plant extracts	AU2004246728	Raw materials, semipermeable nanofiltration membrane, partially dried starting material, supercritical CO_2 extraction	Fruits, vegetables, herbs, grasses	Brewer, 2004 [95]

(*continued*)

Table 11.2 (*Continued*)

Title	Patent Number	Method	Raw Materials	References
Supercritical carbon dioxide extraction of carotenoids from natural materials using a continuous co-solvent	US2005266132	Raw materials grinding (0.2 to 2 mm), drying (<10% moisture), powder + oil SFE co_2 (35 to 100 °c / 10 to 100 mpa / 0.5 to 3.0 l/min)	Carrots, tomatoes, marine algae	Temelli and Sun, 2005 [96]
Method of extracting carotenoids and edible glycerol from *Dunaliella salina*	CN101107991	Optimized culture of *Dunaliella salina* Concentrate with hollow-fiber film method centrifugal separation, dehydration, and drying carbon dioxide with supercritical method	*Dunaliella salina*	Zhen *et al.*, 2008 [97]
Method for extraction and concentration of carotenoids using supercritical fluids	US7329789	Supercritical gas: dimethyl ether, Optional second step, supercritical gas: CO_2	Algae-derived materials, marine organisms, vegetables	Schonemann *et al.*, 2008 [98]
Method for extracting carotenoids from tobacco leaf by overcritical co_2	CN101209985	Supercritical CO_2, column chromatographic separation	Tobacco leaves	Mingqin & Jinxia, 2008 [99]
Dense gas means for extraction of solute from solids	US2008251454	Inclined single auger or multiple augers in a pressurized chamber, continuously refilled biphasic dense gas mixed with raw materials Solute + gas and liquid phases at the bottom, insoluble components + vapor phase at the top	Soybean, rapeseed (canola), corn, palm sunflower, jatropha, corn germ, safflower, cotton, flax, peanut, olive, coconut, woody material, animal matter	Waibel *et al.*, 2008 [100]
Methods for processing crustacean material [46]	CA2421820	Enzymes having phospholipase activity in an aqueous liquid Separation, inactivation, or removal of added enzymes	Crustacean materials	Nielsen, 2002 [101]
Increasing bioavailability of carotenoids	CA2448125	Esterase + cellulase + protease + pectinase, emulsifier, detection assay for determining the efficiency of the esterase	Red pepper, apple, apricot, avocado, citrus fruit, mango, nectarine, papaya, peach, persimmon, plum, potato, pumpkin, tangerine, zucchini	Levy *et al.*, 2002 [102]

AU, Australia; CA, Canada; CN, China; DE, Germany; ES, Spain; JP, Japan; KR, South Korea; RU, Russia; SFE, supercritical fluid extraction ; UA, Ukraine; US, United States).

on *cis-trans*-isomerization of β-carotene in carrot juice produced on a pilot plant scale and in β-carotene-containing preparations have been studied by Marx *et al.* [42]. The authors observed that pasteurization and sterilization at 121 °C caused only minor isomerization, whereas sterilization at 130 °C and blanching resulted in increased formation of *cis*-isomers. Furthermore, it was found that dissolution of crystalline carotenes by cellular lipids during blanching of carrots can be used as the prerequisite for isomerization. In a similar approach, addition of grapeseed oil to the coarse mash enhanced isomerization in both unheated and heat-preserved carrot juices. Based on model preparations containing crystalline β-carotene, the authors were able to present a pronounced stability during heating, whereas thermal treatment of β-carotene dissolved in toluene resulted in temperature-dependent isomerization. It is assumed that the carotene-stabilizing principles observed in carrot juice can be related to chromoplast fragments as the core, coated by water-insoluble juice constituents such as pectin, cellulose, and protein that prevent carotenes from being dissolved in neutral lipids upon moderate heating.

By 1993, an ethanol–pentane solvent extraction method and a supercritical CO_2 extraction procedure were being compared for a subsequent HPLC determination of α- and β-carotene in vegetables [43]. The analyzed samples included carrots, collard greens, turnips, turnip greens, mustard greens, broccoli florets, zucchini, and squash. It was found that homogenization of the samples prior to extraction significantly improved recovery of the carotenoids. A combination of static and dynamic modes of extraction with ethanol as modifier, performed at 338 atm and 40 °C, was necessary to achieve optimum recovery with the supercritical fluid procedure. Applying the supercritical CO_2 technique, the carotene content was 23% higher when compared to results obtained by liquid extraction. Only corn and carrots contained detectable levels of α-carotene, and, in both cases, liquid extraction yielded slightly higher results. Whereas liquid extractions needed approximately 90 minutes, the supercritical fluid procedure could be performed within 30 minutes.

Gao *et al.* [44] developed a supercritical CO_2 method enhanced by ultrasound for the extraction of lutein esters from marigold (*Tagetes erecta*). The effects of extraction parameters, including particle size of matrix, temperature, pressure, flow rate of CO_2, and ultrasonic conditions consisting of power, frequency, and irradiation time/interval on the yield of lutein esters, were studied with single-factor experiments. The results showed that the yield of lutein esters increased significantly with the presence of ultrasound ($p < 0.05$). Optimal yield of lutein esters (690 mg 100 g^{-1}) was obtained for a particle size fraction of 0.245–0.350 mm, extraction pressure of 32.5 MPa, temperature of 55 °C, and CO_2 flow rate of 10 kg h^{-1} with ultrasonic power of 400 W, ultrasonic frequency of 25 kHz, and ultrasonic irradiation time/interval of 6/9 s.

Barth *et al.* [45] also applied SFE to optimize the isolation of carotenoids from freeze-dried carrots and compared the SFE results with those obtained by traditional solvent extraction (TSE) methods. To optimize SFE for carotenoids, a factorial experiment was conducted with varying temperature of the sample chamber (30, 40, or 50 °C), different pressure of the extraction fluid (300, 400, or 500 atm), and various co-solvent modifications (5 or 10% ethanol). The optimum conditions for extraction of α-carotene and β-carotene by SFE were 50 °C, 300 atm, and 10% co-solvent ethanol. Total provitamin A activity (α- plus β-carotene) was greater in SFE than in TSE studies. The time required for SFE was 1 h, whereas for the TSE procedure 6 hours were needed. Therefore, the authors recommend SFE as a reliable and improved method for extraction of carotenoids from carrot tissue.

Howe and Tanumihardjo performed biofortification of maize with α-carotene to improve the vitamin A status in vitamin A–deficient populations where maize is a staple crop [46].

The main objective of their work was to evaluate different carotenoid extraction methods and to adapt them for application in countries growing biofortified maize. The most reproducible method based on coefficient of variation and extraction efficiency was a modification of Kurilich and Juvik's method [47]. Furthermore, it was found that heat and saponification are necessary to release carotenoids from biofortified maize. In order to get satisfying results also for maize samples with high oil content, addition of base has been proved to ensure complete saponification. The described method was found to be applicable for lutein, zeaxanthin, α-cryptoxanthin, and α-carotene.

A powerful SFE method for the isolation of all-*trans*-lycopene from tomatoes using CO_2 at 40 °C without any modifiers has been described by Gomez-Prieto *et al.* [48]. This method allows minimizing the risk of degradation via isomerization and oxidation of health-promoting ingredients, such as lycopene. The effects of different experimental parameters on the solvating power of the supercritical fluid are evaluated in terms of both the selectivity achievable in the process and the yield of the extraction of all-*trans*-lycopene. The isolated fractions contain 88% all-*trans*-lycopene and 12% *cis*-lycopene.

Another approach aiming to extract lycopene and α-carotene from tomato paste waste using supercritical carbon dioxide has been described by Baysal *et al.* [49]. To optimize the extraction process with regard to increased amounts of lycopene and α-carotene, a factorial designed experiment was conducted. The factors assessed were temperature of the extractor (35, 45, 55, and 65 °C), pressure of the extraction fluid (200, 250, and 300 bar), addition of co-solvent (5, 10, and 15% ethanol), extraction time (1, 2, and 3 h), and CO_2 flow rate (2, 4, and 8 kg/h). The individual amounts of lycopene and α-carotene in the tomato paste waste, extracts, and residues were determined by HPLC. A maximum of 53.93% of lycopene was extracted in 2 h (CO_2 flow rate = 4 kg/h) at 55 °C and 300 bar, with the addition of 5% ethanol as a co-solvent.

A similar SFE method has been presented for the extraction of lycopene from tomato peel by-product using the indigenous oil from tomato seed that has been obtained along with the tomato peel [50]. The authors determined the effects of temperature, pressure, and CO_2 flow rate on lycopene recovery from tomato peel in the presence of tomato seed oil as a co-solvent to enhance the supercritical CO_2 solvating power for lycopene and β-carotene extraction (Figure 11.4). In this context, they found that the presence of tomato seed oil can significantly improve the extraction yield of lycopene.

Furthermore, a beneficial role in the stability of lycopene due to its fatty acid content could be identified. However, increasing temperature (70, 80, and 90 °C) caused a slightly decrease in the recovery of β-carotene, whereas the amount of lycopene increased at the same time [50]. The optimum process conditions for lycopene extraction were obtained using the following parameters: temperature 90 °C, pressure 40 MPa, particle size 1.05±0.10 mm, and a ratio of tomato peel to seed of 37:63. Under these conditions, 56% of lycopene could be extracted from the tomato peel, whereas 44% of this carotenoid remained in both the pipeline and the solid matrix. The authors stress that the presence of fatty acid content in the tomato seed oil improved the recovery of lycopene extracted from 18% to 56%.

Another research group also performed SFE of tomato seeds and skins obtained as by-products from the industrial processing of tomatoes [51]. Here, the extracts were analyzed for their content of lycopene, α-carotene, β-carotene, α-tocopherol, γ-tocopherol, and δ-tocopherol by HPLC, and the amounts compared to a chemically extracted control. The SFE experiments were carried out using CO_2 at seven temperatures (range, 32–86 °C) and six pressures (range, 13.78–48.26 MPa). The authors also studied the effect of CO_2 flow rate and volume on the extraction yield. It was found that the percentage of lycopene extracted increased with elevated temperature and pressure to a maximum recovery of 38.8% (obtained at 86 °C and 34.47 MPa). Optimal conditions for extraction of lycopene from 3 g

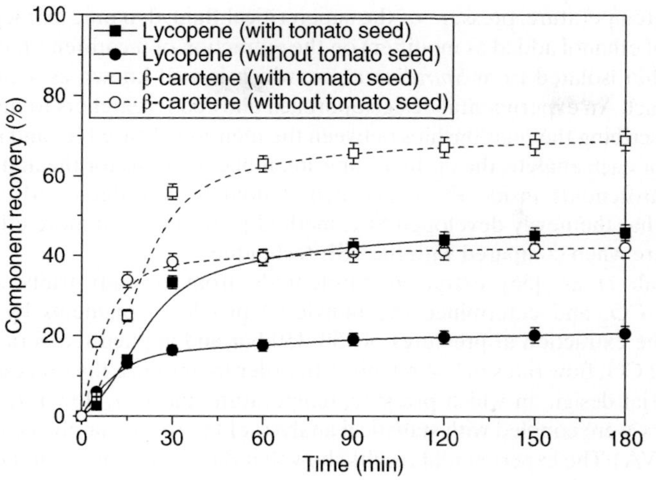

Figure 11.4 Effect of tomato seed oil as co-solvent on the recovery of lycopene and β-carotene at 90 °C, 40 MPa, and 3 ml min^{-1}. (Reproduced with permission from Machmudah *et al.*, 2012 [50]. © Elsevier.)

of raw material were determined to be 86 °C, 34.47 MPa, and 500 mL of CO_2 at a flow rate of 2.5 mL/min. Applying these conditions, an extraction yield of 61.0% of lycopene could be obtained.

The influence of some operative parameters of supercritical carbon dioxide extraction employed for the isolation of lycopene and β-carotene from the pulp and skins of ripe tomatoes have been evaluated by Cadoni *et al.* [52]. The extractions were conducted at pressures and temperatures ranging from 2500 to 4000 psi and from 40 to 80 °C, respectively. The extracted product at 4000 psi and 80 °C contained about 65% of lycopene and 35% of β-carotene. Lycopene and β-carotene showed a different solubility in the supercritical fluid depending on the individual process parameters. Applying optimal operative parameters, the authors were able to obtain a product that contained 87% lycopene and 13% β-carotene.

Madavalappil and Swaminathan [53] patented a new method using the SFE method to isolate the carotenoid fraction from marigold flowers. In a first step, they performed an anaerobic fermentation pretreatment to promote fixation and enrichment of the target substances, followed by dehydration through an eco-friendly drying process. At the end, they obtained a dried meal that could be pelletized and subsequently extracted with food-grade solvents such as n-hexane.

Vagi *et al.* [54] extracted chlorophylls and carotenoids from marjoram (*Origanum majorana*) applying the supercritical carbon dioxide technique. They studied the effects of extraction pressure and temperature on the yield of the pigments by applying a 32 full factorial design with three repeated tests in the center of the design. According to the applied extraction methods, different amounts of each pigment were determined. The highest levels of carotenoids and chlorophylls were found in the samples obtained by alcoholic Soxhlet extraction applying a laboratory and pilot plant apparatus. When supercritical CO_2 was applied, the highest amounts of pigment substances were extracted at 450 bar pressure and 50 °C temperature.

Another useful application of supercritical CO_2 extraction has been published by Careri *et al.* [55]. The authors developed a procedure to investigate the effects of various process parameters (temperature, pressure of the supercritical fluid, dynamic extraction time, and percentage of ethanol added as modifier) on the extraction of β-carotene, β-cryptoxanthin, and zeaxanthin isolated from *Spirulina* algae, which is well known as a carotenoid-rich dietary product. An experimental design approach allowed researchers to find polynomial functions describing the relationships between the mentioned variables and responses and to identify, for each analyte, the optimal experimental conditions for the individual SFE of the three carotenoids inside the experimental domain considered. Also, the authors highlighted that the newly developed SFE method proved to be a more effective extraction procedure when compared with the TSE technique.

Machmudah *et al.* [56] extracted carotenoids from rosehip fruits also applying supercritical CO_2 and determined the individual profile of pigments by HPLC. They performed the extraction at pressures of 150–450 bar and applied temperatures between 40–80 °C and CO_2 flow rates of 2–4 ml min^{-1}. In order to optimize the process conditions, a full 33-factorial design, in which pressure, temperature and CO_2 flow rate were used as design factors, were coupled with statistical analysis of the results, applying analysis of variance (ANOVA). The experimental results show that the maximum amount of carotenoids extracted was obtained at 80 °C, 450 bar, and 4 ml min^{-1}. According to the HPLC results obtained, the carotenoids extracted contain lycopene and β-carotene as main components, and additionally a small amount of lutein. The amount of lycopene, β-carotene, and lutein extracted were 1.180–14.37 mg g^{-1} feed, 0.154–1.017 mg g^{-1} feed, and 1.258–16.84 g g^{-1} feed, respectively. The authors were able to demonstrate that temperature mainly influenced the extraction yield of carotenoids, whereas for lycopene extracted, all variables (temperature, pressure, and CO_2 flow rate) had a more or less similar influence. Furthermore, the authors discovered that the mean extraction rate constant of total carotenoids increased with increasing pressure and temperature, reaching levels of (3.344–5.851) × 10^{-3} min^{-1}.

Macias-Sanchez *et al.* [3] described the extraction of carotenoids and chlorophylls using CO_2 modified with ethanol as a co-solvent. The extraction of both plant pigments was performed using freeze-dried powders of the three microalgae *Nannochloropsis gaditana*, *Synechococcus* sp., and *Dunaliella salina* as raw materials. They applied the following processing conditions: pressures of 200, 300, 400, and 500 bar; and temperatures of 40, 50, and 60 °C. The highest extraction yields of carotenoids and chlorophyll with CO_2 and 5% ethanol from *N. gaditana* were obtained at 500 bar and 60 °C. In the case of the microalga *D. salina*, the maximum yields for both pigments were obtained at 400 bar and 60 °C, the same operating temperature as for *N. gaditana*. With regard to *Synechococcus* sp., the highest carotenoid extraction yields were achieved at 300 bar and 50 °C. The authors found that optimal carotenoid–chlorophyll ratios were obtained by using SFE with co-solvent instead of using conventional extraction. The largest amount of carotenoids was extracted from *D. salina* due to the higher total content of carotenoids present in this microalga compared to the other two.

A novel method to separate *cis* and *trans* isomers of β-carotene from a freeze-dried powder (Figure 11.5) obtained from the algae *Dunaliella bardawil* applying SFE has been introduced by Gamlieli-Bonshtein *et al.* [57]. The solubility of the 9-*cis* isomer was found to be nearly four times higher than that of the all-*trans* isomer. When SFE was applied to a carotenoid concentrate, the authors obtained 39% recovery of β-carotene at the initial extraction stages and achieved 80% purity of the 9-*cis*-isomer. Contrary to that, extraction from freeze-dried algae was slower and provided less recovery and purity of the *cis*-isomer.

Another fast and selective extraction method has been developed by Guedes *et al.* [58] to isolate food-grade pigments and antioxidants from microalgae. The study describes the influence of pressure, temperature, CO_2 flow rate, and a polar co-solvent upon the yields of carotenoids and chlorophylls in SFE of *Scenedesmus obliquus* biomass. The highest

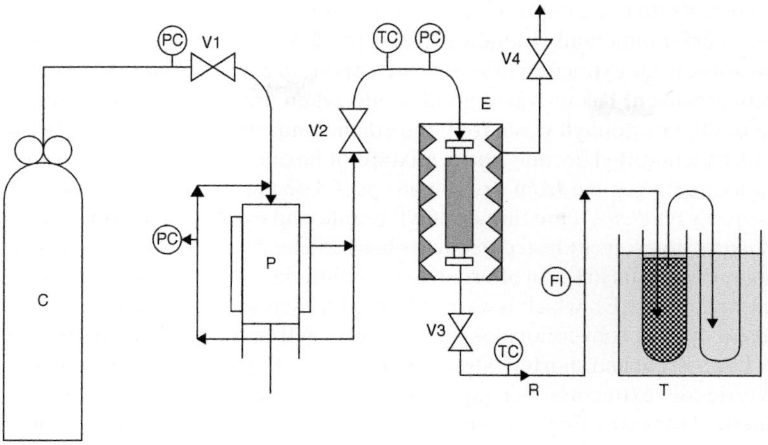

Figure 11.5 Schematic flow diagram of the experimental supercritical fluid extraction (SFE) apparatus used for isolation of carotenoids from the algae *Dunaliella bardawil*. C, cylinder for supply of liquid CO_2; V1–V4, valves; P, high-pressure pump; E, extractor cell; R, restrictor; T, collection glass tube. (Reproduced with permission from Gamlieli-Bonshtein *et al.*, 2002 [57]. © Wiley.)

carotenoid yield was obtained applying 250 bar and 60 °C, whereas optimal conditions for extraction of chlorophyll were found at 4:3 g CO_2 min^{-1}. Using ethanol as co-solvent for liquid CO_2, generally an increased extraction yield could be achieved except for chlorophyll c. The authors observed a remarkable selectivity under the described operating conditions, and they stress that the new extraction methods may enable easy separation and purification of numerous plant pigments.

Studies related to carotenoid extraction are mainly based on single-solvent extraction. In this context, it has been found that ethyl lactate works efficiently for solvent extraction of both *cis* and *trans* isomers of lycopene [59]. Commonly used solvents in most extraction processes show adverse effects on human health and cannot be removed completely from the product. Such solvents, therefore, are not acceptable as raw materials for food or cosmetic products. Most nonpolar solvents that possess high extraction efficiencies are considered to be toxic. Solvents used in various patents for extracting lycopene include hexane, ethyl acetate, methylene chloride, methanol, ethanol, propanol, and acetone [60, 61]. At present, ethyl acetate is most commonly applied for extracting carotenoids that will be used in the food industry; it isolates β-carotene and lutein more effectively than the other polar solvents mentioned here, but unfortunately it is less efficient in extracting the all-*trans* isomer of lycopene. Furthermore, it is not considered to be environmentally friendly, and it is highly flammable. In order to find alternatives, ethyl lactate was identified as a useful solvent for carotenoid extraction because of its solubility in both aqueous and organic solvents. It is an environmentally friendly substance produced from fermentation of carbohydrate feedstocks and is available from the corn and soybean industries. Furthermore, it has a relatively high flashpoint and is colorless, environmentally benign, and completely biodegradable in CO_2 and water. Due to its miscibility with both hydrophilic and hydrophobic substances, the authors suggest ethyl lactate as an efficient solvent for extraction of carotenoids, including their stereoisomeric forms.

The uses of hexane and ethanol in several vegetable matrices have been evaluated for quantification of carotenoids such as lycopene and α- and β-carotene [33]. However, many of these solvents do not comply with regulations for human consumption. One alternative is the use of environmentally friendly solvents [60, 62]. Ethyl lactate has been proved as an excellent solvent for extraction of *trans-cis*-lycopene, β-carotene, and astaxanthin. The use of ethanol as solvent has provided good results when used for the extraction of carotenoids, besides the xantophyll waste from the ethanol industry. Some investigations compare the use of hexane, ethyl acetate, and a mixture of hexane, acetone, and ethanol (50:25:25, v/v/v) to extract lycopene from dry tomato peel. For the extraction of astaxanthin from *Hematococcus pluvialis*, a mixture of ethyl acetate and ethanol (1:1, v/v) was found to be the best extraction solvent tested due to its high efficiency and low toxicity compared with other organic solvents [63]. An alternative to traditional extraction methods is pressurized liquid extraction (PLE), which is currently used to extract biologically active substances. This system applies conventional solvents at elevated temperatures and pressures, but it requires less solvent and shorter extraction times, resulting in a more efficient and environmentally friendly extraction technique. The use of ethanol in PLE is described as a very useful method for extracting zeaxanthin from *Chlorella ellipsoidea*, a green microalga that contains more than nine times of the total zeaxanthin level than that of red pepper [64]. The same process has been applied to isolate carotenoids from carrot by-products using pressurized hot ethanol [65].

Freeze-dried samples of the microalga *Chlorella vulgaris* were extracted with supercritical CO_2 at temperatures of 40 and 55 °C and pressures up to 35 MPa [66]. The authors performed the studies on whole and crushed algae. The extraction yields of carotenoids and other lipids increased with pressure, and the carotenoid fraction in the oil was also greater at higher pressures.

Aiming to improve the yield and selectivity of lutein in the extract obtained by supercritical carbon dioxide extraction, Ruen-ngam *et al.* [67] applied a pretreatment process using alcohol for the removal of chlorophyll a, chlorophyll b, and β-carotene from *C. vulgaris.* After this treatment, supercritical carbon dioxide extraction was carried out in a pressure range between 20 and 40 MPa and a temperature range between 40 and 80 °C. Ethanol and methanol were used as modifier solvents, of which ethanol was found to be more suitable for the elution and pretreatment process. The authors recognized that the amount of lutein in the extract increased with pressure but decreased with extraction temperature. The amount of lutein in the extract was significantly enhanced at an entrainer flow rate up to 0.4 ml min^{-1}, reaching a maximum at around 53±0.01%. Increasing the ethanol flow rate further to 0.5 ml min^{-1} reduced the amount of lutein. Moreover, using ethanol as modifier, the amount of lutein in the extract increased 28 times, compared to CO_2 extraction without entrainer. Ethanol was found to enhance the polar characteristics of the solvent, resulting in an enhancement of lutein solubility. The presence of the ethanol entrainer significantly improved the solubility, but it could be seen that a very high amount of modifier limited the mass transfer diffusion. In some cases, a two-phase system was observed (liquid and supercritical fluid), resulting in a lower amount of lutein in the extract. The highest recovery percentage and the selectivity of lutein were around 52.9±0.02% and 43.1±0.02%, respectively, obtained from supercritical carbon dioxide extraction with pretreatment and ethanol as entrainer at 40 MPa and 40 °C.

Carotenoids from the microalgae *Spirulina maxima* were obtained with CO_2 supercritical fluid extraction [68]. The effects of pressure and temperature on the yield and chemical composition of the extracts were studied. The experiments were conducted at temperatures of 20–70 °C and pressures of 15–180 bar. The solvent mass flow rate was 3.33×10^{-5} kg s^{-1}. Statistical analysis showed that neither the temperature nor the pressure significantly influenced the total carotenoid yield, but both the temperature and the pressure affected the extraction rate, and the effect of the temperature prevailed over that of the pressure. Generally, the extracts contained comparatively high amounts of fatty acids and carotenes, but at 100 bar and 45 °C the extract contained no carotenes. As expected, process temperatures higher than 50 °C degraded the carotenes significantly.

Pu *et al.* [69] extracted astaxanthin with flaxseed oil (FO) from shrimp (*Litopenaeus setiferus*) by-products. In this context, they determined the kinetics of flaxseed oil oxidation containing different amounts of astaxanthin (FAO) and degradation substances of this carotenoid compound. Furthermore, they determined the individual content of free fatty acids, peroxide value, fatty acid methyl ester profiles, and color. The amount of extractable astaxanthin in the shrimp by-products was 4.83 mg 100 g^{-1} of shrimp waste. A similar α-linolenic content has been analyzed in FOA and FO samples, but the oxidation rate of FOA samples was lower compared to that of FO. When FO and FOA were heated to 30 °C, both oils exhibited minimal lipid oxidation with increasing heating time, whereas FO, when heated to 40, 50, and 60 °C, had a higher lipid oxidation rate than FOA with increasing heating time from 0 to 4 h. Therefore, astaxanthin showed clearly effective antioxidant properties in flaxseed oil when it was heated from 40 to 60 °C. The rate of astaxanthin degradation in FOA samples was significantly influenced by temperature. Both FO and FOA showed minimal lipid oxidation at 30 °C with increasing time, whereas FO had a higher oxidation at 40–60 °C than FOA with increasing heating time from 0 to 4 h. The authors were able to demonstrate that astaxanthin could effectively reduce lipid oxidation in FO when it is heated from 40 to 60 °C. The degradation of astaxanthin during heating was successfully described by first-order reaction kinetics. Astaxanthin was stable in FOA at 30 and 40 °C, but had substantial degradation at 50 and 60 °C. Finally, the authors point out that by-products generated from the shrimp-peeling process are a good source to obtain high-quality astaxanthin, which can be used as a natural colorant and antioxidant ingredient in human food and other industrial applications.

In a similar approach, Mezzomo *et al.* [70] used residues of pink shrimp (*Penaeus brasiliensis* and *Penaeus paulensis*) waste as raw material to obtain carotenoid-enriched extracts. They investigated different pretreatments and extraction methods such as Soxhlet, maceration, and ultrasound. Different organic solvents and even vegetable oil have been applied as extraction solvents. Cooking associated with milling and drying provided the extracts richest in the carotenoid fraction. The extracts were evaluated in terms of yield, individual carotenoid profile, total carotenoid content, UV-visible scanning spectrophotometry, and mid-Fourier transform infrared spectroscopy. The authors demonstrate that shrimp waste can provide carotenoid-enriched extracts, containing particularly astaxanthin, in concentrations up to 252 g astaxanthin g^{-1} extract. For maceration, the most appropriate solvents were acetone and a mixture of hexane and isopropanol (50:50, v/v).

Recently, Almahy *et al.* [71] developed a solid–liquid extraction technique for leaching natural colorants from plant materials for applications in plant research applying boiling and solvent extraction. They used water, methanol, and acidified methanol as solvent to extract the carotenoid fraction from carrot and studied the influence of ultrasound on the yield of the individual natural substances in comparison with a magnetic stirring process as control. It was found that the application of ultrasound-assisted extraction can increase the yield of dyes from different parts of various plant resources. The reason for the improvement could be due to better leaching of natural dye materials from plant cell membranes and mass transfer to the solvent, supported by ultrasound. The results indicate that there is about 12–100% improvement in yield of extract obtained due to the use of ultrasound as compared to magnetic stirring at 45 °C. The authors assumed that this novel technique can be employed effectively for the extraction of pigments from various plant resources, and they recommended the process as an eco-friendly method in the current situation of global environmental concern.

In recent years, research into the application of enzymatic treatments in vegetable matrices to obtain the release of valuable plant substances has increased remarkably [72]. It has been shown that the application of enzymatic treatments in carrot and dried pumpkin improves the attractiveness of dehydrated products. Usually, the disintegration of the cell wall structure accelerates metabolic changes, forming undesirable colors and flavor substances. But this is not observed in enzymatically treated vegetable matrices, because here the carotenoids released from cellular structures by pectinase and cellulase are still bound to proteins so they keep their state, which provides stability to the highly unsaturated pigment structure. In this context, it also has been observed that the use of enzyme mixtures generated from cultures of microorganisms can reduce the processing time dramatically when compared to treatments in which commercial enzymes are used. Therefore, enzymatic treatments as an alternative approach in the extraction process also have been used by Barzana *et al.* [73]: prior to the use of solvents, they applied different pretreatments to the plant matrix to increase cell wall permeability, facilitating the mechanisms of diffusion and mass exchange between the immiscible phases during the leaching process. They found a clear correlation between these applications of enzymatic pretreatment and the extraction yield of carotenoids. Several of their experiments showed that complex substrates were hydrolyzed under a combination of different enzymes. The authors mentioned in this context that the use of raw enzymes has some advantages over the use of commercial enzymes because of their cost-effectiveness rate and a substantial reduction in processing time. In industrial processes, some microorganisms are known for their production of cellulolytic enzymes, like *A. terreus* with an enzyme activity of 0.688 U mg^{-1} of protein [74]. *Aspergillus niger* is considered as one of the most complete multienzyme producers to produce cellulases, hemicellulases, glucoamylases, and pectinases, showing enzymatic activities of 0.99, 15.86, 13.37, and 7.62 U mg^{-1} of protein, respectively [75]. For the described enzymatic treatments, water has been identified as the most appropriate solvent; however, although it allows the enzymatic hydrolysis to take place, an excess of this solvent can slow the extraction process because it may prevent the necessary contact with the vesicles of intracellular lipids leading to carotenoids. Generally, a rapid adsorption of the enzyme accelerates the lysis of the cell wall, leading to an increase in the extraction yield. This is why agitation plays an important role in enzymatic treatments [76].

11.5 Conclusions

This chapter presented various options used for the isolation and production of carotenoids from natural sources. Most of the individual studies demonstrate that sample pretreatments performed prior to the extraction process are essential for optimal yield of carotenoids. Furthermore, it becomes clear that a successful extraction is largely influenced by the sample matrix and the carotenoid profile present therein. Beside supercritical CO_2 extraction, other powerful and environmentally friendly technologies (e.g. pressurized liquid extraction, extraction assisted by enzymes, microwave, or ultrasound) also are applied to isolate carotenoids from higher plants, algae, fungi, yeasts, and seafood waste. Generally, more research is needed in the near future to get more accurate knowledge of carotenoid bioavailability from various food materials in order to develop food-based strategies for long-term alleviation of vitamin A deficiency around the world. In this context, environmentally friendly and cheap production of natural carotenoid extracts can make an important contribution to improve the worldwide supply of these bioactive substances.

11.6 Perspectives

In order to obtain more reliable and consistent results regarding carotenoid bioavailability, it will be necessary to improve the existing knowledge, reconsidering the *in vitro* conditions to simulate more precisely both human digestion and absorption in additional accurately designed case studies. Furthermore, integrated approaches would be helpful for identifying the key factors for carotenoid release and absorption from various food matrices. Thus, data received from different surveys could be more easily compared with each other and would be also available for bioavailability studies of other nutrients or evaluations of various food functionalities. Generally, the use of "green" separation techniques such as supercritical CO_2 extraction will further increase in the near future. It also can be assumed that other safe and environmentally friendly organic solvents applicable for isolation of carotenoids from food materials (e.g., ethyl lactate and ethanol) will get more potential for future use in this context. Last but not least, enzymatic pretreatments (e.g., the use of pectinase or cellulase) prior to the application of solvents in vegetable matrices will help to release carotenoids from cellular structures, thus improving the yield of the whole extraction process.

References

1. G. E. Bartley and P. A. Scolnik, "Plant carotenoids: pigments for photoprotectin, visual attraction, and human health," *Plant Cell*, **7**, 1027–38 (1995).
2. O. Montero, M. D. Macias-Sanchez, C. M. Lama, L. M. Lubian, C. Mantell, M. Rodriguez, and E. M. de la Ossa, "Supercritical CO_2 extraction of β-carotene from a marine strain of the cyanobacterium *Synechococcus* species," *J. Agric. Food Chem.*, **53**, 9701–7 (2005).
3. M. D. Macias-Sanchez, C. M. Serrano, M. R. Rodriguez, E. M. de la Ossa, E. M. Lubian, and O. Montero, "Extraction of carotenoids and chlorophyll from microalgae with supercritical carbon dioxide and ethanol as co-solvent," *J. Separation Sci.*, **31**, 1352–62 (2008).
4. G. Britton and F. Khachik, "Carotenoids in food," in G. Britton, S. Liaaen-Jensen, and H.P. Pfander (Eds.), *Carotenoids, nutrition and health*, vol. **5**, Basel: Birkhäuser, 2009, pp. 45–66.
5. M. I. Minguez-Mosquera and D. Hornero-Méndez, "Changes in provitamin A during paprika processing," *J. Food Protect.*, **60**, 853–7 (1997).
6. J. J. M. Castenmiller and C. E. West, "Bioavailability and bioconversion of carotenoids. *Ann. Rev. Nutr.*, **18**, 19–38 (1998).
7. J. C. Bauernfeind, "Carotenoid vitamin A precursors and analogs in foods and feeds," *J. Agric. Food Chem.*, **20**, 456–73 (1972).
8. A. Bonora, S. Pancaldi, R. Gualandri, and M. P. Fasulo, "Carotenoid and ultrastructure variations in plastids of *Arum italicum* Miller fruit during maturation and ripening," *J. Exper. Botany*, **51**, 873–84 (2000).
9. A. L. Vasquez-Caicedo, P. Sruamsiri, R. Carle, and S. Neidhart, "Accumulation of all-*trans*-β-carotene and its 9-*cis* and 13-*cis* stereoisomers during postharvest ripening of nine Thai mango cultivars," *J. Agric. Food Chem.*, **53**, 4827–35 (2005).
10. B. Camara and J. Brangeon, "Carotenoid metabolism during chloroplast to chromoplast transformation in *Capsicum annuum* fruit," *Planta*, **151**, 359–64 (1981).
11. P. D. Fraser and P. M. Bramley, "The biosynthesis and nutritional uses of carotenoids," *Prog. Lipid Res.*, **43**, 228–65 (2004).

12. S. Voutilainen, T. Nurmi, J. Mursu, and T. H. Rissanen, "Carotenoids and cardiovascular health," *Amer. J. Clin. Nutr.,* **83**, 1265–71 (2006).

13. A. V. Rao and S. Agarwal, "Role of lycopene as antioxidant carotenoid in the prevention of chronic diseases: a review," *Nutr. Res.,* **19**, 305–23 (1999).

14. E. Giovannucci, "A review of epidemiologic studies of tomatoes, lycopene, and prostate cancer," *Exper. Biol. Med.*, **227**, 852–9 (2002).

15. R. S. Parker, J. E. Swanson, C. You, A. J. Edwards, and T. Huang, "Bioavailability of carotenoids in human subjects," *Proc. Nutr. Soc.*, **58**, 155–62 (1999).

16. P. Borel, "Factors affecting intestinal absorption of highly lipophilic food microconstituents (fat-soluble vitamins, carotenoids and phytosterols)," *Clin. Chem. Lab. Med.*, **41**, 979–94 (2003).

17. E. H. Harrison, "Mechanisms involved in the intestinal absorption of dietary vitamin A and provitamin A carotenoids," *Biochim. Biophys. Acta*, **1821**, 70–77 (2012).

18. K. H. van het Hof, I. A. Brouwer, C. E. West, E. Haddeman, R. P. Steegers-Theunissen, M. Dusseldorp, J. A. Weststrate, T. K. Eskes, and J. G. Hautvast, "Bioavailability of lutein from vegetables is 5 times higher than that of β-carotene," *Amer. J. Clin. Nutr.*, **70**, 261–8 (1999).

19. D. Kostic, W. S. White, and J. A. Olson, "Intestinal absorption, serum clearance, and interactions between lutein and β-carotene when administered to human adults in separate or combined oral doses," *Amer. J. Clin. Nutr.,* **62**, 604–10 (1995).

20. K. H. van het Hof, C. E. West, J. A. Weststrate, and J. G. Hautvast, "Dietary factors that affect the bioavailability of carotenoids," *J. Nutr.,* **130**, 503–6 (2000).

21. C. L. Rock, J. L. Lovalvo, C. Emenhiser, M. T. Ruffin, S. W. Flatt, and S. J. Schwartz, "Bioavailability of β-carotene is lower in raw than in processed carrots and spinach in women," *J. Nutr.,* **128**, 913–16 (1998).

22. R. M. Schweiggert, C. B. Steingass, A. Heller, P. Esquivel, and R. Carle, "Characterization of chromoplasts and carotenoids of red and yellow fleshed papaya (*Carica papaya* L.)," *Planta,* **234**, 1031–44 (2011).

23. R. M. Schweiggert, R. E. Kopec, M. G. Villalobos-Gutierrez, J. Högel, S. Quesada, P. Esquivel, S. J. Schwartz, and R. Carle, "Carotenoids are more bioavailable from papaya than from tomato and carrot in humans: a randomized cross-over study," *British J. Nutr.,* **111**, 490–8 (2014).

24. R. M. Schweiggert, D. Mezger, F. Schimpf, C. B. Steingass, and R. Carle, "Influence of chromoplast morphology on carotenoid bioaccessibility of carrot, mango, and tomato," *Food Chem.,* **135**, 2736–42 (2012).

25. C. M. Metzler and D. C. Huang, "Statistical methods for bioavailability and bioequivalence," *Clin. Res. Pract. Drug Regul. Affairs*, **1**, 109–32 (1983).

26. W. Stahl, H. van den Berg, J. Arthur, A. Bast, J. Dainty, and R. M. Faulks, *et al.*, "Bioavailability and metabolism," *Mol. Aspects Med.*, **23**, 39–101 (2002).

27. World Health Organization (WHO), "Global prevalence of vitamin A deficiency in populations at risk 1995–2005," in *WHO Global Database on Vitamin A Deficiency*, Geneva: WHO, 2009, pp. 1–19.

28. V. Böhm, "Lycopene and heart health," *Mol. Nutr. Food Res.*, **56**, 296–303 (2012).

29. M. Perrut, "Supercritical fluid applications: Industrial developments and economic issues," *Indian Engin. Chem. Res.,* **39**, 4531–4535 (2000).

30. J. Shi, M. LeMageur, and M. Bryan, "Lycopene from tomatoes," in J. Shi, G. Mazza, and M. LeMageur (Eds.), *Functional foods: biochemical process aspects*, Boca Raton, FL: CRC Press, 2002, pp. 135–67.

31. K. Schiedt and S. Liaaein-Jensen, "Isolation and analysis," in G. Britton, S. Liaaen-Jensen, and H. Pfander (Eds.), *Carotenoids*, vol. 1A, *Isolation and analysis*, Basel: Birkhäuser, 1995, pp. 81–108.
32. F. Khachik, G. R. Beecher, and N. F. Whitaker, "Separation, identification, and quantification of the major carotenoid and chlorophyll constituents in extracts of several green vegetables by liquid chromatography," *J. Agric. Food Chem.*, **34**, 603–16 (1986).
33. A. K. Taungbodhitham, G. P. Jones, M. L. Wahlqvist, and D. R. Briggs, "Evaluation of extraction method for the analysis of carotenoids in fruits and vegetables," *Food Chem.*, **63**, 577–84 (1998).
34. R. E. Wrolstad, T. E. Acree, E. A. Decker, M. H. Penner, D. S. Reid, S. J. Schwartz, C. F. Shoemaker, D. Smith, and P. Sporus (Eds.), *Handbook of food analytical chemistry: pigments, colorants, flavors, texture, and bioactive food components*, Hoboken, NJ: Wiley, 2005.
35. K. Zosel, "Process for recovering caffeine," US3806619, 1974.
36. D. R. J. Laws, N. A. Bath, C. S. Ennis, and A. G. Wheldon, "Hop extraction with carbon dioxide," US4218491, 1980.
37. E. Riggi, C. Patane, and G. Ruberto, "Content of carotenoids at different ripening stages in processing tomato in relation to soil water availability," *Austral. J. Agric. Res.*, **59**, 384–53 (2008).
38. E. Riggi and G. Avola, "Quantification of the waste stream from fresh tomato packing-houses and its fluctuations: implications for waste management planning," *Resources Conserv. Recyc.*, **54**, 436–41 (2010).
39. B. Demmig-Adams and W. W. Adams III, "Antioxidants in photosynthesis and human nutrition," *Science*, **298**, 2149–53 (2002).
40. S. Aparicio, S. Halajian, R. Alcalde, B. Garcia, and J. M. Leal, "Liquid structure of ethyl lactate, pure and water mixed, as seen by dielectric spectroscopy, solvatochromic and thermophysical studies," *Chem. Phys. Lett.*, **454**, 49–55 (2008).
41. A. Chandra and N. G. Nair, "Supercritical fluid carbon dioxide extraction of α- and β-carotene from carrot (*Daucus carota* L.)," *Phytochem. Anal.*, **8**, 244–6 (1997).
42. M. Marx, M. Stuparic, A. Schieber, and R. Carle, "Analytical, nutritional and clinical methods: effects of thermal processing on *trans–cis*-isomerization of β-carotene in carrot juices and carotene-containing preparations," *Food Chem.*, **83**, 609–17 (2003).
43. R. Marsili and D. Callahan, "Comparison of a liquid solvent extraction technique and supercritical fluid extraction for the determination of α- and β-carotene in vegetables," *J. Chromat. Sci.*, **31**, 422–8 (1993).
44. Y. Gao, B. Nagy, X. Liu, B. Simandi, and Q. Wang, "Supercritical CO_2 extraction of lutein esters from marigold (*Tagetes erecta* L.) enhanced by ultrasound," *J. Supercrit. Fluids,* **49**, 345–50 (2009).
45. M. M. Barth, C. Zhou, K. M. Kute, and G. A. Rosenthal, "Determination of optimum conditions for supercritical fluid extraction of carotenoids from carrot (*Daucus carota* L.) tissue," *J. Agric. Food Chem.*, **43**, 2876–8 (1995).
46. J. A. Howe and S. A. Tanumihardjo, "Evaluation of analytical methods for carotenoid extraction from biofortified maize (*Zea mays* sp.)," *J. Agric. Food Chem.*, **54**, 7992–7 (2006).
47. A. C. Kurilich and J. A. Juvik, "Quantification of carotenoid and tocopherol antioxidants in *Zea mays*," *J. Agric. Food Chem.*, **47**, 1948–55 (1999).
48. M. S. G. Gomez-Prieto, M. M. Caja, M. Marta Herraiz, and G. Santa-Maria, "Supercritical fluid extraction of all-*trans*-lycopene from tomato," *J. Agric. Food Chem.*, **51**, 3–7 (2003).

49. T. Baysal, S. Ersus, and D. A. J. Starmans, "Supercritical CO_2 extraction of α-carotene and lycopene from tomato paste waste," *J. Agric. Food Chem.*, **48**, 5507–11 (2000).
50. M. Machmudah, Z. S. Winardi, M. Sasaki, M. Goto, N. Kusumoto, and K. Hayakawa, "Lycopene extraction from tomato peel by-product containing tomato seed using supercritical carbon dioxide," *J. Food Engin.*, **108**, 290–6 (2012).
51. N. L. Rozzi, R. K. Singh, R. A. Vierling, and B. A. Watkins, "Supercritical fluid extraction of lycopene from tomato processing byproducts," *J. Agric. Food Chem.*, **50**, 2638–43 (2002).
52. E. Cadoni, M. R. de Giorgi, E. Medda, and G. Poma, "Supercritical CO_2 extraction of lycopene and β-carotene from ripe tomatoes," *Dyes Pigments*, **44**, 27–32 (2000).
53. K. P. Madavalappil and S. Swaminathan, "Isolation and purification of carotenoids from marigold flowers," AU2006331246, 2006.
54. E. Vagi, B. Simandi, H. G. Daood, A. Deak, and J. Sawinsky, "Recovery of pigments from *Origanum majorana* L. by extraction with supercritical carbon dioxide," *J. Agric. Food Chem.*, **50**, 2297–301 (2002).
55. M. Careri, L. Furlattini, A. Mangiaa, M. Muscia, E. Anklamb, A. Theobaldb, and C. von Holst, "Supercritical fluid extraction for liquid chromatographic determination of carotenoids in *Spirulina pacifica* algae: a chemometric approach," *J. Chromatog. A*, **912**, 61–71 (2001).
56. S. Machmudah, Y. Kawahito, M. Sasaki, and M. Motonobu Goto, "Process optimisation and extraction rate analysis of carotenoids extraction from rosehip fruit using supercritical CO_2," *J. Supercrit. Fluids*, **44**, 308–14 (2008).
57. I. Gamlieli-Bonshtein, E. Korn, and S. Cohen, "Selective separation of *cis-trans* geometrical isomers of β-carotene via CO_2 supercritical fluid extraction," *Biotechnol. Bioengin.*, **80**, 169–74 (2002).
58. A. C. Guedes, M. S. Gião, A. A. Matias, A. V. M. Nunes, M. E. Pintado, C. M. M. Duarte, and F. X. Malcata, "Supercritical fluid extraction of carotenoids and chlorophylls a, b and c," *J. Food Engin.*, **116**, 478–82 (2013).
59. B. K. Ishida and M. H. Chapman, "Carotenoid extraction from plants using a novel, environmentally friendly solvent," *J. Agric. Food Chem.*, **57**, 1051–9 (2009).
60. M. Kawaragi, T. Kuraishi, H. Shirasawa, N. Takada, N. Takada, Y. Katsumi, and S. Kojima, "Method for collecting tomato pigment and its application," US5871574, 1999.
61. M. Zelkha, M. Ben-Yehuda, D. Hartal, Y. Raveh, and N. Garti, "Industrial processing of tomatoes and product thereof," US5837311, 1998.
62. W. Wu, M. Lu, and L. Yu, "A new environmentally friendly method for astaxanthin extraction from *Xanthophyllomyces dendrorhous*," *Euro. Food Res. Technol.*, **232**, 463–7 (2011).
63. J. Liu, H. Wu, C. Zhao, Y. Xiao, M. Zhou, and X. Liu, "Determination of astaxanthin in *Haematococcus pluvialis* by first-order derivative spectrophotometry," *AOAC Int.*, **94**, 1752–61 (2011).
64. K. Song, C. Kwang, S. Dae, C. Donghwa, and P. Cheol, "Optimization of pressurized liquid extraction of zeaxanthin from *Chlorella ellipsoidea*," *J. Appl. Phycol.*, **24**, 725–30 (2012).
65. A. Mustafa, L. Mijangos, and C. Turner, "Pressurized hot ethanol extraction of carotenoids from carrot by-products," *Molecules*, **17**, 1809–18 (2012).
66. R. L. Mendes, H. L. Fernandes, J. P. Coelho, E. C. Reis, J. M. S. Cabral, J. M. Novais, and A. F. Palavra, "Supercritical CO_2 extraction of carotenoids and other lipids from *Chlorella vulgaris*," *Food Chem.*, **53**, 99–103 (1995).

67. D. Ruen-ngam, A. Shotipruk, P. Pavasant, S. Machmudah, and M. Goto, "Selective extraction of lutein from alcohol treated *Chlorella vulgaris* by supercritical CO_2," *Chem. Engin. Tech.*, **35**, 255–60 (2012).

68. A. P. R. F. Canela, P. T. V. Rosa, M. O. M. Marques, M. Angela, and A. Meireles, "Supercritical fluid extraction of fatty acids and carotenoids from the microalgae *Spirulina maxima*," *Indian Engin. Chem. Res.*, **41**, 3012–18 (2002).

69. J. Pu, P. J. Bechtel, and S. Sathivel, "Extraction of shrimp astaxanthin with flaxseed oil: Effects on lipid oxidation and astaxanthin degradation rates," *Biosys. Engin.*, **107**, 364–71 (2010).

70. N. Mezzomo, B. Maestri, R. Lazzaris dos Santos, M. Maraschin, R. S. Sandra, and S. R. S. Ferreira, "Pink shrimp (*P. brasiliensis* and *P. paulensis*) residue: influence of extraction method on carotenoid concentration," *Talanta*, **85**, 1383–91 (2011).

71. H. A. Almahy, M. A. Ali, and A. A. Ali, "Extraction of carotenoids as natural dyes from the *Daucus carota* L. (carrot) using ultrasound in Kingdom of Saudi Arabia," *Res. J. Chem. Sci.*, **3**, 63–66 (2013).

72. D. Konopacka, "The effect of enzymatic treatment on dried vegetable color," *Drying Tech.*, **24**, 1173–8 (2006).

73. E. Barzana, D. Rubio, I. R. Santamaria, O. Garcia, F. Garcia, V. E. Ridaura, and A. Lopez, "Enzyme-mediated solvent extraction of carotenoids from marigold flower *(Tagetes erecta)*," *J. Agric. Food Chem.*, **50**, 4491–6 (2002).

74. S. Y. Mirzaakhmedov, Z. F. Ziyavitdinov, Z. R. Akhmedova, A. B. Saliev, D. T. Ruzmetova, K. B. Ashurov, D. Fessas, and S. Iametti, "Isolation, purication and enzymatic activity of cellulase components," *Chem. Natural Comp.*, **43**, 594–7 (2007).

75. J. Wang, G. Bai, and X. Liang, "Optimization of multienzyme production by two mixed strains in solid-state fermentation," *Appl. Microb. Biotechn.*, **73**, 533–40 (2006).

76. J. L. Navarrete-Bolaños, H. Jiménez-Islas, E. Botello-Alvarez, R. Rico-Martínez, and O. Paredes-López, "Improving xanthophyll extraction from marigold flower using cellulolytic enzymes," *J Agric Food Chem.*, **52**, 11, 3394–8 (2004).

77. E. Riggi, "Recent patents on the extraction of carotenoids," *Rec. Patents Food, Nutr. Agric.*, **2**, 75–82 (2010).

78. B. S. Engelhardt, S. P. Adu-Peasah, C. M. Ruecker, and G. T. Veeder, "Solventless extraction process," CA2397655, 2001.

79. S. Lee Hyoung and G. A. Coates, "Separating juice from pulp of grapefruit using aqueous solution; slurrying; ultrafiltration," US2003091704, 2003.

80. M. Hoffman, D. Baugh, M. Ahern, and D. Walsh, "Pigment extraction system and method," US2004176475, 2004.

81. M. Kagan and S. Braun, "Process for extracting carotenoids and for preparing feed materials," CA2395319, 2001.

82. J. H. Wolf, M. Sibeijn, and A. Schaap, "Isolation of carotenoid crystals," CA2396167, 2001.

83. M. Zelkha and T. Sedlov, "Carotenoid extraction process," US2003044499, 2003.

84. V. O. Postoienko, O. M. Postoienko, A. L. Boiko, and M. Y. Kucherenko, "Method for producing carotenoid concentrate from green mass of plant material," UA73556, 2004.

85. M. R. Rusnack and S. D. Allen, "Process for extracting carotenoids from fruit and vegetable processing waste," AU2004287701, 2004.

86. V. A. E. Mukhin, V. J. E. Novikov, L. A. Shapovalova, and O. A. Sheveleva, "Method for production of fat-soluble carotenoid complex from hydrobios and waste," RU22278556, 2006.

87. S. E. Rey, "Production of lycopene enriched antioxidants," ES2241503, 2005.

88. S. Ishikawa, A. Tsubokura, and K. Hirasawa, "Process for production of carotenoids," JP2007319015, 2007.
89. B. K. Ishida, M. H. Chapman, S. S. Randhava, and S. S. Randhava, "Extraction of carotenoids from plant material," US20097572468, 2009.
90. J. Shi, "Separation of carotenoids from fruits and vegetables," CA2305091, 2001.
91. B. S. Chun and S. G. Hong, "Method for extracting chlorophyll and carotenoid pigments from seaweeds, crustacean, echinodermata using supercritical and subcritical carbon dioxides with entrainer," KR20020000660, 2002.
92. S. E. Rey, R. A. Gonzales, G. J. F. Gonzalez, C. F. J. Gomez, B. M. J. Garcia, and M. V. De Espinosa Tena, "Method of preparing lycopene-enriched formulations that are free of organic solvents, formulations thus obtained, compositions comprising said formulations and use of the same," AU2369002, 2002.
93. A. D. Mackenzie, J. B. Grey, and O. J. Catchpole, "Extraction process for separation of lipophilic compounds from urea-containing solutions," CA2483191, 2003.
94. L. B. Crombie, "Supercritical fluid extraction, two different pressures; separates beta-carotene and lutein," US20046737552, 2004.
95. G. Brewer, "A process and apparatus for modifying plant extracts," AU2004246728, 2004.
96. F. Temelli and M. Sun, "Supercritical carbon dioxide extraction of carotenoids from natural materials using a continuous co-solvent," US2005266132, 2005.
97. C. Zhen, Y. Mingde, D. Jie, W. Yulong, H. Husheng, and L. Ji, "Method of extracting carotenoid and edible glycerol from *Dunaliella salina*," CN101107991, 2008.
98. H. Schonemann, A. Gudinas, K. Williams, P. Wetmore, and V. Krukonis, "Method for extraction and concentration of carotenoids using supercritical fluids," US2008146851, 2008.
99. Z. Mingqin and L. Jinxia, "Method for extracting carotinoid from tobacco leaf by overcritical CO_2 and application of the carotinoid in perfuming cigarette," CN101209985, 2008.
100. B. J. Waibel, W. C. Morton, and S. M. Cope, "Dense gas means for extraction of a solute from solids," US2008251454, 2008.
101. P. M. Nielsen, "Procédés de traitement de matière crustacée," CA2421820, 2002.
102. A. Levy, J. Kanner, and R. Granit, "Increasing bioavailability of carotenoids," CA2448125, 2002.

12

Carotenoid Production by Bacteria, Microalgae, and Fungi

Ralf Martin Schweiggert and Reinhold Carle

Institute of Food Science and Biotechnology, Hohenheim University, Stuttgart, Germany

12.1 Introduction

Carotenoids represent an important group of natural pigments throughout all biological kingdoms, and they play essential roles in photoprotection, light harvesting, pollinator attraction, and species-specific coloration. Besides their ultraviolet (UV) irradiation and visible-light absorbing properties, a number of highly important biological functions have been associated with their antioxidant properties, their role in the biosynthesis of hormones, and their function as direct precursors of vitamin A [1]. Although the beneficial health properties of several carotenoids (e.g., β-carotene) as provitamin A and photoprotective agents are widely accepted [1, 2], further potential health effects are the subject of current investigations. For instance, the carotenoid lycopene, the red pigment of tomato fruits, is among the most powerful known natural antioxidants. Because the consumption of lycopene-rich foods has been associated with a 30–40% reduction in prostate cancer [3], a causal relationship to lycopene is discussed [4], in particular because it was found in biologically active concentrations in the human prostate [5]. Similarly, the carotenoids lutein and zeaxanthin are found in circa 500-fold higher concentrations in the macula lutea of the human retina than in other tissues. Moreover, lutein and zeaxanthin account for 66–77% of the total carotenoids in human brain tissue [6]. Supported by epidemiological trials, the frequent intake of lutein and zeaxanthin has therefore been associated with a reduced risk of age-related degenerative diseases, such as macular degeneration, cataract, and the decline of cognitive functions in the elderly [6, 7].

Besides health-related aspects, carotenoids are widely applied by the food industry as coloring foodstuffs. For this purpose, the commercially most important carotenoids are β-carotene and astaxanthin. β-carotene adds color to beverages, dairy products,

Carotenoids: Nutrition, Analysis and Technology, First Edition. Edited by Agnieszka Kaczor and Malgorzata Baranska.

confectionery, and many other commodities, whereas astaxanthin is widely applied as feed additive in salmon and trout aquacultures as well as in chicken and quail farming. Carotenoids are valued as feed additives to improve and standardize the color of flesh and egg yolks [8]. In total, food, feed, and pharmaceutical companies achieve significant sales with carotenoids, which are estimated at a total market volume of $786 million [9]. Although only a few carotenoids are commercially applied, over 600 different, naturally occurring carotenoids are known to date, and the highest diversity can be found among microorganisms. Beyond the as-yet-unknown functions of such microbial carotenoids, their biotechnological production holds enormous potential due to rapid microbial growth rates and extremely high carotenoid concentrations, creating serious competition with carotenoids from chemical synthesis or extraction from plant materials. For better understanding of their enormous potential, biosynthesis of microbial carotenoids will be outlined in this chapter, and information on particularly carotenoid-rich microorganisms will be subsequently reviewed. In the final section, modern biotechnological processes for the production of the most important carotenoids (β-carotene, astaxanthin, lutein, zeaxanthin, and lycopene) will be described.

12.2 Microbial biosynthesis of carotenoids

More than 100 million tons of carotenoids are annually biosynthesized and found in an enormous diversity of organisms across all biological kingdoms [10]. Although animals are unable to biosynthesize carotenoids and derive them from their diet, a variety of carotenoids is biosynthesized by higher plants, which use carotenoids for photosynthesis, photoprotection, and pollinator attraction. However, although less obvious, the highest diversity of carotenoids is biosynthesized by algae, yeasts, fungi, and bacteria, including extremophilic archaea as well as non-photosynthetic and photosynthetic eubacteria. Investigations into the gene clusters of bacteria from the genera *Pantoea* (syn. *Erwinia*) and *Myxococcus* were of utmost importance for an understanding of carotenoid biosynthesis in general [11]. However, the most prominent representatives of carotenogenic microorganisms are presumably the cyanobacteria. According to the endosymbiotic theory, the biosynthetic capability of an ancient cyanobacterial species has been transferred to algae and plants by their "immigration" into the respective eukaryotic cell. Subsequent extensive gene transfers and metabolic interactions led to a close and vital association of the endosymbiont to the host organism. The resulting cellular organelles were the plastids, such as chloroplasts of higher plants. These organelles are surrounded by membranes, contain their own DNA, and segregate by cell division similar to their bacterial ancestors [12]. Therefore, carotenogenic genes from plants, algae, and cyanobacteria often show high homology, and large genetic dissimilarities to genes of bacteria and fungi are frequently observed [10].

In general, biosynthesis of all carotenoids follows the isoprenoid biosynthetic pathway. Isoprenoid compounds are biosynthesized from the basic C_5-elements isopentenyl diphosphate (IDP) and its isomer, dimethylallyl diphosphate (DMADP). For a long time, the mevalonate pathway was considered to be the only route to IDP and DMADP and, thus, for all isoprenoid compounds in all living organisms. IPP biosynthesis starts with acetyl-CoA to yield mevalonic acid (MVA), which then is phosphorylated, decarboxylated, and dehydrated to IDP and DMADP (Figure 12.1A).

Investigations of this pathway were mostly conducted with noncarotenogenic organisms like yeasts and mammalian liver, focusing on the elucidation of sterol biosynthesis. Later, similar work was conducted with carotenogenic organisms, confirming that the

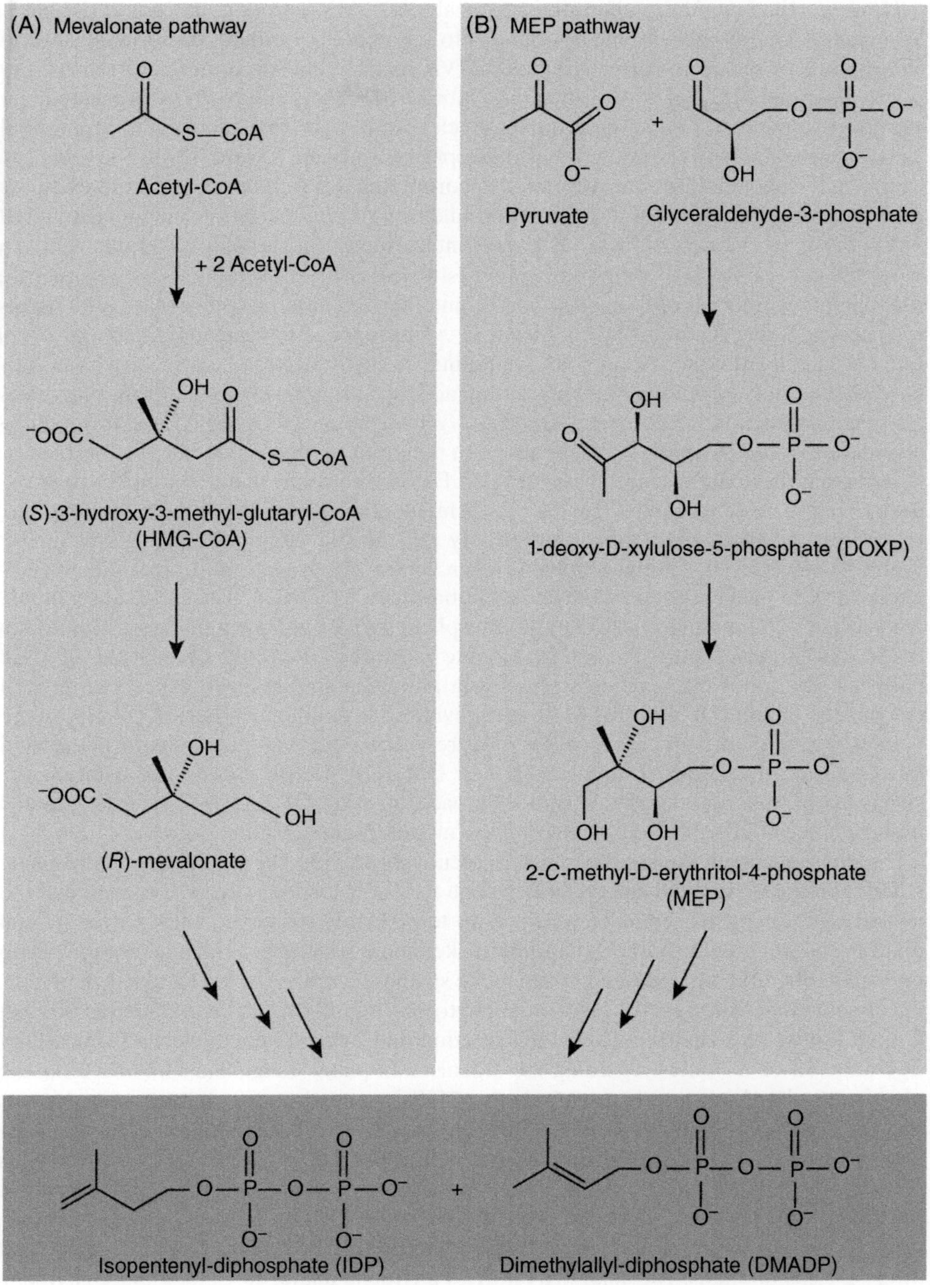

Figure 12.1 Biosynthetic pathways to IDP and DMADP.

same pathway was feeding carotenoid biosynthesis. For instance, isotopically labeled acetate proved to be an efficient precursor of β-carotene in the molds *Phycomyces blakesleanus* and *Mucor hiermalis*, in the protist *Euglena gracilis*, and in carrot root (*Daucus carota* L.) [10].

However, the first doubts about the universal role of MVA arose as early as in the 1950s. Whereas $^{14}CO_2$ was heavily incorporated into carotenoids in many bacteria, algae, and chloroplasts of plants, isotopically labeled MVA and acetate were not or were only very poorly integrated [13, 14]. At the same time, labeled MVA was efficiently incorporated into sterols, triterpenoids, and sesquiterpenes. Such results were first ascribed to a potential lack of permeability of the bacterial or chloroplast membrane toward MVA. Nevertheless, isotopically labeled IDP was very well incorporated into chloroplast carotenoids. As a consequence of these and other contradictory results, an MVA-independent IDP biosynthesis in chloroplasts was proposed. Interestingly, this second metabolic route to biosynthesize isoprenoid compounds was first discovered in bacteria and, subsequently, found in plant embryos of *Gingko biloba* L., and then in numerous other plants and bacterial species. Today, the non-MVA pathway is even proposed to represent the major route to carotenoids and other isoprenoid compounds in many bacteria, particularly in cyanobacteria and in chloroplasts of plants and algae [10]. It is noteworthy that this pathway is also essential to pathogenic eubacteria (e.g., *Mycobacterium tuberculosis*), and the detailed elucidation of this biosynthetic route has great potential for the development of new drugs, in particular due to its absence in humans [15]. Furthermore, knowledge about this pathway has proved to be a prerequisite for successful metabolic engineering of the isoprenoid flux toward an enhanced carotenoid productivity [16]. In the nonmevalonate pathway, IPP synthesis starts by the initial condensation reaction of pyruvate and glyceraldehyde-3-phosphate to yield 1-deoxy-D-xylulose-5-phosphate (DOXP), which is subsequently converted to 2-*C*-methyl-D-erythritol-4-phosphate (MEP), as shown in Figure 12.1B. Due to these two intermediates, the nonmevalonate pathway is often called the DOXP or MEP pathway. The following reaction steps and in particular the involved genes and derived enzymes to obtain IDP and DMADP were reviewed in detail recently [15].

Irrespective of the metabolic route, IDP represents the key precursor of carotenoid biosynthesis. After isomerization of IDP to DMADP, prenyl transferases catalyze the subsequent condensation of one molecule each of DMADP and IDP to form geranyl diphosphate (GDP), the C_{10}-precursor of the monoterpenes (Figure 12.2A).

The subsequent addition of IDP units consecutively provides the C_{15}-farnesyl diphosphate (FDP) and the C_{20}-geranylgeranyl diphosphate (GGDP), respectively. GGDP synthase and its corresponding gene sequence were shown to be highly conserved among bacteria and plants. Subsequently, the basic C_{40} carotenoid skeleton is synthesized by condensation of two molecules of GGDP as catalyzed by phytoene synthase (crtB in bacteria and Psy in plants), yielding the first, colorless C_{40}-carotenoid phytoene (Fig. 12.2A). A central double bond at C15,15′ is introduced in the course of this reaction, and, interestingly, its stereochemical configuration (*Z* or *E*) varies regarding the organism. In plants, fungi, and some bacteria, the phytoene isolated was mostly or entirely the (15*Z*)-isomer, although all further carotenoids had the (15*E*)-configuration. In some bacteria such as *Mycobacterium* and *Halobacterium* species as well as *Cellulomonas dehydrogenans*, the phytoene predominantly occurred in its (*all-E*) form. Although GGDP is the direct precursor of phytoene and, thus, that of the most common C_{40} carotenoids, FDP represents the substrate for an analogous series of rare C_{30} carotenoids found in non-phototrophic bacteria (e.g., in *Staphylococcus aureus* and *Streptococcus faecium*). The similarly colorless phytoene-analogon C_{30}-4,4′-diapophytoene (dehydrosqualene) is derived from two molecules of FDP. Subsequently, desaturation reactions of phytoene and dehydrosqualene lead to the consecutive formation of colored derivatives, namely, phytofluene, ζ-carotene, neurosporene, and lycopene (common C_{40} pathway) and 4,4′diapophytofluene, 4,4′diapo-ζ-carotene, 4,4′diapo-neurosporene, and 4,4′diapo-lycopene (C_{30} pathway in bacteria; Figure 12.2B), respectively.

A variety of C_{45}- and C_{50}-carotenoids was found in some Gram-positive Eubacteria and Archaea. They are biosynthesized by the normal C_{40}-carotenoid pathway, and the additional

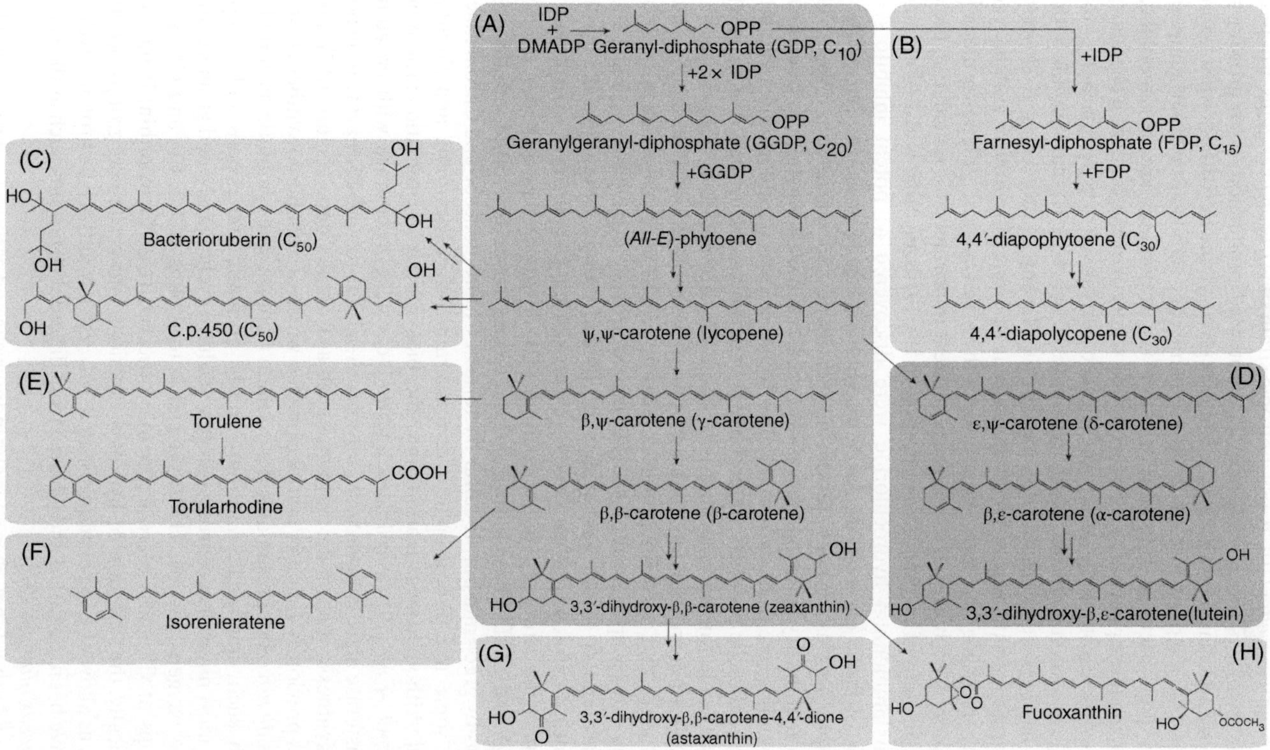

Figure 12.2 Major biosynthetic routes to carotenoids in microorganisms.

introduction of C_5-units occurs at a later stage, such as during the cyclization of lycopene (see Figure 12.2C). The most prominent examples are bacterioruberin, its derivatives from the *Halobacterium* and *Arthrobacter* species, and the "C.p. 450" from *Curtobacterium flaccumfaciens* pvar. *poinsettia* [10]. A psychotropic strain of *Arthrobacter agilis*, isolated from the Antarctic sea ice, showed increased C_{50}-carotenoid production when growing at low temperatures. Particularly, bacterioruberin and its glycosylated derivatives were assumed to enhance their cold adaption by contributing to membrane stabilization at low temperatures. By analogy, other bacteria containing C_{45}- and C_{50}-carotenoids are extremophilic, most likely producing these pigments to cope with their respective environmental challenges [17].

Besides acyclic carotenoids, mono- and dicyclic derivatives of particularly C_{40}- but also C_{45}- and C_{50}-carotenoids are frequently encountered, whereas C_{30}-carotenoids with cyclic end groups have not been described in nature [10]. Recently, however, an *Escherichia coli* strain was equipped with genes for 4,4′-diapo-neurosporene biosynthesis and the lycopene cyclase crtY, producing detectable quantities of the novel cyclic C_{30}-diapo-torulene [18].

Investigations with bacterial strains were of great importance for elucidating the mechanism of cyclization of carotenoid end groups. In the 1970s, nicotine and 2-(4-chlorophenylthio)triethylammonium hydrochloride were discovered as potent inhibitors of the biosynthesis of cyclic carotenoids. After nicotine treatment of a *Mycobacterium* and a *Flavobacterium* species normally producing β-carotene and zeaxanthin, respectively, the accumulation of the acyclic lycopene was observed. When washing the cells free of nicotine and resuspending them in growth media, lycopene was readily converted into the corresponding dicyclic products. Later, further experiments confirmed that lycopene was the major substrate for the biosynthesis of cyclic C_{40}-carotenoids [10]. Such inhibitors of lycopene cyclization are used for commercial lycopene production by the fungus *Blakeslea trispora*, a fungus that normally produces β-carotene. The chemical mechanism proposed for lycopene end-group cyclization leads to the three basic ring types: β, γ, and ε. The most common carotenoids of the human diet are β- and ε-ring carotenoids like β-carotene (β,β-carotene), α-carotene (β,ε-carotene), β-cryptoxanthin (3-hydroxy-β,β-carotene), lutein (3,3′-dihydroxy-β,ε-carotene), and zeaxanthin (3,3′-dihydroxy-β,β-carotene), as shown in Figure 12.2A and 12.2D. These basic β-, γ-, and ε-rings can be converted into the aromatic ϕ and χ rings by green and purple sulfur bacteria of Chlorobioaceae and Chromatiaceae as well as by some non-phototrophic *Brevibacterium*, *Mycobacterium*, and *Streptomyces* species [10]. Although investigations into the biosynthesis of aromatic carotenoids are scarce, Krügel *et al.* [19] described a unique β-carotene desaturase with an additional methyl transferase activity from *Streptomyces griseus*. The described enzyme is responsible for the biosynthesis of aromatic carotenes such as isorenieratene (Figure 12.2F); isorenieratene was previously found in marine sponges, which are unable to synthesize aromatic carotenoids *de novo* but presumably derive them from specific symbiotic bacteria [20].

Although such monocyclic and, particularly, aromatic end groups rather represent exceptions, most naturally occurring carotenoids have cyclic β and ε end groups containing at least one oxygen function. Hydroxyl and keto groups at C2, C3, and C4 as well as epoxy groups at C5 and C6 are frequently observed (e.g., fucoxanthin; Figure 12.2H). Biosynthetically, the insertion of hydroxyl functions into cyclic end groups occurs after cyclization, as shown by experiments with a *Flavobacterium* [21]. β-carotene hydroxylase enzymes have been identified and isolated from different organisms, such as the green alga *Haematococcus pluvialis* [22].

In yeasts and other fungi, characteristic monocyclic and carboxylic carotenoids like torulene and torularhodin are frequently encountered. In *Rhodotorula* species, the biosynthetic monocyclization of lycopene results in the formation of γ-carotene, which is subsequently desaturated to torulene. Torulene is hydroxylated and oxidized by a mixed-function oxidase to yield the carboxylic torularhodin (Figure 12.2E). In *Xanthophyllomyces* species (= sexual state of *Phaffia*), the γ-carotene is transformed to β-carotene and, via other intermediates, to their major pigment astaxanthin, as shown in Figure 12.2G [23]. The production of astaxanthin, the commercially second most important carotenoid, by these *Xanthophyllomyces* and *Haematococcus* species is described below. A number of excellent reviews about the extensive knowledge on carotenoid biosynthesis is available for further information elsewhere [10–12, 24–26].

12.3 Carotenoid-rich microorganisms

12.3.1 Microalgae

Although the estimated number of existing microalgae species ranges from 200,000 to 800,000, only about 35,000 species of microalgae have so far been described [27]. Microscopically small representatives (microalgae) were described within all algal classes [28]. Prior to polymerase chain reaction and next-generation sequencing techniques, the characterization of carotenoids and their biosynthetic intermediates has been used for their chemosystematic classification [28, 29], although their extreme diversity substantially complicated this attempt.

In general, carotenoid biosynthesis in algae occurs in plastids, evolutionarily representing reduced cyanobacteria according to the widely accepted endosymbiotic theory. Such "primary plastids" are found in the diverse groups of green and red algae as well as the small group of glaucophytes. The photosynthetically active plastids of the microscopic glaucophytes (Glaucophyta) contain chlorophyll *a*, several carotenoids, and highly characteristic relics of a peptidoglycan wall, which are very similar to the peptidoglycan of their suggested cyanobacterial ancestors. About 5000–6000 species of red algae (Rhodophyta) are known today, ranging from coccoid nonflagellated cells to multicellular and large marine algae. Characteristic components of red algae plastids are chlorophyll *a*, several carotenoids, and light-harvesting phycobiliproteins containing the accessory pigment phycoerythrin. The green algae (Chlorophyta and Charophyta) are a similarly diverse group that are abundantly encountered in marine and freshwater environments. Their plastids are highly similar to those of land plants and other members of the Chloroplastida group. These plastids contain chlorophyll *a* and *b*, and several carotenoids highly similar to those found in green parts of land plants, but they lack the red algae–specific phycobiliproteins. Although there has been some controversy, phylogenetic studies have shown that the above-mentioned three groups were monophyletic, and the current scientific consensus is that an ancient cyanobacterium was taken up by an eukaryotic ancestor during a single endosymbiotic event. The endosymbiont was genetically reduced and integrated into its host and, subsequently, the above-described three major lineages of Archaeplastida (Glaucophyta, Rhodophyta, and Chloroplastida) evolved. Plastids from the majority of today's eukaryotes are related to this origin [30]. The photosynthetic amoeboid *Paulinella chromatophora* is a still controversially discussed exception, which was just recently shown to have taken on a different cyanobacterium as an endosymbiont [31].

The uptake and retention of a primary algal cell by another eukaryotic lineage are called a *secondary endosymbiotic event*. This process has led to a large diversity of plastids among numerous algal lineages. For instance, chlorarachniophytes and euglenids acquired secondary plastids from at least two different green algal lineages. Haptophytes, cryptomonads, heterokonts, dinoflagellates, and apicomplexans acquired secondary plastids from different red algal lineages. Highlighting the importance of this secondary endosymbiotic event, over 50 percent of the presently described protist species are estimated to contain secondary red algal plastids [30].

In addition to secondary endosymbiotic events, a subsequent plastid loss or the transformation of photosynthetic plastids to cryptic non-photosynthetic plastids occurred in many heterotrophic lineages. An even more complex evolutionary history was revealed in dinoflagellates (Dinophyta), a large group of partly photosynthetic flagellated protists. Dinoflagellates are found among marine plankton but also in freshwater environments, and a few species are known to have acquired plastids by the uptake of a red algal lineage, which already contained a secondary plastid [30]. Little information is available about such tertiary plastids and, particularly, their causal relationship to the biosynthesis of the typical dinoflagellate carotenoids. For instance, dinoflagellates of the *Peridinium* genus produce the unique C_{37}-carotenoid peridinin (Figure 12.3) as a primary pigment, and their tertiary endosymbiont was shown to be of unusual Chrysophyceaen algal origin [32].

In contrast, the dinoflagellate *Karenia* spp. were shown to contain the similarly unique carotenoid gyroxanthin (Figure 12.3) as well as several characteristic fucoxanthin derivatives.

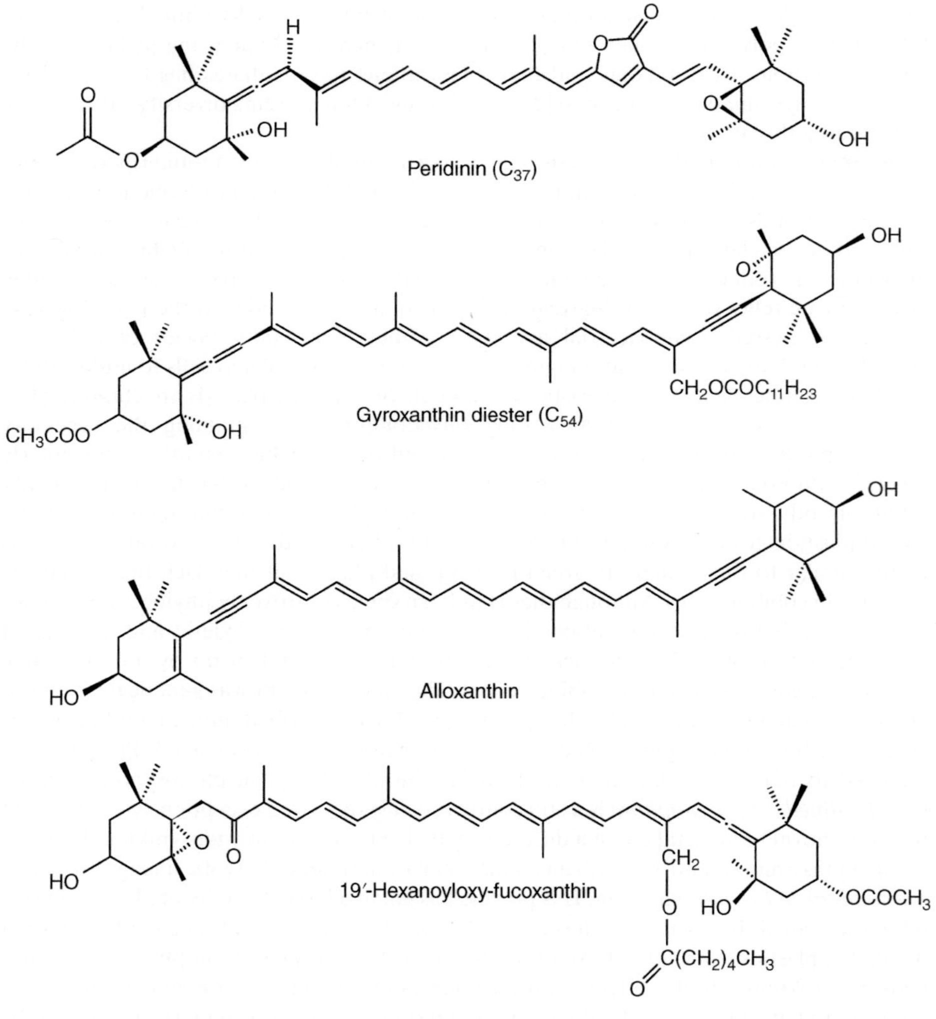

Figure 12.3 Unique carotenoids in microalgae.

Their endosymbiont was shown to be of a prymnesiophyceaen algal origin. Therefore, the unique gyroxanthin diester was used as an early marker of harmful *Karenia brevis* outbreaks, the so-called Florida red tides. Such dinoflagellates produce large amounts of brevetoxins with deleterious effects on commercial-aquacultural fisheries and public health, and, thus, an early detection of its outbreaks proved to be most helpful [33].

Other characteristic carotenoids are exclusively found in algae. The distribution of carotenoids and chlorophylls in algae was previously compiled by Takaichi [34]. For instance, the alleneic (C=C=C) carotenoid fucoxanthin is only found in brown algae and other heterokonts (Heterokontophyta), and 19′-acyloxy-fucoxanthin derivatives such as 19′-hexanoyloxy-fucoxanthin (Fig. 12.3) are also present in Haptophyta and Dinophyta. These fucoxanthin-containing algae and the Cryptophyta contain chlorophyll *c* as a further characteristic trait. Similarly, acetylenic (C≡C) carotenoids were solely reported in algae. For instance, alloxanthin (Figure 12.3), crocoxanthin, and monadoxanthin are typical pigments of Cryptophyta, and diadinoxanthin and diatoxanthin were described in Heterokontophyta, Haptophyta, Dinophyta, and Euglenophyta [34].

12.3.2 Yeasts and filamentous fungi

In contrast to algae, much fewer yeasts and fungi are known to produce carotenoids. The yeasts of the genera *Rhodotorula*, *Rhodosporidium*, *Sporobolomyces*, and *Xanthophyllomyces* (*Phaffia*) have been studied extensively [35], whereas most work on fungal carotenoids was carried out on *P. blakesleanus*, *B. trispora*, and *Neurospora crassa*. Fungi and yeasts exclusively utilize the classical mevalonate pathway for the biosynthesis of isoprenoid compounds. A characteristic fungal product of this pathway is ergosterol, and the accumulation of carotenoids often depends on the exposure to light [10]. Apart from illumination, carotenoid biosynthesis in several members of the Mucorales was enhanced or initiated during sexual interaction of different mating-type strains. The most prominent and commercially important representative member of the Mucorales is *B. trispora*. The organism was discovered in 1904 by Blakeslee, who made the fundamental observation that zygotes were not formed when the fungus was grown from one spore. Blakeslee showed that two mycelia different in sex are required for sexual reproduction, naming the phenomenon heterothallism and the mycelia (+) and (−) [36]. Furthermore, he noted developing coloration when (+) and (−) mycelia were combined. By analogy to many members of the order Mucorales, the sexual activity of *B. trispora* is accompanied by a substantially increased accumulation of carotenoids. In 1968, van den Ende confirmed the trisporic acids B and C (Figure 12.4) to induce carotenogenesis in *B. trispora*; they are considered "sex hormones", as they also induce the formation of gametangia in *Mucor mucedo*. The quantities of carotenoids obtained after external stimulation of a (−) mycelia culture of *B. trispora* are similar to those found in mated cultures [37]. As described further in this chapter, *B. trispora* is used for the commercial production of β-carotene and lycopene today.

Generally, the most abundant carotenoids in yeast and fungi are β-carotene, γ-carotene, and other carotenes. A short overview is provided in Table 12.1.

Nevertheless, several specific und unique carotenoids were found in yeasts and fungi, such as the carboxylic carotenoids neurosporaxanthin (e.g., in *Neurospora crassa*; Fig. 12.4) as well as torulene and torularhodin (in *Rhodotorula* spp.; Fig. 12.2E).

Being of commercial interest, as described further in this chapter, the heterobasidiomycetous yeast *Xanthophyllomyces dendrorhous* (*Phaffia rhodozyma*) naturally produces astaxanthin, although its concentration in the microorganism highly depends on the strain

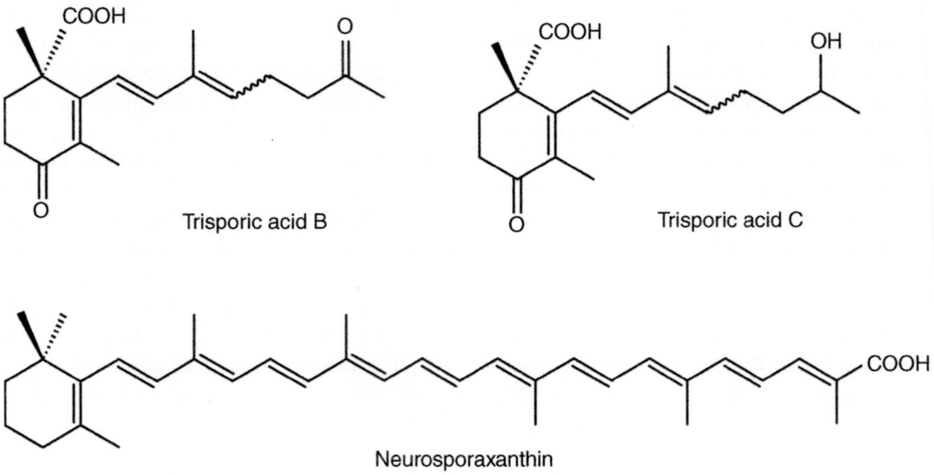

Figure 12.4 Trisporic acids B and C and a typical fungal carotenoid.

Table 12.1 Distribution of carotenoids in yeasts and fungi.

Order	Abundant Carotenoids	Occasional Carotenoids
Phycomycetes	β-carotene, γ-carotene	Other carotenes
Ascomycetes	β-carotene, γ-carotene	Lycopene, neurosporaxanthin, aleuriaxanthin, plectaniaxanthin, phillipsiaxanthin
Heterobasidiomycetes	β-carotene, γ-carotene, astaxanthin	Other carotenes and simple hydroxycarotenoids
Hymenomycetes	β-carotene, γ-carotene	Other carotenes, torularhodin, simple hydroxycarotenoids, keto-carotenoids
Deuteromycetes	β-carotene, γ-carotene, torulene, torularhodin	Lycopene, other carotenes, neurosporaxanthin, plectaniaxanthin, astaxanthin, keto-carotenoids

Source: Liaaen-Jensen [29].

and environmental factors [38]. As also described further, astaxanthin production processes using *Xanthophyllomyces* sp. were significantly improved in recent decades and might soon gain commercial importance.

12.3.3 Bacteria

Carotenoid-producing bacteria can be classified into anoxygenic phototrophic, oxygenic phototrophic, and non-phototrophic bacteria. Anoxygenic photosynthetic bacteria possess a light-harvesting photosystem based on the accessory pigments bacteriochlorophyll and several carotenoids. More than 50 genera with about 130 species of anoxygenic phototrophoic bacteria have been described to produce around 100 different carotenoids. The chemical structures of most of these carotenoids are different from those found in algae, higher plants, fungi, and non-photosynthetic bacteria. For instance, they are most often acyclic compounds with hydroxyl or methoxy groups at C-1, and also with carbonyl functions at rare positions. If cyclic, aromatic rings are frequently observed, for instance in chlorobactene (Figure 12.5).

Unusual C_{30} carotenoids as well as carotenoid glycosides, sulfates, and carboxyl and hydroxyl derivatives are characteristic of particular bacterial genera, as described in

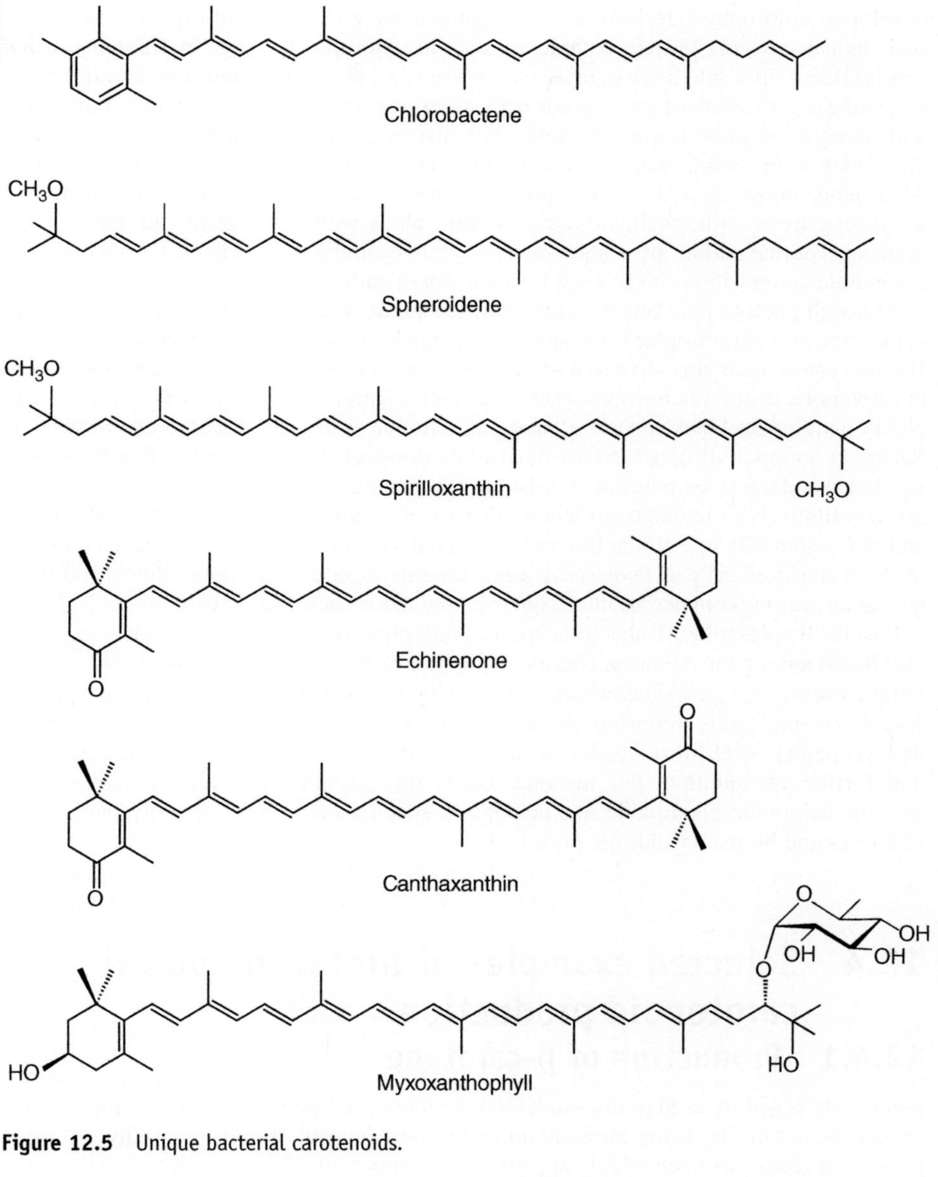

Figure 12.5 Unique bacterial carotenoids.

great detail by Takaichi [39], who also reviewed the five known pathways leading to this enormous diversity. For instance, the anoxygenic purple bacteria contain typical acyclic carotenoids like spirilloxanthin and spheroidene (Fig. 12.5), whereas both green-sulfur and green-filamentous bacteria contain rare derivatives of β-carotene and γ-carotene such as isorenieratene and chlorobactene [40].

Oxygenic phototrophic bacteria are exclusively represented by cyanobacteria (Cyanophyta), sometimes also called *blue-green algae*. Besides the production of oxygen during photosynthesis, they differ from anoxygenic phototrophic bacteria by producing phycobiliproteins and chlorophyll *a* instead of bacteriochlorophylls. The prokaryotes of the Prochlorophyta are an exception, as they produce chlorophylls *a* and *b* but lack phycobiliproteins [29]. Mostly thriving in low-light habitats, a few cyanobacteria have developed chlorophyll derivatives with significantly red-shifted absorption maxima in their light-harvesting protein complexes, such as chlorophyll *d* (e.g., in *Halomicronema* spp. [41]) and chlorophyll *f* (e.g., in *Acaryochloris* spp. [42]). Furthermore, all cyanobacteria biosynthesize a variety of carotenoids with structures similar to those found in both algae and anoxygenic phototrophic bacteria. For instance, bacteria-characteristic carotenoid glycosides were found, and, at the same time, common dicyclic β-ring carotenoids (e.g., β-carotene) occur as part of their photosystems. Several derivatives of the carotenoid glycosides myxoxanthophyll and oscillaxanthin, along with keto-carotenoids like echinenone and canthaxanthin, are unique carotenoids of cyanobacteria (Figure 12.5). Thus, their carotenoid composition can be used for their classification [29, 40].

Although phototrophic bacteria utilize carotenoids as part of their light-harvesting protein complexes, non-phototrophic carotenoid-containing bacteria do not conduct photosynthesis. Because carotenoids also serve as a protectant against photo-oxidative damage, biosynthesis of carotenoids in non-phototrophic bacteria is often a light-induced process. Prominent examples of light-induced biosynthesis are non-phototrophic bacteria of the *Myxococcus* spp. and *Streptomyces* spp., both of which have been used extensively for investigations into the genetic regulation and transcriptional initiation of carotenogenic gene clusters. In contrast, *Paracoccus* spp. constitutively accumulate carotenoids that are of commercial interest, such as astaxanthin and zeaxanthin [43]. In 2007, the European Food Safety Authority (EFSA) considered the use of dried sterilized cells of *Paracoccus carotinifaciens* as safe for feeding salmon and trout, indicating growing commercial interest in this production route of feed carotenoids [44].

Besides the described Eubacteria species, non-phototrophic carotenogenic species are also found among the Archaea. Thermoacidophilic *Sulfolobus* spp. were described to form unique zeaxanthin glycosides, whereas several halophilic species (*Halobacterium* spp. and *Haloferax* spp.) were reported to accumulate astaxanthin, β-carotene, canthaxanthin, and lycopene [43]. However, technical difficulties impair their biotechnological cultivation and further exploitation. For instance, corrosion-resistant materials are required for growing halophilic, alkaliphilic, and acidophilic species, and, most frequently, the production rates and biomass yields are poor [45].

12.4 Selected examples of biotechnological carotenoid production

12.4.1 Production of β-carotene

β-carotene is widely used in the food, feed, cosmetic, and pharmaceutical industries due to its potent coloring traits, antioxidant properties, and provitamin A activity. Its use in foods and feeds has been widely approved by competent authorities worldwide. In the

European Union, β-carotene and β-carotene-rich preparations require labeling as *E 160a*, which comprises two subcategories: E 160a (i) mixed carotenes, and E 160a (ii) β-carotene. Mixed carotenes are further divided into plant carotenes and algal carotenes. Plant carotenes need to be "obtained by solvent extraction of natural strains of edible plants, carrots, vegetable oils, grass, alfalfa (lucerne), and nettle", containing "carotenoids of which β-carotene accounts for the major part" [46]. The extraction of carotenoids from crude palm oil (*Elaeis guineensis* Jacq.) is a commercially utilized example, commonly involving alkaline saponification of a specific carotene-rich oil fraction, and subsequent solvent-assisted carotene extraction [47]. Eventually, crystallization at lowered temperatures may be carried out to remove noncarotenoid impurities [48]. Algal carotenes are obtained from the halophilic green alga *Dunaliella salina*, mostly containing E- and Z-isomers of β-carotene in different ratios ranging from 50:50 to 71:29 [46].

In contrast, pure β-carotene (E 160a (ii)) comprises at least 96% (*all-E*)-β-carotene, and it may be derived synthetically or originate from the fungus *B. trispora* [46]. However, more than 90% of commercialized β-carotene is still derived from chemical synthesis because biotechnological production is associated with several disadvantages, such as poor process control in open ponds, high nutrient consumption with low efficiency in bioreactors, contamination problems, and difficult optimal nutrient requirements [49].

Nevertheless, carotenoid production with *B. trispora* is currently carried out at the industrial scale, and several companies are expecting significant growth rates within the next decade, in particular because substantial technical and scientific progress enabled a more efficient carotenoid production using this fungus. As described in Section 12.3.2, a prerequisite for carotenoid accumulation by *B. trispora* is the presence of both (+) and (−) mating types, which disp trisporic acids—fungal sexual hormones. Moreover, carotenoid production also increased after the addition of structurally similar chemical enhancers, such as abscisic acid, β-ionone, α-ionone, and vitamin A [50]. The addition of citrus oils, citrus pulp, and molasses was found to exert a surprising carotenoid-enhancing effect similar to that of β-ionone [51, 52]. Span 20 and geraniol were reported to intensely increase carotenoid production in mated *B. trispora* [53, 54]. Reports are available on the systematic optimization of growth media [55] as well as on the optimum mixing ratio of 30:1 of the (−) and (+) types [56]. Several bioreactor systems, such as stirred-tank and airlift reactors, have been investigated [57, 58], and solutions to technical problems such as foam formation and excessive dissolved oxygen have enabled processes that enhance yields up to fivefold higher than those of conventional systems [59].

Unicellular flagellate green microalgae belonging to *Dunaliella* spp. (Chlorophyta and Chlorophyceae), which are naturally occurring in media with very high salt concentrations of up to 35%, are further important sources of "natural" β-carotene. According to Ben-Amotz and Avron [60], *Dunaliella* represents the only eukaryotic photosynthetic organism that is found in significant numbers in saline lakes such as the Dead Sea in Israel and the Great Salt Lake in Utah, United States. In contrast to other algae, it lacks a rigid polysaccharide cell wall. Instead, the thin elastic plasma membrane is covered by a flexible mucilaginous coat. The absence of a rigid cell wall allows rapid cell volume changes in response to extracellular changes in osmotic pressure. A further response to high salinity is the massive accumulation of β-carotene within its chloroplasts. As a result, the commonly green algae appear rather red due to their extremely high β-carotene content reaching up to 10% of dry weight. For comparison, the β-carotene levels of most other algae are around 0.3%, according to Ben-Amotz and Avron [60]. Most interestingly, despite the high concentration, crystals of β-carotene are not observed in the chloroplasts of highly pigmented *Dunaliella*. Besides (*all-E*)-β-carotene, the algae also accumulate high amounts of (9*Z*)-β-carotene, which is an oily substance when purified or concentrated and, therefore, is believed to aid the solubilization of its (*all-E*)-isomer in the algae chloroplasts [60]. Up to 50% of the total β-carotene from *Dunaliella* may be present as its (*Z*)-isomer [46]. Such lipid-dissolved β-carotene may be expected to be highly bioavailable, as has been previously shown by comparing the bioavailability of solid-crystalline β-carotene from carrots to that of lipid-dissolved and liquid-crystalline β-carotene from papaya [61, 62]. In agreement with this hypothesis, Ben-Amotz *et al.* reported a 10-fold higher bioavailability of the algal carotene when feeding equivalent doses of β-carotene from a *Dunaliella* supplement and synthetic (*all-E*)-β-carotene [63]. Large-scale β-carotene production by *Dunaliella* is mostly carried out in outdoor cultivation ponds. These ponds are relatively shallow (10–25 cm deep) in order to meet optimum surface–volume ratios. Thereby, the cells are exposed to the highest possible intensity of photosynthetically effective irradiation, which is required for maximum β-carotene yield. Both nonmixed and paddle-wheel mixed ponds are suitable for production, whereas the use of airlifts or centrifugal pumps may damage the fragile cell wall of *Dunaliella* algae [60].

β-carotene accumulation is maximized under high salt concentrations, high light intensity, and slow growth rates. High salt concentrations close to saturation (>27%) allow simultaneous limitation of the growth rate and, at the same time, effectively keep halotolerant predatory protozoa and competitor algae deprived [49]. In intensive cultivation facilities, growth rate limitations are achieved by limiting nutrients in the bioreactor (e.g., by depriving nitrogen or carbon dioxide supply). Recently, a modern gentle airlift loop bioreactor has been described for the cultivation of *D. salina*, providing controlled CO_2 supply for growth regulation [64]. Furthermore, the use of light-emitting diodes (LEDs) has been shown to allow control of both growth and carotenoid accumulation rates. The combination of a red and blue LED at a ratio of 75% and 25%, respectively, yielded the highest growth rates, whereas increasing proportions of blue light was shown to foster β-carotene and lutein accumulation [65].

Other microorganisms have been examined for their applicability to industrial β-carotene production. For instance, fungi strains from *Mucor* spp. (e.g., *Mucor circinelloides*) biosynthesize appreciable amounts of β-carotene when exposed to blue light. Furthermore, *Phycomyces blakesleeanus* has been investigated, producing carotenoids when exposed to intersexual hormones. To date, however, β-carotene production from *Mucor*, *Phycomyces*, or other microorganisms has not been able to compete with the established manufacture from *Blakeslea* or *Dunaliella*.

12.4.2 Production of astaxanthin

Astaxanthin can be considered the second most important carotenoid after β-carotene, and about 29% of total carotenoid sales are allotted to astaxanthin [66]. Currently, its use for the aquacultural production of salmon and trout is by far the most significant application, because this carotenoid provides the orange-red coloration to the flesh of these fish. Astaxanthin is also fed to chicken and quails to improve and standardize the color of flesh and egg yolks [8]. Furthermore, antiaging, anti-inflammatory, and sunproofing properties have been proven for astaxanthin. Although these health-beneficial assumptions have not yet been translated into reliable and legal health claims, the importance of astaxanthin as a dietary supplement is increasing. By analogy to β-carotene, the overwhelming proportion of astaxanthin is derived from chemical synthesis. The enormous market value of synthetic astaxanthin was estimated to be more than $200 million in 2011. The most promising natural sources of astaxanthin are the yeast *X. dendrorhous* and the microalga *H. pluvialis*. Astaxanthin-rich biomass from *X. dendrorhous* (= *Phaffia rhodozyma*) has been approved for trout and salmon farming by the European Union. Recently, the production cost of astaxanthin by *H. pluvialis* in improved large-scale outdoor photobioreactors was estimated to be $718 per kg in 2011, which might even underprice the cost of chemical synthesis, which has an estimated cost of $1000/kg [67]. More importantly, the use of food and feed additives from natural sources is a demand of many consumers, and, thus, microbial astaxanthin synthesis is expected to gain importance.

Commercial cultivation methods for *H. pluvialis* have been developed, and a total yield of 1.5–3.0% astaxanthin (of dry weight) has been achieved. Both closed photobioreactors and open culture ponds are being successfully used for *Haematococcus* cultivation by a two-phase process. First, the reproduction of vegetative cells is enhanced by near-optimum growing conditions, including the control of temperature, pH, and nutrient levels, if possible. After reaching a sufficient cellular density, the microalgae is exposed to environmental and nutrient stress to induce massive astaxanthin accumulation. For instance, the salinity of the medium might be increased, as well as the temperature or light intensity. The vegetative *Haematococcus* cells will transform into so-called hematocysts within two or three days, and after 3–5 more days maximum astaxanthin concentrations (1.5–3.0% of dry weight) are reached. Subsequently, the cells are harvested by settling or centrifugation, eventually combined with ethoxyquin or other antioxidants, dried, and then cracked by milling to ensure maximum bioavailability for their use as a feed supplement. Excellent photographs of the microalgae and an outdoor cultivation site are available from Lorenz and Cysewski [68].

Besides the microalga *Haematococcus*, the astaxanthin-producing yeast *X. dendrorhous* appears to be a further promising microorganism providing several advantages. The yeast does not require light for growth and accumulation of astaxanthin, its principal carotenoid. Moreover, it metabolizes many kinds of saccharides under both aerobic and anaerobic conditions and reproduces at relatively high growth rates [69]. Its modesty regarding the substrate enables the utilization of industrial by-products, such as malt waste and residues from mustard production [70, 71]. Schmidt *et al.* [66] have recently compiled an overview of growth media suitable for *Xanthophyllomyces* cultivation. The moderately psychrophilic yeast grows at temperatures from 0 to 27 °C (optimum: 18–22 °C) at a pH value between 5 and 6. Because oxygen is required for astaxanthin biosynthesis, a sufficient but nonabundant supply of oxygen ensured high carotenoid yields. Inadequate oxygen supply fostered β-carotene instead of astaxanthin biosynthesis, whereas oversupply led to reduced growth rates. By analogy to the above-described *Haematococcus* process, cultivation is typically divided into a cell growth phase and a subsequent maturation phase [66]. The astaxanthin content of wild strains of *X. dendrorhous* was reported to be 200–400 μg/g of dry yeast, and an increase by a factor of 10–50 would be necessary to become competitive with astaxanthin from *Haematococcus* or even from chemical synthesis. Thus, encouraging attempts to genetically improve *Xanthophyllomyces* strains by metabolic engineering have been pioneered in the past decade by Visser *et al.* [72]. By upregulating phytoene synthase and lycopene cyclase, a significantly increased accumulation of β-carotene and echinone was achieved, indicating that the oxygenation reactions might be rate limiting [72]. More recently, Sandmann and coworkers combined a chemical mutagenic approach with systematic genetic pathway improvements, thereby yielding a strain that produced more than 5000 μg astaxanthin per gram of dry weight [73]. One year later, the same group reported further improvements, obtaining up to 9000 μg per gram of dry weight by metabolic engineering. This encouraging success will significantly enhance the economic importance of biotechnologically produced astaxanthin soon.

12.4.3 Production of lycopene

Frequent dietary uptake of lycopene has been associated with several health benefits. For instance, several epidemiological trials associated the consumption of lycopene-rich foods with a 30–40% risk reduction of prostate cancer incidence [3], although several research groups claimed the need for further studies in order to maintain a causal association to lycopene [4]. Besides further potential health benefits described in the literature, lycopene recently gained enormous attention from the food colorant industry, because it may be used for the replacement of the natural red colorant carmine. The replacement of carmine has been of interest since lycopene producers promotionally highlighted its origin from a louse (*Dactylopius coccus* Costa), thus effectively provoking disgust by the customer. In 2009, the European Commission approved various applications of lycopene of synthetic origin as well as from tomato oleoresins and *B. trispora*, respectively, as a novel food ingredient for coloring food and as a food supplement (see [74–76]). By analogy, US Food and Drug Administration (FDA) regulations allow lycopene usage from these sources within the United States, where GRAS (generally recognized as safe) status was granted for corresponding products during the years 2003–2006 [77].

In contrast to β-carotene, lycopene yields and purities obtained by chemical synthesis were reported to be poor, particularly its isomeric purity [78]. Carotenoids extracted from tomato, however, naturally contain high proportions (>91%) of (*all-E*)-lycopene [79]. Thus, efficient commercial processes are based on the extraction from plant sources and on biotechnological approaches. Besides tomato, other plant sources are under current investigation (Table 12.2).

Extremely high concentrations were found in gac fruit arils (up to 190 mg lycopene/100 g of fresh weight [FW]) and autumn olives (up to 54 mg/100 of FW), whereas lower concentrations comparable to tomato were observed in red carrots (6.5 mg/100 g of FW), pink guava (5.2 mg/100 g of FW), and red-fleshed papaya (4.3 mg/100 g of FW; see Table 12.2). Several promising lycopene-producing microorganisms such as *Streptomyces chrestomyceticus*, *B. trispora*, *P. blakesleanus*, and a genetically modified *Flavobacterium* sp. have also been investigated, without reaching industrial production (except for *B. trispora*) [52]. As described here, common strains accumulate mostly β-carotene and only minor amounts of lycopene. For high lycopene production, *B. trispora* strains either without lycopene cyclase activity or supported by chemical lycopene cyclase inhibitors are required. Examples for

Table 12.2 Examples of plant foods rich in lycopene.

Source	Latin Plant Name	Total Lycopene in mg/100 g Fresh Weight	Ref.
Autumn olive	*Elaeagnus umbellata* Thunb.	15.1–54.0	[90]
Buffalo berry	*Shepherdia argentea* [Pursh] Nutt.	18.2–36.0	[91]
Gac fruit aril	*Momordica cochinchinensis* Spreng.	34.8–190.2	[92, 93]
Red-fleshed papaya	*Carica papaya* L.	2.1–4.3	[94]
Red carrot	*Daucus carota* L.	6.5	[92]
Tomato (raw)	*Lycopersicon esculentum* L.	3.5–17.2	[79, 95]
Pink guava	*Psidium guajava* L.	5.2	[92]
Watermelon	*Citrullus lanatus* (Thunb.) Matsum. & Nakai	4.5	[92]

such inhibitors are several tertiary amines, aminomethyl pyridines, imidazole, pyridine, morpholine, quinolone [52], nicotine [80], piperidine, and vitamin A acetate [53]. In recent years, significant progress was made in the fermentative production of lycopene by *B. trispora*, yielding up to 156–578 mg lycopene per liter [54, 81]. López-Nieto *et al.* [52] developed a process for semi-industrial lycopene production in an 800 L bioreactor, including a careful medium optimization and the application of lycopene cyclase inhibitors. Besides *B. trispora*, blue-light illuminated mutant strains of *P. blakesleanus*, metabolically engineered *E. coli*, and the above-mentioned microorganisms were proposed for lycopene production. However, to date, none of these microorganisms was shown to be able to compete with the outstanding lycopene production rates of *B. trispora*.

12.4.4 Production of lutein and zeaxanthin

Commercial sources of lutein and zeaxanthin are of high interest due to their use as feed and food supplements. Lutein and zeaxanthin specifically accumulate in the macula of the human retina at concentrations of up to 500-fold higher than in human blood serum and other tissues. Their presence in the macula is related to effects protecting against the development of cataract and macular degeneration. Moreover, high consumption of lutein- and zeaxanthin-rich food was related to the maintenance of cognitive functions in the elderly and, possibly, a lowered incidence of Alzheimer's disease [6]. In addition, there is still controversy whether lutein and zeaxanthin meet the three substantial criteria of a conditionally essential nutrient, because dietary lack of lutein and zeaxanthin resulted in structural abnormalities in the retina of primates. However, in order to classify lutein and zeaxanthin as conditionally essential nutrients, controlled clinical trials are required to provide clear-cut evidence in humans first [82]. Although lutein has been approved for food and feed uses in many countries for a long period, the placing on the market of synthetic zeaxanthin as a novel food ingredient in food supplements was authorized in the European Union only in 2013 [83]. According to Fernández-Sevilla, lutein sales in the United States, where it is largely applied as a food colorant and ingested as food and feed supplements, amounted to circa \$150 million in 2010 [84]. Other market reports stated a total market value of lutein of circa \$233 million in 2010, closely surpassing that of astaxanthin [9]. Interestingly, chemical synthesis of lutein was described to be an outstandingly expensive process [84], and, thus, commercial lutein is almost exclusively derived from the petals of marigold flowers (*Tagetes erecta* L.). After extraction with organic solvents such as hexane, an oleoresin containing mostly lutein esters is obtained, whereas free lutein can be derived after alkaline saponification and subsequent solvent extraction, eventually followed by recrystallization to enhance purity [85]. Regarding their biotechnological production, several lutein-producing microalgae have been examined as the most promising sources. Lutein production from marigold was recently compared in detail to its production from the microalgae *Murielopsis* sp., *Chlorella* sp., and *Scenedesmus* sp. by Fernández-Sevilla *et al.* [84]. The same authors carried out highly promising experiments in 4,000 and 28,000 L photobioreactors, showing enhanced lutein yields under increased illumination conditions. The addition of stress-inducing chemicals such as H_2O_2 and sodium hypochlorite was reported to exert a moderate effect on lutein yield. As compared to the production of lutein from marigold (*Tagetes* sp.), a major obstacle for obtaining carotenoids from the above-mentioned Chlorophycean microalgae is their thick and hard cell walls, which need to be broken up by energy- and cost-intensive procedures, such as milling, ultrasound, microwave, freeze–thaw cycles, or the addition of chemical agents. Further procedures are analogous to the marigold process (i.e., they include saponification and solvent-assisted carotenoid extraction) [84].

Altough several processes for the biotechnological production of lutein are currently under investigation, information on biotechnological zeaxanthin production is still scarce. For instance, *Flavobacterium* spp. have been reported to be a microbial source of zeaxanthin, producing up to 190 mg zeaxanthin per liter of cell culture. Zeaxanthin from *Flavobacterium* spp. has been proposed for uses in the cosmetic, food, and feed industries [86]. In addition, Singh *et al.* [87] reported the isolation of a fast-growing strain of microalgae (*Chlorella saccharophila*), containing zeaxanthin and β-carotene at a ratio of circa 75:25. Chinese wolfberries (*Lycium barbarum* L.) and the husks of Chinese lantern (*Physalis alkekengi* L.) are among the richest natural sources of zeaxanthin, which might be of particular interest as biological starting material, as the latter are commonly discarded [88]. The importance of "natural" zeaxanthin might increase substantially in the future, as it is similarly found in the human macula and neural system. In contrast to lutein, only minor amounts of zeaxanthin are part of the common human diet, thus making its supplementation potentially interesting.

12.5 Perspectives and conclusions

In response to the continuously increasing demand for natural carotenoids, feasibility of their production by microorganisms has already reached industrial scale, as described in this chapter. For a few examples, namely, astaxanthin production, the biotechnological process is already competitive with chemical synthesis, owing to substantial genetic and mutagenic improvements of the producing organism. At the same time, optimized microalgal cultivation allows astaxanthin production without using genetically modified organisms. Lycopene is a carotenoid of increasing importance due to its health-beneficial properties and its potential to replace synthetic and animal-derived dyes, such as red azo-dyes and carmine, respectively. Lycopene production by *B. trispora* ruled out the attempts for its chemical synthesis, particularly due to the achievable high isomeric purity. In addition, this organism is already being used for the commercial production of natural β-carotene, and extensive knowledge about process control is available. The β-carotene process appears to be easily adaptable to lycopene production by the addition of lycopene cyclase inhibitors. The microalga *Dunaliella* has also been applied for the large scale β-carotene production, and cultivation systems have been optimized during the past few decades. The derived products are particularly interesting, because their high proportion of up to 50% (*Z*)-isomers and their lipid-dissolved physical state result in a superior total β-carotene bioavailability. However, chemical synthesis of β-carotene still dominates the market. The "hard-to-synthesize" carotenoid lutein is almost exclusively obtained from the extraction of *T. erecta* petals, although biotechnological processes for lutein production are currently under development. A similar development is expected for zeaxanthin, a carotenoid that is found in high concentrations in the retina and neural tissues of humans. Because Western diets are commonly low in zeaxanthin, the need for dietary supplements may increase as knowledge about this carotenoid and its biological functions expands.

Carotenoids aside, further food grade pigments from microbial sources have recently entered, or are about to enter, the markets, such as *Monascus* pigments, hydroxyanthraquinoids (Arpink red; e.g., from *Penicillium oxalicum*), and riboflavin from *Ashbya gossypii*. As previously highlighted by Dufosse *et al.* [89], the successful marketing of any pigment from microbial sources highly depends on its acceptability by the consumers, regulatory approval, and the essentially required capital investment to allow the product to leap from research facilities to the market. The food industry's major concerns often are related to the duration and high cost of the extensive required toxicity studies as well as the enormous investments of building and operating indoor fermentation facilities [89].

The worldwide demand for "naturally" produced food, feed, and cosmetic ingredients has provided great opportunities for biotechnological processes, and a scientifically and economically bright future might be expected for microbial pigments. Looking at the astonishing diversity of algae, yeasts, fungi, and bacteria, many discoveries regarding the production of carotenoids and beyond are certainly yet to be made.

References

1. G. Britton, "Functions of intact carotenoids," in G. Britton, S. Liaaen-Jensen, and H. Pfander, (eds.), *Carotenoids*, vol. 4, *Natural functions*, Basel: Birkhäuser, 2008, pp. 189–236.
2. R. Goralczyk and K. Wertz, "Skin photoprotection by carotenoids," in G. Britton, S. Liaaen-Jensen, and H. Pfander, (eds.), *Carotenoids*, vol. 5, *Nutrition and Health*, Basel: Birkhäuser, 2009, pp. 335–62.
3. E. Giovannucci, "Tomatoes, tomato-based products, lycopene, and cancer: review of the epidemiologic literature," *J. Natl. Cancer Inst.*, **91**, 317–31 (1999).
4. M. Y. Wei and E. L. Giovannucci, "Lycopene, tomato products, and prostate cancer incidence: a review and reassessment in the PSA screening era," *J. Oncol.*, **2012**, 1–7 (2012).
5. S. K. Clinton, C. Emenhiser, S. J. Schwartz, D. G. Bostwick, A. W. Williams, B. J. Moore, and J. W. Erdman Jr., "Cis-trans lycopene isomers, carotenoids, and retinol in the human prostate," *Cancer Epidem. Biomar.*, **5**, 823–33 (1996).
6. E. J. Johnson, "A possible role for lutein and zeaxanthin in cognitive function in the elderly," *Am. J. Clin. Nutr.*, **96**, 1161–5 (2012).
7. W. Schalch, J. T. Landrum, and R. A. Bone, "The eye," in G. Britton, S. Liaaen-Jensen, and H. Pfander, (eds.), *Carotenoids*, vol. 5, *Nutrition and Health*, Basel: Birkhäuser, 2009, pp. 301–34.
8. P. Bhosale and P. S. Bernstein, "Microbial xanthophylls," *Appl. Microbiol. Biotechnol.*, **68**, 445–55 (2005).
9. BCC Research, "The global market for carotenoids," 2011, http://www.bccresearch.com/market-research/food-and-beverage/carotenoids-global-market-fod025d.html (last accessed January 20, 2015).
10. G. Britton, "Overview of carotenoid biosynthesis," in G. Britton, S. Liaaen-Jensen, and H. Pfander, (eds.), *Carotenoids*, vol. 3, *Biosynthesis and metabolism*, Basel: Birkhäuser, pp. 13–140.
11. G. Sandmann, "Molecular evolution of carotenoid biosynthesis from bacteria to plants," *Physiol. Plantarum*, **116**, 431–40 (2002).
12. M. H. Walter and D. Strack, "Carotenoids and their cleavage products: biosynthesis and functions," *Nat. Prod. Rep.*, **28**, 663–92 (2011).
13. M. Rohmer, "The discovery of a mevalonate-independent pathway for isoprenoid biosynthesis in bacteria, algae and higher plants," *Nat. Prod. Rep.*, **16**, 565–74 (1999).
14. K. J. Treharne, E. I. Mercer, and T. W. Goodwin, "Incorporation of [14C] carbon dioxide and [2-14C] mevalonic acid into terpenoids of higher plants during chloroplast development," *Biochem. J.*, **99**, 239–45 (1966).
15. T. Gräwert, M. Groll, F. Rohdich, A. Bacher, and W. Eisenreich, "Biochemistry of the non-mevalonate isoprenoid pathway," *Cell. Mol. Life Sci.*, **68**, 3797–814 (2011).

16. P. C. Lee and C. Schmidt-Dannert, "Metabolic engineering towards biotechnological production of carotenoids in microorganisms," *Appl. Microbiol. Biotechnol.*, **60**, 1–11 (2003).
17. N. J. C. Fong, M. L. Burgess, K. D. Barrow, and D. R. Glenn, "Carotenoid accumulation in the psychrotrophic bacterium *Arthrobacter agilis* in response to thermal and salt stress," *Appl. Microbiol. Biotechnol.*, **56**, 750–6 (2001).
18. P. C. Lee, A. Z. R. Momen, B. N. Mijts, and C. Schmidt-Dannert, "Biosynthesis of structurally novel carotenoids in *Escherichia coli*," *Chem. Biol.*, **10**, 453–62 (2003).
19. H. Krügel, P. Krubasik, K. Weber, H. P. Saluz, and G. Sandmann, "Functional analysis of genes from *Streptomyces griseus* involved in the synthesis of isorenieratene, a carotenoid with aromatic end groups, revealed a novel type of carotenoid desaturase," *Biochim. Biophys. Acta—Mol. Cell Biol. Lipids*, **1439**, 57–64 (1999).
20. T. Matsuno, "Aquatic animal carotenoids," *Fisheries Sci.*, **67**, 771–83 (2001).
21. J. C. B. McDermott, D. J. Brown, G. Britton, and T. W. Goodwin, "Alternative pathways of zeaxanthin biosynthesis in a *Flavobacterium* species: experiments with nicotine as inhibitor," *Biochem. J.*, **144**, 231–43 (1974).
22. H. Linden, "Carotenoid hydroxylase from *Haematococcus pluvialis*: cDNA sequence, regulation and functional complementation," *Biochim. Biophys. Acta—Gene Struct. Expr.*, **1446**, 203–12 (1999).
23. G. I. Frengova and D. M. Beshkova, "Carotenoids from *Rhodotorula* and *Phaffia*: yeasts of biotechnological importance," *J. Ind. Microbiol. Biotechnol.*, **36**, 163–80 (2009).
24. G. A. Armstrong, "Genetics of eubacterial carotenoid biosynthesis: a colorful tale," *Ann. Rev. Microbiol.*, **51**, 629–59 (1997).
25. G. Britton, S. Liaaen-Jensen, and H. Pfander, "Synthesis from a different perspective: how nature does it," in G. Britton, S. Liaaen-Jensen, and H. Pfander, (eds.), *Carotenoids*, vol. 3, *Biosynthesis*, Basel: Birkhäuser, 1998, pp. 1–147.
26. P. D. Fraser and P. M. Bramley, "The biosynthesis and nutritional uses of carotenoids," *Prog. Lipid Res.*, **43**, 228–65 (2004).
27. V. Ebenezer, L. K. Medlin, and J. Ki, "Molecular detection, quantification, and diversity evaluation of microalgae," *Mar. Biotechnol.*, **14**, 129–42 (2012).
28. S. Liaaen-Jensen and A. G. Andrewes, "Microbial carotenoids," *Annu. Rev. Microbiol.*, **26**, 225–48 (1972).
29. S. Liaaen-Jensen, "Carotenoids in chemosystematics," in G. Britton, S. Liaaen-Jensen, and H. Pfander, (eds.), *Carotenoids*, vol. 3, *Biosynthesis*, Basel: Birkhäuser, 1998, pp. 217–47.
30. P. J. Keeling, "The endosymbiotic origin, diversification and fate of plastids," *Phil. Trans. R. Soc. B Biol. Sci.*, **365**, 729–48 (2010).
31. E. C. M. Nowack, M. Melkonian, and G. Glöckner, "Chromatophore genome sequence of *Paulinella* sheds light on acquisition of photosynthesis by eukaryotes," *Curr. Biol.*, **18**, 410–18 (2008).
32. T. Bjørnland, F. T. Haxo, and S. Liaaen-Jensen, "Carotenoids of the Florida red tide dinoflagellate *Karenia brevis*," *Biochem. Syst. Ecol.*, **31**, 1147–62 (2003).
33. D. F. Millie, O. M. Schofield, G. J. Kirkpatrick, G. Johnsen, P. A. Tester, and B. T. Vinyard, "Detection of harmful algal blooms using photopigments and absorption signatures: a case study of the Florida red tide dinoflagellate, *Gymnodinium breve*," *Limnol. Oceanogr.* **42**, 1240–51 (1998).
34. S. Takaichi, "Carotenoids in algae: distributions, biosyntheses and functions," *Mar. Drugs*, **9**, 1101–18 (2011).

35. P. Buzzini, "Production of yeast carotenoids by using agro-industrial by-products," *Agro Food Industry Hi-Tech*, **12**, 7–10 (2001).

36. A. F. Blakeslee, "Sexual reproduction in the Mucorineae," *Proc. Amer. Acad. Arts Sci.*, **40**, 205–319 (1904).

37. H. van den Ende, "Relationship between sexuality and carotene synthesis in *Blakeslea trispora*," *J. Bacteriol.*, **96**, 1298–303 (1968).

38. Z. Liu, J. Zhang, Y. Zheng, and Y. Shen, "Improvement of astaxanthin production by a newly isolated *Phaffia rhodozyma* mutant with low-energy ion beam implantation," *J. Appl. Microbiol.*, **104**, 861–72 (2008).

39. S. Takaichi, "Carotenoids and carotenogenesis in anoxygenic photosynthetic bacteria," in H. A. Frank, A. J. Young, G. Britton, and R. J. Cogdell, (eds.), *The photochemistry of carotenoids: advances in photosynthesis*, vol. **8**, Dordrecht: Kluwer Academic, 1999, pp. 39–69.

40. S. Takaichi and M. Mochimaru, "Carotenoids and carotenogenesis in cyanobacteria: unique ketocarotenoids and carotenoid glycosides," *Cell Mol. Life Sci.*, **64**, 2607–19 (2007).

41. H. Miyashita, H. Ikemoto, N. Kurano, K. Adachi, M. Chihara, and S. Miyachi, "Chlorophyll d as a major pigment," *Nature*, **383**, 402 (1996).

42. M. Chen, Y. Li, D. Birch, and R. D. Willows, "A cyanobacterium that contains chlorophyll f: a red-absorbing photopigment," *FEBS Lett.*, **586**, 3249–54 (2012).

43. H. Takano, D. Asker, T. Beppu, and K. Ueda, "Genetic control for light-induced carotenoid production in non-phototrophic bacteria," *J. Ind. Microbiol. Biotechnol.*, **33**, 88–93 (2006).

44. European Food Safety Agency (EFSA), EFSA Panel on Additives and Products or Substances Used in Animal Feed, "Safety and efficacy of Panaferd-AX (red carotenoid-rich bacterium *Paracoccus carotinifaciens*) as feed additive for salmon and trout," *The EFSA Journal*, **546**, 1–30 (2007).

45. C. Schiraldi, M. Giuliano, and M. De Rosa, "Perspectives on biotechnological applications of archaea," *Archaea*, **1**, 75–86 (2002).

46. Commission of the European Communities, "Commission Directive 2008/128/EC of 22 December 2008 laying down specific purity criteria concerning colours for use in foodstuffs," *Off. J. Eur. Union*, **6**, 20–63 (2009).

47. M. Nitsche, W. Johannisbauer, and V. Jordan, "Process for obtaining carotene from palm oil," US Patent No. US08/913,710, 1999, 1–5.

48. F. Khachik, "Process for purification and crystallization of palm oil carotenoids," US Patent No. US10/332,700, 2006, 1–7.

49. R. Raja, S. Hemaiswarya, and R. Rengasamy, "Exploitation of *Dunaliella* for β-carotene production," *Appl. Microbiol. Biotechnol.*, **74**, 517–23 (2007).

50. S. Dandekar, V. V. Modi, and U. K. Jani, "Chemical regulators of carotenogenesis by *Blakeslea trispora*," *Phytochemistry*, **19**, 795–8 (1980).

51. A. Ciegler, G. E. Nelson, and H. H. Hall, "Enhancement of β-carotene synthesis by citrus products," *Appl. Microbiol.*, **11**, 128–31 (1963).

52. M. J. López-Nieto, J. Costa, E. Peiro, E. Méndez, M. Rodríguez-Sáiz, J. L. De La Fuente, W. Cabri, and J. L. Barredo, "Biotechnological lycopene production by mated fermentation of *Blakeslea trispora*," *Appl. Microbiol. Biotechnol.*, **66**, 153–9 (2004).

53. S. M. Choudhari, L. Ananthanarayan, and R. S. Singhal, "Use of metabolic stimulators and inhibitors for enhanced production of β-carotene and lycopene by *Blakeslea trispora* NRRL 2895 and 2896," *Bioresour. Technol.*, **99**, 3166–73 (2008).

54. Y. Shi, X. Xin, and Q. Yuan, "Improved lycopene production by *Blakeslea trispora* with isopentenyl compounds and metabolic precursors," *Biotechnol. Lett.*, **34**, 849–52 (2012).
55. S. Choudhari and R. Singhal, "Media optimization for the production of β-carotene by *Blakeslea trispora*: a statistical approach," *Bioresour. Technol.*, **99**, 722–30 (2008).
56. K. Böhme, C. Richter, and R. Pätz, "New insights into mechanisms of growth and β-carotene production in *Blakeslea trispora*," *Biotechnol. J.*, **11**, 1080–4 (2006).
57. M. Varzakakou, T. Roukas, E. Papaioannou, P. aKotzekidou, nd M. Liakopoulou-Kyriakides, "Autolysis of *Blakeslea trispora* during carotene production from cheese whey in an airlift reactor," *Prep. Biochem. Biotechnol.*, **41**, 7–21 (2011).
58. F. Mantzouridou, T. Roukas, and P. Kotzekidou, "Optimization of β-carotene production from synthetic medium by *Blakeslea trispora* in a stirred tank reactor and relationship between morphological changes and pigment formation," *Food Biotechnol.*, **16**, 167–87 (2002).
59. S. W. Kim, I. Y. Lee, J. C. Jeong, J. H. Lee, and Y. H. Park, "Control of both foam and dissolved oxygen in the presence of a surfactant for production of β-carotene in *Blakeslea trispora*," *J Microbiol. Biotechnol.*, **9**, 548–53 (1999).
60. A. Ben-Amotz and M. Avron, "The biotechnology of cultivating the halotolerant alga *Dunaliella*," *Trends Biotechnol.*, **8**, 121–6 (1990).
61. R. M. Schweiggert, R. E. Kopec, M. G. Villalobos-Gutierrez, J. Högel, S. Quesada, P. Esquivel, S. J. Schwartz, and R. Carle, "Carotenoids are more bioavailable from papaya than from tomato and carrot in humans: a randomised cross-over study," *Br. J. Nutr.*, **111**, 490–8 (2014).
62. R. M. Schweiggert, D. Mezger, F. Schimpf, C. B. Steingass, and R. Carle, "Influence of chromoplast morphology on carotenoid bioaccessibility of carrot, mango, papaya, and tomato," *Food Chem.*, **60**, 2577–85 (2012).
63. A. Ben-Amotz, S. Mokady, S. Edelstein, and M. Avron, "Bioavailability of a natural isomer mixture as compared with synthetic all-trans-β-carotene in rats and chicks," *J. Nutr.*, **119**, 1013–19 (1989).
64. K. Ying, D. J. Gilmour, Y. Shi, and W. B. Zimmerman, "Growth enhancement of *Dunaliella salina* by microbubble induced airlift loop bioreactor (ALB): the relation between mass transfer and growth rate," *J. Biomater. Nanobiotechnol.*, **4**, 1–9 (2013).
65. W. Fu, O. Guomundsson, G. Paglia, G. Herjólfsson, O. S. Andrésson, B. O. Palsson, and S. Brynjólfsson, "Enhancement of carotenoid biosynthesis in the green microalga *Dunaliella salina* with light-emitting diodes and adaptive laboratory evolution," *Appl. Microbiol. Biotechnol.*, **97**, 2395–403 (2013).
66. I. Schmidt, H. Schewe, S. Gassel, C. Jin, J. Buckingham, M. Hümbelin, G. Sandmann, and J. Schrader, "Biotechnological production of astaxanthin with *Phaffia rhodozyma/Xanthophyllomyces dendrorhous*," *Appl. Microbiol. Biotechnol.*, **89**, 555–71 (2011).
67. J. Li, D. Zhu, J. Niu, S. Shen, and G. Wang, "An economic assessment of astaxanthin production by large scale cultivation of *Haematococcus pluvialis*," *Biotechnol. Adv.*, **29**, 568–74 (2011).
68. R. T. Lorenz and G. R. Cysewski, "Commercial potential for *Haematococcus* microalgae as a natural source of astaxanthin," *Trends Biotechnol.*, **18**, 160–7 (2000).
69. Y. Yamane, K. Higashida, Y. Nakashimada, T. Kakizono, and N. Nishio, "Influence of oxygen and glucose on primary metabolism and astaxanthin production by *Phaffia rhodozyma* in batch and fed-batch cultures: Kinetic and stoichiometric analysis," *Appl. Environ. Microbiol.*, **63**, 4471–8 (1997).

70. W. P. Cheung, "Carotenoid production by *Phaffia rhodozyma* with industrial waste as substrate," Hong Kong Polytechnic University Dissertations, 2004, http://hdl.handle.net/10397/2936 (last accessed January 20, 2015).

71. J. Tinoi, N. Rakariyatham, and R. L. Deming, "Utilization of mustard waste isolates for improved production of astaxanthin by *Xanthophyllomyces dendrorhous*," *J Ind. Microbiol. Biotechnol.*, **33**, 309–14 (2006).

72. H. Visser, A. J. J. Van Ooyen, and J. C. Verdoes, "Metabolic engineering of the astaxanthin-biosynthetic pathway of *Xanthophyllomyces dendrorhous*," *FEMS Yeast Res.*, **4**, 221–31 (2003).

73. S. Gassel, H. Schewe, I. Schmidt, J. Schrader, and G. Sandmann, "Multiple improvement of astaxanthin biosynthesis in *Xanthophyllomyces dendrorhous* by a combination of conventional mutagenesis and metabolic pathway engineering," *Biotechnol. Lett.*, **35**, 565–9 (2013).

74. European Commission, "Commission decision of 23 April 2009 authorising the placing on the market of lycopene as a novel food ingredient under Regulation (EC) No 258/97 of the European Parliament and of the Council (notified under document number C(2009) 2975)," *Off. J. Eur. Union*, **106**, 55–9 (2009).

75. European Commission, "Commission decision of 28 April 2009 authorising the placing on the market of lycopene from *Blakeslea trispora* as a novel food ingredient under Regulation (EC) No 258/97 of the European Parliament and of the Council (notified under document number C(2009) 3039)," *Off. J. Eur. Union*, **111,** 31–4 (2009).

76. European Commission, "Commission decision of 28 April 2009 authorising the placing on the market of lycopene oleoresin from tomatoes as novel food ingredient under Regulation (EC) No 258/97 of the European Parliament and of the Council," *Off. J. Eur. Union*, **109**, 47–50 (2009).

77. US Food and Drug Administration (FDA), "GRAS notice No. 185, 173, 156, and 119," GRAS Notices Database, 2014, http://www.accessdata.fda.gov (last accessed September 20, 2014).

78. H. Ernst, "Recent advances in industrial carotenoid synthesis," *Pure Appl. Chem.*, **74**, 2213–26 (2002).

79. R. M. Schweiggert, C. B. Steingass, A. Heller, P. Esquivel, and R. Carle, "Characterization of chromoplasts and carotenoids of red and yellow fleshed papaya (*Carica papaya* L.)," *Planta*, **234**, 1031–44 (2011).

80. B. J. Mehta, I. N. Obraztsova, and E. Cerdá-Olmedo, "Mutants and intersexual heterokaryons of *Blakeslea trispora* for production of ß-carotene and lycopene," *Appl. Environ. Microbiol.*, **69**, 4043–8 (2003).

81. J. Wang, X. Liu, R. Liu, H. Li, and Y. Tang, "Optimization of the mated fermentation process for the production of lycopene by *Blakeslea trispora* NRRL 2895 (+) and NRRL 2896 (−)," *Bioproc. Biosys. Eng.*, **35**, 553–64 (2012).

82. R. D. Semba and G. Dagnelie, "Are lutein and zeaxanthin conditionally essential nutrients for eye health?" *Med. Hypotheses*, **61**, 465–72 (2003).

83. European Commission, "Commission decision of 22 January 2013 authorising the placing on the market of synthetic zeaxanthin as a novel food ingredient under Regulation (EC) No 258/97 of the European Parliament and of the Council (notified under document C(2013)110)," *Off. J. Eur. Union*, **21**, 32–3 (2013).

84. J. M. Fernández-Sevilla, F. G. Acién Fernández, and E. Molina Grima, "Biotechnological production of lutein and its applications," *Appl. Microbiol. Biotechnol.*, **86**, 27–40 (2010).

85 F. Khachik, "Process for isolation, purification, and recrystallization of lutein from saponified marigold oleoresin and uses thereof," US Patent No. US08/210,009, 1995, 1–6.

86. L. Dufossé, "Microbial production of food grade pigments," *Food Technol. Biotechnol.*, **44**, 313–21 (2006).

87. D. Singh, M. Puri, S. Wilkens, A. S. Mathur, D. K. Tuli, and C. J. Barrow, "Characterization of a new zeaxanthin producing strain of *Chlorella saccharophila* isolated from New Zealand marine waters," *Bioresour. Technol.*, **143**, 308–14 (2013).

88. P. Weller and D. E. Breithaupt, "Identification and quantification of zeaxanthin esters in plants using liquid chromatography-mass spectrometry," *J. Agric. Food Chem.*, **51**, 7044–9 (2003).

89. L. Dufossé, M. Fouillaud, Y. Caro, S. A. S. Mapari, and N. Sutthiwong, "Filamentous fungi are large-scale producers of pigments and colorants for the food industry," *Curr. Opin. Biotechnol.*, **26**, 56–61 (2014).

90. I. M. Fordham, B. A. Clevidence, E. R. Wiley, and R. H. Zimmerman, "Fruit of autumn olive: a rich source of lycopene," *HortScience*, **36**, 1136–7 (2001).

91. K. M. Riedl, K. Choksi, F. J. Wyzgoski, J. C. Scheerens, S. J. Schwartz, and R. N. Reese, "Variation in lycopene and lycopenoates, antioxidant capacity, and fruit quality of buffaloberry (*Shepherdia argentea* [Pursh]Nutt.)," *J. Food Sci.*, **78**, C1673–9 (2013).

92. J. K. Collins, P. Perkins-Veazie, and W. Roberts, "Lycopene: from plants to humans," *HortScience*, **41**, 1135–44 (2006).

93. H. Aoki, N. T. M. Kieu, N. Kuze, K. Tomisaka, and N. V. Chuyen, "Carotenoid pigments in gac fruit (*Momordica cochinchinensis* Spreng)," *Biosci. Biotechnol. Biochem.*, **66**, 2479–82 (2002).

94. R. M. Schweiggert, C. B. Steingass, P. Esquivel, and R. Carle, "Chemical and morphological characterization of Costa Rican papaya (*Carica papaya* L.) hybrids and lines with particular focus on their genuine carotenoid profiles," *J. Agric. Food Chem.*, **60**, 2577–85 (2012).

95. D. M. Barrett and G. Anthon, "Lycopene content of california-grown tomato varieties," *Acta Hort.*, **542**, 165–73 (2001).

13

Impact of Stress Factors on Carotenoid Composition, Structures, and Bioavailability in Microbial Sources

Agnieszka Kaczor[a,b] and Marta Z. Pacia[a,b]

[a]*Faculty of Chemistry, Jagiellonian University, Krakow, Poland*
[b]*Jagiellonian Centre for Experimental Therapeutics (JCET), Jagiellonian University, Krakow, Poland*

13.1 Introduction

The market value of commercially used carotenoids was estimated at nearly $1.2 billion in 2010 and is predicted to grow to $1.4 billion in 2018 [1]. Only a small percentage of these pigments is obtained from *de novo* producers: some species of algae, yeasts, bacteria, and fungi. However, already about 20–30% of the total β-carotene market is related to natural pigment sources [2]. The culture of *Dunaliella salina*, which is the most important source for natural production of β-carotene, is adapted to produce this pigment on a commercial scale in Australia, China, the United States, and Israel [3]. Astaxanthin is commercially obtained from *Haematocuccus pluvialis* microalgae in Sweden, Israel, and the United States [3]. Also, several other algae and yeasts (e.g., *Xanthophyllomyces dendrorhous*, *Blakeslea trispora*, *Phycomyces blakesleeanus*, *Rhodotorula* spp., and *Chlorella*) are rich sources of various carotenoids [4].

Numerous factors affect carotenoid production in these natural biomanufactures, including light, temperature, media composition, pH, and the presence of chemical compounds. The action of these agents multidirectionally changes the total carotenoid content, pigment composition, and relative isomeric content, affecting also their accessibility and

Carotenoids: Nutrition, Analysis and Technology, First Edition. Edited by Agnieszka Kaczor and Malgorzata Baranska.

bioavailability. This review summarizes results of relatively recent works related to the above issues.

Microbial synthesis of carotenoids and various optimization strategies of pigments production are discussed in Chapter 12.

13.2 Light

White-light illumination is one of the most widely studied factors influencing volumetric production of carotenoids in algae, bacteria, and fungi, associated both with altered growth of the microorganisms and increased activation of carotenoid biosynthetic enzymes [5]. Although typically illumination increases the cellular carotenoid content, depending on the illumination scheme (continuous, cyclic), chosen light intensity, and presence of other influencing factors (temperature, metal ions, chemical compounds, etc.), the carotenoids' composition, level, and isomeric content vary in a rather wide range. Irradiance conditions (studied in the 20–1250 μmol m^{-2} s^{-1} range) had a significant effect on carotene production by *D. salina* (*Ds*) with maximal fivefold improvement of the cellular carotenoid content [6]. The increased carotene production was related to the suppressed algal growth and was irradiance dependent, that is, low irradiances promoted the 9-*cis* isomer accumulation contrarily to high-irradiance conditions that favored all-*trans* carotene [6]. These results are somehow contradictory to the early works of Ben Amotz *et al.* [7, 8], who demonstrated that the ratio of the 9-*cis* and all-*trans* β-carotene isomers in *Dunaliella bardawil* (*Db*), equal to about 1 in the high-light-irradiance conditions, was about 10-fold decreased in the low-irradiance conditions. Nevertheless, a long exposure of *Db* to high-intensity blue light (2000 μmol m^{-2} s^{-1}, 500–580 nm) resulted in the stereoisomer-dependent degradation of β-carotene with faster degradation of the 9-*cis* form than the all-*trans* isomer [8].

Also, a study of outdoor cultivation of *Ds* in a closed tubular photoreactor showed over 30% net increase in both β-carotene and lutein levels and demonstrated that the 9-*cis*-β-carotene level raised during light period with the all-*trans*-isomer level unchanged until sunset (about 6 p.m.) [9]. The apparent influence of solar irradiance (maximally 460 μmol m^{-2} s^{-1}) on the *cis*-β-carotene accumulation (47 and 60% of total β-carotene before sunrise and in the afternoon–evening, respectively) affected significantly the *cis*-to-*trans* β-carotene ratio during the day–night cycle [9].

The above-mentioned studies demonstrate that usage of different irradiation conditions or/and algal strains result in different isomeric composition of β-carotene. Also, determination of which produced β-carotene forms are more beneficial on human health is not straightforward.

Deming *et al.* [10] reported that the all-*trans* β-carotene isomer is more bioavailable than the 9- and 13-*cis* isomers after a single oral dose in gerbils. Also, a longer administration of β-carotene isomers in humans brought similar conclusions. The preferential serum absorption of all-*trans* β-carotene over 9-*cis* β-carotene was noticed (14 days of daily administration of 40 mg synthetic or *Db*-derived carotenoid) [11]. These results were confirmed by the study of Tamai *et al.* [12], who found higher levels of both the 9-*cis* and all-*trans* forms of β-carotene in plasma, platelets, and mononuclear cells of healthy human males after administration of synthetic carotene compared to *Db*-derived samples containing approximately equal amounts of the all-*trans* and 9-*cis* forms (44 weeks daily administration of 60 mg synthetic, *Db*-derived carotenoid, or placebo). However, observed increased human serum concentrations of all-*trans*, and not 9-*cis*, β-carotene, upon ingestion of a natural isomer mixture obtained from *Ds* (Betatene) might have various reasons: preferential absorption of the all-*trans* form, rapid distribution of the 9-*cis* isomer into the tissues, or the presence of isomerase activity processing 9-*cis* to all-*trans* β-carotene conversion [13]. This and other reports demonstrate that many controversies have arisen around bioproperties of synthetic all-*trans* versus "natural" *cis-trans* isomeric mixtures of this pigment [14], and the question if algal β-carotene is more beneficial than the synthetic one still waits for a clear answer.

One of the most promising biosources of another carotenoid—the "superantioxidant" astaxanthin—is the green microalga *Haematococcus pluvialis* (*Hp*), one of the most commonly studied models for carotenoid production. Astaxanthin accumulation takes place in *Hp* upon various stress factors, among others high irradiance [15–19]. *Hp* with maximal total content of 22.7 mg per gram of the biomass was pointed out as the most efficient astaxanthin producer in strong light conditions (350 μmol m^{-2} s^{-1}, optimal sodium acetate content), followed by *Neochloris wimmeri*, *Protosiphon botryoides*, *Scotiellopsis oocystiformis*, *Chorella zofingiensis*, and *Scenedesmus vacuolatus* (19.3, 14.3, 10.9, 6.8, and 2.7 mg astaxanthin g^{-1} biomass, respectively) [20]. Astaxanthin content in *Hp,* grown on a Fe^{2+}-rich acetate medium, considerably increased upon illumination, with the high light intensity being favored over low, and continuous illumination being more efficient than light-dark cycles. Additionally, blue (370–480 nm) light was a more effective stimulus than red (>530 nm) light for astaxanthin overproduction [16]. The increase of the astaxanthin concentration in *Hp* upon illumination is accompanied with the higher expression of astaxanthin biosynthesis genes—lycopene cyclase, phytoene synthase, phytoene desaturase, and carotenoid hydroxylase—and, in turn, is correlated with the redox state of the photosynthetic electron transport [21, 22]. Nevertheless, it seems that astaxanthin is produced as a result of a photoprotection process rather than is itself a protective agent [23]. From the morphological point of view, irradiance of *Hp* cells leads to alteration from the green motile cells to cyst forms. This change is associated with the drastic change of the carotenoid pool. Whereas lutein (70%) and the xanthophyll cycle pigments (i.e., violaxanthin, antheraxanthin, zeaxanthin, and β-carotene) are the most abundant components of green motile cells [24], astaxanthin is the main pigment in cysts. Raman imaging was applied to study the relative concentration and distribution of three pure components (astaxanthin, β-carotene, and chlorophyll) in morphotypes of *Hp* cells upon noninductive and inductive conditions (cells induced to accumulate astaxanthin by suspending in nitrate-depleted medium and exposure to continuous high light [~350 μmol m^{-2} s^{-1}] for several days) [25]. Applied methodology enabled following the process of carotenoids formation in live cells and obtaining information about their distribution (Figure 13.1, Color Supplement).

Carotenoids accumulation in *Hp* was also studied from the kinetic point of view [26]. In the first phase of carotenoid accumulation (up to 5 h of irradiation with 1100 μmol m^{-2} s^{-1}), β-carotene is linearly consumed, whereas astaxanthin is synthesized in the following sequence: non-esterified, monoesterified, and finally di-esterified [26]. Consumed β-carotene is of photosynthetic origin (light-harvesting complex), in opposition to phase II (24 h of irradiation with 1100 μmol m^{-2} s^{-1}) when ongoing *de novo* synthesis of β-carotene (astaxanthin's precursor) takes place. Initially, in phase II, free and monoesterified astaxanthin is produced, followed by diesters amassing [26]. As the accumulated pigment is predominantly esterified, fatty acid synthesis is associated with astaxanthin accumulation [26]. Five fatty acids (oleic, linoleic, linolenic, palmitic, and stearic) were found in esterified astaxanthin in different proportions depending on the number of esters groups, irradiance time, and conditions [24]. Oleic and saturated (palmitic and stearic) were the main fatty acids found in monoesters and diesters, respectively [24, 27, 28].

It is known that astaxanthin oral bioavailability (in humans) can be enhanced in the presence of fat [29]. Deposition of natural astaxanthin fatty acid esters from *Hp* and the synthetic racemic pigment in rainbow trout brought no significant differences in the white

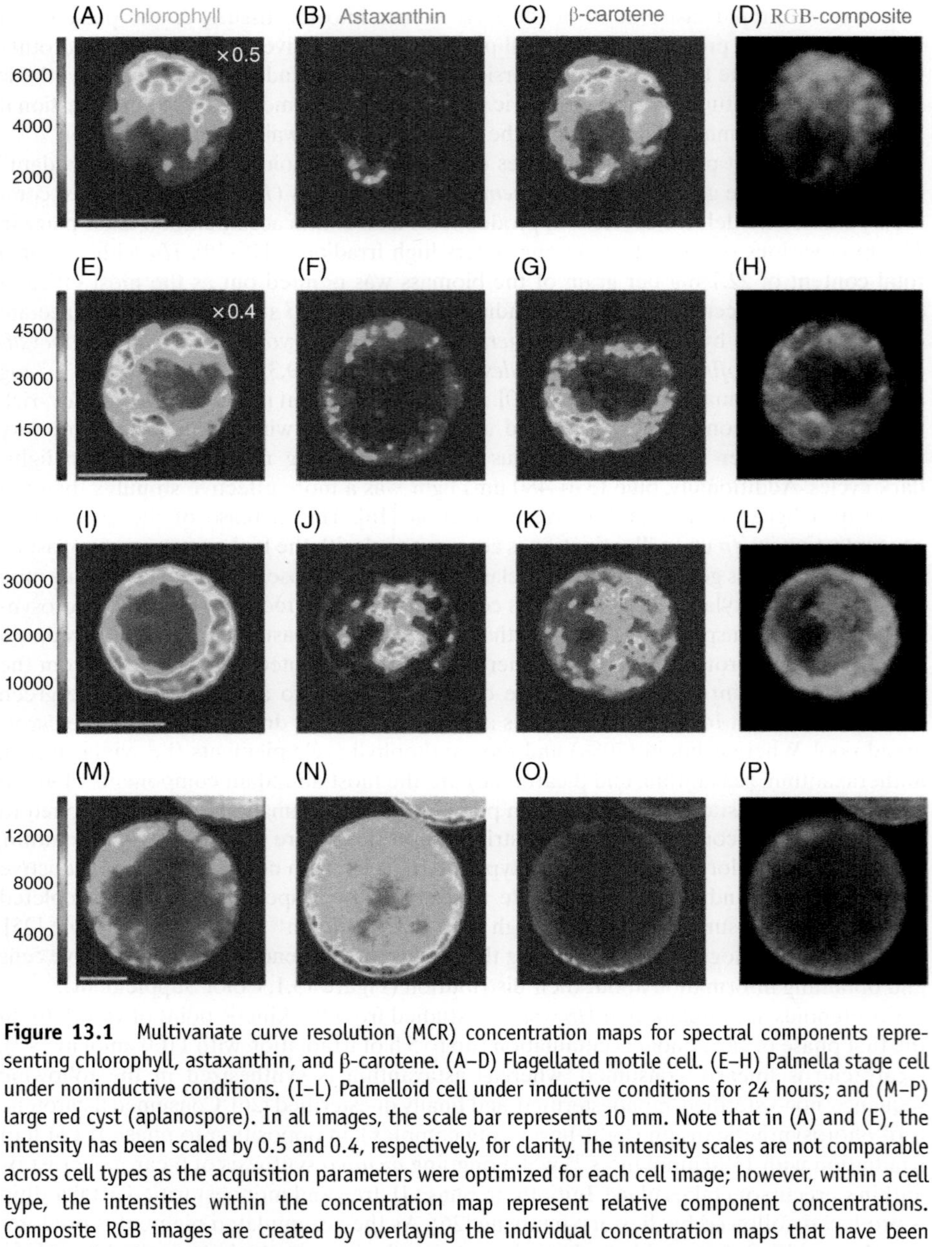

Figure 13.1 Multivariate curve resolution (MCR) concentration maps for spectral components representing chlorophyll, astaxanthin, and β-carotene. (A–D) Flagellated motile cell. (E–H) Palmella stage cell under noninductive conditions. (I–L) Palmelloid cell under inductive conditions for 24 hours; and (M–P) large red cyst (aplanospore). In all images, the scale bar represents 10 mm. Note that in (A) and (E), the intensity has been scaled by 0.5 and 0.4, respectively, for clarity. The intensity scales are not comparable across cell types as the acquisition parameters were optimized for each cell image; however, within a cell type, the intensities within the concentration map represent relative component concentrations. Composite RGB images are created by overlaying the individual concentration maps that have been pseudo-colored, as indicated in the image titles [25]. Figure reprinted upon Creative Commons Attribution License (CCAL). (*See insert for color representation of the figure.*)

muscle after 6 weeks of feeding [30]. Contrarily, absorption of astaxanthin by rainbow trout (56 days of feeding, 50 mg kg^{-1}) was not as efficient when it was fed with a mixture of esters (astaxanthin from *Hp*) as opposed to being fed with the non-esterified form (free, synthetic astaxanthin) [31].

Another very important source of astaxanthin is the yeast *Xanthophyllomyces dendrorhous* (*Xd*, the sexual state of *Phaffia rhodozyma*), potentially a more convenient source of pigments due to easier large-scale production of yeasts compared to algae [32]. It was demonstrated that all studied *Xd* strains have increased pigment-producing capability. Upon moderate white-light illumination, the final astaxanthin content was significantly strain-dependent, yet the 1.2–2.9-fold increase of the pigment content was detected in illuminated cultures relative to the dark-grown ones [33]. Contrarily, Hwan and Johnson [34] observed an overall decrease in the total carotenoid content and considerable alterations of the pigment composition (astaxanthin, phoenicoxanthin, 3-hydroxy-echinenone, 3,3′-dihydroxy-3′,4′-didehydro-β,ψ-caroten-4-one, β-zeacarotene, and β-carotene) and isomeric pool (*trans*/*cis* astaxanthin) in the light-grown conditions compared to the control, depending on the light wavelength and yeast strain. Vazquez [35] also denoted significant differences in the carotenoid composition in six *Xd* strains grown in light (500 lux) and in the dark, although for all strains the total carotenoid level and the astaxanthin content increased, contrarily to 3,3′-dihydroxy-3′,4′-didehydro-β-ψ-caroten-4-one, echinenone, 3-hydroxyechinenone, and cantaxanthin, whose content changes were strain-dependent. It can be concluded that the light influence on carotenoids production in *Xd* is considerably strain-dependent and, further, that systematic studies are necessary to obtain firm conclusions about this phenomenon.

Different stereoisomers of astaxanthin are formed in various carotenoid sources. For instance, the pigment in *Hp* and *Xd* is optically pure: (3S,3′S) and (3R,3′R) isomers, respectively; whereas the synthetic xanthophyll is the mixture of three forms: (3S,3′S), (*meso*), and (3R,3′R) in the 1:2:1 ratio. A single administration of the mixture of esters—95.2% all-*trans*-, 1.2% 9-*cis*-, and 3.6% 13-*cis*-astaxanthin, which is a mixture of (3R,3′R)-, (*meso*), and (3S,3′S)-astaxanthin in the 31:49:20 ratio—resulted in considerable selective accumulation of the *cis*- isomers over all-*trans*-astaxanthin in the plasma (with the proportions of ~70 and 30%, respectively). The (3R,3′R) optical isomer was also accumulated selectively in the plasma compared to other forms ((3R,3′R)-, (*meso*)-, and (3S,3′S)-astaxanthin in the 54:40:6 ratio) [36]. These results indicate that a selective process increases the relative proportion of *cis*- and (3R,3′R) isomers of astaxanthin compared to the all-*trans*-astaxanthin and *meso*/(3S,3′S) forms before uptake in the blood [36]. Selective absorption of the *cis*-isomers compared to all-*trans*-astaxanthin after a single-dose pigment ingestion, during blood uptake [37], was also observed by Osterlie *et al.*, without detecting changes is the optical isomers ratio. It was also reported that all three optical isomers are equally well resorbed by fish [38].

Carotenoid production by *Rhodotorula glutinis* depends on the mutual influence of white light and anaerobic or aerobic conditions [39]. The level of torularhodin, a specific carotenoid for *Rhodotorula* spp., can be increased at a cost of growth following exposure to low-intensity white light [40]. Bhosale and Gadre reported that *Rhodotorula* also can be a valuable source of β-carotene as illumination with white light in the late exponential growth phase led to a 58% increase in the β-carotene level in a β-carotene-producing mutant of *R. glutinis* [41]. Few other reports indicating the influence of illumination on carotenoid production in other microorganisms have been published [42–46].

Various studies seeking further commercialization and intensification of microbial carotenoid production by illumination have been recently undertaken. A quite simple but effective way is development of a proper selection method to obtain microbial mutants of increased carotenoid productivity. A variation of this method based on eliminating β-carotene-poor algae using high-intensity (200 W m^{-2}) blue light was applied in the case of *Db*, resulting in a circa sixfold increase of β-carotene production in the mutants [47]. Various types of photoreactor constructions were tested, for instance a considerable (maximal 7.6-fold enhancement) increase of the intracellular β-carotene concentration in *Ds* was obtained in a flat-panel photobioreactor run in turbidostat mode upon high-irradiance conditions (2×1000 μmol m^{-2} s^{-1}) [28]. An example of a quite different tactic resulting in carotenoid overproduction is the study of Steinbrenner and Sandmann [48], who applied site-directed mutagenesis in carotenoid biosynthesis enzyme phytoene desaturase in *Hp*. Under light stress conditions, one of the studied *Hp* mutants showed enhanced accumulation of astaxanthin, whose level after 48 h of exposure to high light was 26% higher compared to the native alga [48].

13.3 Temperature

As temperature is one of the key factors for controlling growth of the organisms, the effects of temperature on the pigmentation of algae have been noticed since the 1950s [49]. For many carotenoid producers, including their commercial sources the *Dunaliella* and *Haematococcus* spp., temperature is the most important factor controlling cell growth and pigment production [5].

In *Db* culture, decreasing the temperature from 30 to 10 °C resulted in a twofold increase of the β-carotene content with no significant changes in other carotenoids. Additionally, it was noticed that the decrease of the temperature selectively increased 9-*cis* carotene content more than twice compared to the all-*trans* isomer [50].

Orset and Young's study [51] of carotenoid production in *Ds* upon the temperature increase demonstrated that, at low-irradiance conditions (120 μmol m^{-2} s^{-1}), a low temperature did not affect total carotenoid accumulation, although it resulted in the selective increase of the α-carotene (7.5-fold with the temperature decrease from 34 to 17 °C) and *cis*-β-carotene level. These changes were interconnected with the decrease of all-*trans* β-carotene content (the level of the 9-*cis*-form increased relatively to all-*trans*-β-carotene about 10% between 17 and 34 °C, but no significant changes in the isomer population of α-carotene were noticed). At high-irradiance conditions (1000 μmol m^{-2} s^{-1}), α-carotene was also selectively accumulated upon the temperature decrease, but, in this case, the total pigment amassing was also promoted by low temperatures [51]. Similarly to the low-irradiance conditions, the ratio of the 9-*cis* to all-*trans* forms of β-carotene increased with the temperature decrease (twofold between 19 and 30 °C), and so did the ratio of the 9-*cis* to all-*trans* forms of α-carotene [51].

The above-mentioned study is one of scarce examples of the research devoted to the study of non-β isomers of carotene. Therefore, it is worth noticing that a recent momentous work (human serum concentration: 16,573 adults, 13.9 years duration) demonstrated that the serum α-carotene concentrations were inversely associated with the risk of death from all causes, among others cardiovascular diseases and cancer [52]. This conclusion explains the fact that although high consumption of fruits and vegetables was associated with low risks of many chronic diseases (among others, cancer, cardiovascular diseases, and type 2 diabetes mellitus), results from randomized trials were unable to unambiguously link the consumption of β-carotene supplements with the risk of chronic diseases [53–56]. As the α- to β-carotene ratio in *Dunaliella* can be quite easily controlled (at least to some extent) by using temperature [51], it may be of potential future interest to use this factor to further optimize α-carotene production.

The influence of the temperature on carotenoid production in outdoor *Ds* cultures in the tubular photobioreactor was tested. The temperature was (1) kept at 25 °C throughout the day, (2) oscillating between 17 and 25 °C, and (3) in the range of 17–30 °C (no temperature control), and the obtained results showed that the constant temperature conditions are favorable (the productivity ratio of β-carotene equaled 2.9:1.6:1 for a, b, and c, respectively) [9].

A β-carotene level was shown to increase exponentially in the temperature range of 4–37 °C in the aerobic mycelium *Mucor rouxii* (from ca. 10 to 170 μg g^{-1} dry weight), showing the twofold increase in 37 °C compared to its usual growth temperature (28 °C) [57].

A very interesting example of temperature influence on carotenoids production is the behavior of recombinant *Sacharomyces cerevisiae* expressing carotenogenic genes from *Xd*. The recombinant Sc-EYBI cells were reported to synthesize massively higher (258.8 μg g^{-1} dry cell weight) amounts of β-carotene when growing at 20 °C, about 59-fold higher compared to 30 °C. In a modified recombinant (Sc-EYBIH) β-carotene level was further increased to 528.8 μg g^{-1} dry cell weight and was also highly temperature dependent (at 20 °C, 27-fold higher than for cells growing at 30 °C) [58].

This study is an example of using a fast-growing and low-demanding species (*S. cerevisiae*) to obtain quite significant β-carotene content. Further development of carotenoids bioproduction based on recombinant species could result in selectively obtaining other carotenoids with designed properties, for instance higher bioavailability and beneficial effects on human health.

Elevated temperatures may have also a positive effect on some secondary carotenoids production. Astaxanthin accumulation was increased threefold in *Hp* cultivated at 30 °C relatively to 20 °C along with the increased cell encystment [59].

Contrarily, low temperatures resulted in a 50% increase of the total carotenoid level in *Xd* and a change of the relative carotenoid pool [60]. The presence of 10 mM nicotine (inhibitor of the cyclization step in carotenogenesis) in cultures of *Xd* mutants resulted in the accumulation of lycopene and γ-carotene, while the oxidation of β-carotene was inhibited by 10 mM-diphenylamine that was reversible in the low-temperature conditions [60].

The effect of thermal stress was studied in the green alga *Chlorococcum* sp. upon nitrogen starvation conditions [61]. Upon the temperature increase (20–30 °C), the following trends were observed: (1) increase of β-cryptoxanthin (ca. 33-fold), 3′-hydroechinenone (ca. twofold), astaxanthin (ca. twofold), and total carotenoids level (ca. twofold); (2) decrease of β-carotene (ca. fivefold) and cantaxanthin (ca. twofold); and (3) variations of levels of echinenone, adonirubin, and adonixanthin [61].

The temperature also affected the composition of fatty acids and the total carotenoids content in the microalga *Diacronema vlkianum* (*Haptophyceae*) [62]. The total carotenoids content decreased about twofold with a simultaneous increase of the relative concentration of astaxanthin (from ca. 40 to 49%) in 26 °C relatively to 18 °C in the exponential phase of the cell growth [62].

Rather atypical methodology (Raman spectroscopy supported by quantum-chemical calculations) was used to follow changes in the astaxanthin isomers content *in situ* upon the temperature increase in the wide range of temperatures (−100 to 150 °C) [63]. It was proposed that the carotenoid, initially in the form of H-aggregates with the *trans* conformation of both end rings, is released from aggregates and rotamerizes to the more stable gauche forms upon the thermal treatment [63].

The influence of the temperature on the carotenoid level and growth of the microalga *Muriellopsis* sp., a potent lutein producer, was also examined [64]. The lutein per cell level was unchanged in the temperature range of 20–28 °C, followed by about a sixfold increase as the temperature was raised from 28 to 33 °C. Nevertheless, the maximal lutein level in the culture was obtained at 28 °C, due to the maximal cell density at this temperature [64]. The alga *S. almeriensis*, producing up to 76% of lutein in the total carotenoids content, also reacted in a twofold increase of lutein content with the temperature increase from

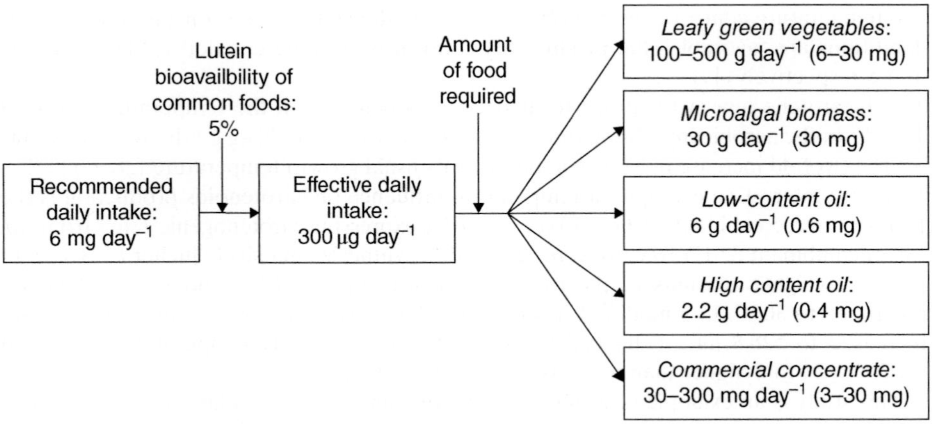

Figure 13.2 Dietary requests of microalgae biomass and lutein concentrates from microalgae compared with other sources taking into account bioavailability. Numbers in parentheses show the total amount of lutein to be ingested to cover the recommended daily dose. Reprinted with permission from Ref. [66].

10 to 30 °C, following a slight drop of lutein upon a further temperature increase to 40 °C (illumination-stimulating solar circle, maximally 1400 μmol m^{-2} s^{-1}) [65].

Microalgae are a potential source of lutein and could be purified and processed similarly to *Marigold oelresin*, which is currently a main source of lutein supplements. Taking into account that some microalgae, particularly *Murielopsis* sp. and *S. almariensis*, have a higher lutein content than *M. oelresin* (Figure 13.2), they can be a very prospective source of lutein, particularly if extraction methods are improved [66].

Significant variations in the carotenoid pool are observed in *R. glutinis* upon temperature changes in the range of 10–40 °C as the proportions of β-carotene–torulene–torularhodin equal 88:9:3 and 65:28:7 at 10 and 40 °C, respectively [41]. The higher content of torulene at higher temperatures is probably caused by the fact that the γ-carotene dehydrogenation and decarboxylation, leading to torulene synthesis, is a temperature-dependent step [5].

These results are in agreement with the previously reported inhibition of the production of torulene and torularhodin and higher β-carotene accumulation in *R. glutinis* cells maintained at 5 °C for 21 days [67]. Also, Buzzini and Martini [68] reported that synthesis of β-carotene and torulene was favored at lower temperatures (25 °C), whereas higher temperatures (35 °C) are better conditions for torularhodin production in *R. glutinis*.

As torulene and torularhodin are used mostly as feed products rather than health supplements, it can be concluded that low-temperature, being the β-carotene-maximizing factor, is of consideration in the large-scale *Rhodotorula* cultures.

Different bacterial strains also accumulate carotenoids upon unfavorable environmental conditions: For example, in the cyanobacterium *Synechococcus* sp., the carotenoid–chlorophyll ratio increased substantially at 15 °C, as compared to cells grown at 38 or 22 °C, due to nitrogen limitation [44]. Also, the low temperature is a stimulant for production of the C_{50} carotenoid bacterioruberin and its glycosylated derivatives in bacterium *Arthrobacter agilis*, isolated from Antarctic sea ice [69]. Two strains of carotenoid-producing thermophilic bacteria similar to *Chloroflexus aurantiacus*, grown at 55 °C and rich in γ-carotene and hydroxy-γ-carotene, and only trace amounts of β-carotene (i.e., the main component of *C. aurantiacus*) were isolated [70].

The temperature influence on the accumulation of carotenoids by microbial cells is quite complicated. Depending on the microorganism, both low and high temperatures can be a carotenoid-stimulating factor. This complicates considerably the optimization of microbial production, as the temperature is rather difficult to control in the outdoor cultures. Nevertheless, knowledge about the temperature influence and analysis of its synergetic or anti-synergetic effects with other factors can be helpful in designing and localizing large-scale microbial carotenoids farms.

13.4 Carbon and nitrogen sources

The carbon source plays a dual role during the microbial fermentation. It is both a major constituent for building cellular material and an important energy source. The influence of different carbon sources on β-carotene production in *B. trispora* cells is presented in Figure 13.3.

The maximum amount of β-carotene (99 mg dm^{-3}) was observed for D-glucose, which can be easily assimilated in the metabolic pathway of β-carotene biosynthesis. The second-best carbon source was fructose, and tapioca dextrins, soluble starch, and maltose resulted in a similar level of β-carotene production (approx. 20–25 mg dm^{-3}). Dextrins, potatoes, sucrose, glycerol, whey, lactose, and molasses were found to be poor substrates with respect to both the cell growth as well as β-carotene production [71].

Regulation of carotenogenesis in the dimorphic fungus *M. rouxii* was also dependent on saccharides used as the carbon source [57]. Among the evaluated saccharides, β-carotene production was the highest for glucose and lower (in decreasing order) for cellobiose, maltose, xylose, lactose, and sucrose. Generally, monosaccharides are the best available carbon source for microorganisms, and in the conditions of their absence the monosaccharides are produced in the medium by digestion of complex sugars whose bioavailability depends on the chemical structure [57].

The effect of chosen organic nitrogen sources on production of β-carotene in *B. trispora* cells is presented in Figure 13.3. A higher yield of β-carotene (90 mg dm^{-3}) was obtained for a yeast extract as compared to a soya peptone and beef extract (approx. 50 mg dm^{-3}).

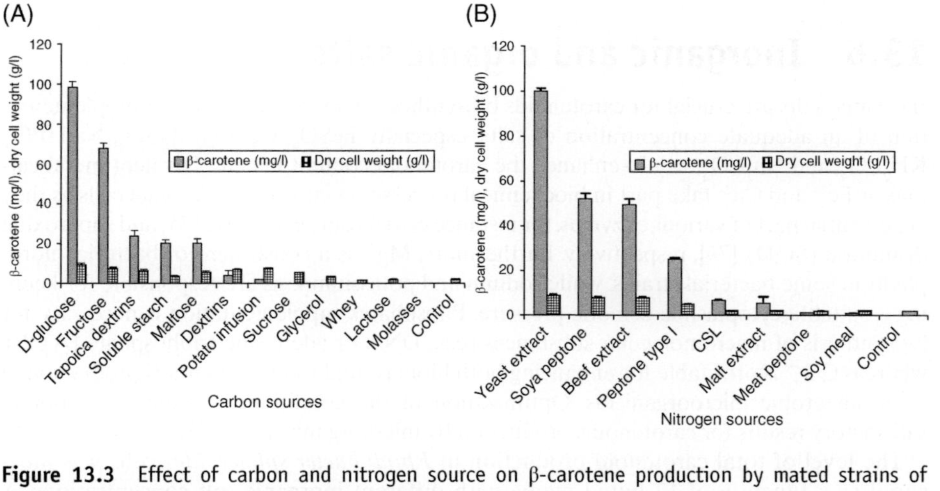

Figure 13.3 Effect of carbon and nitrogen source on β-carotene production by mated strains of *B. trispora*. Reprinted with permission from Ref. [71].

Other screened nitrogen sources resulted in considerably lower β-carotene production [71]. The nitrate concentration of the media is a significant parameter affecting carotenogenesis. The green microalga *Hp* was cultured in different concentrations of sodium nitrate to determine the concentration effect on cell growth and astaxanthin accumulation. The influence of five different concentrations (0.0, 0.75, 1.50, 3.00, and 6.00 mM) of sodium nitrate was evaluated. The highest astaxanthin accumulation was observed for algal cells cultivated in the absence of sodium nitrate [72]. Simultaneously, nitrogen starvation caused retention of division and growth in size in the exposed cells in response to the environmental stress [17, 73]. Under nitrogen starvation, the maximum of astaxanthin accumulation was achieved after 8 days of the experiment, when the amount of chlorophyll per cell decreased significantly [73]. A similar effect was observed when cells of *Hp* grown under optimal conditions were suspended in a phosphate-free medium containing two concentrations of nitrogen: high and low. The phosphate-deprived culture exposed to the high nitrogen concentration produced astaxanthin excessively when compared to cells grown under the low level of nitrogen [17]. An increased secondary carotenoids accumulation (canthaxanthin and astaxanthin) in the green alga *Chlorella zofingiensis* was found to respond to the combined conditions of nitrogen-free medium and high light intensity [43].

13.5 Aerobic versus anaerobic conditions

For yeast, capable of both oxidative phosphorylation and anaerobic fermentation, the environment significantly affects the metabolism, including pigment production capacity. Recently, it was demonstrated in live *Rhodothorula mucilaginosa* cells that carotenoids are not biosynthesized in the anaerobic environment, although they are dominating in the cells cultured in the oxygen atmosphere. Additionally, flavohemoproteins rather than carotenoids are produced in the *Rhodotorula* cells upon the switch of the phenotype to adjust from an anaerobic to aerobic environment [74]. In the live yeast grown in the aerobic conditions, carotenoids are colocalized with lipids, as demonstrated by using high-resolution (lateral ca. 260 nm) Raman imaging (Figure 13.4, Color Supplement).

13.6 Inorganic and organic salts

Inorganic salts are crucial for carotenoids biosynthesis in microbial cells. The supplementation of an adequate concentration of salts, especially $FeSO_4$, $CuSO_4$, $MgSO_4$, Na_2HPO_4, KH_2PO_4, and Na_2CO_3, would enhance the carotenoid content in cells. Divalent metal cations as Fe^{2+} and Cu^{2+} take part in biochemical processes occurring in microbial cells as they are essential part of various enzymes, for instance cytochrome-*c*-oxidase [75] and superoxide dismutase (SOD) [76], respectively. Furthermore, Mg^{2+} is a constituent of bacteriochlorophylls in some bacterial strains, while sodium and potassium ions are responsible for keeping a suitable cytoplasmic osmotic pressure. Phosphates supplementation is necessary for biosynthesis of macromolecular substances (e.g., DNA or adenosine triphosphate [ATP]), whereas CO_3^{2-} is profitable for enhancing both biomass and total carotenoids production in some anaerobic microorganisms. Optimization of the conditions is required to obtain satisfactory results for carotenoids production by microorganisms [71, 75].

The level of total carotenoid production in *Rhodobacter sphaeroides* cells was measured as a function of 12 liquid media with different inorganic salt concentrations. A statistical methodology was applied to find an optimal combination of inorganic salts for

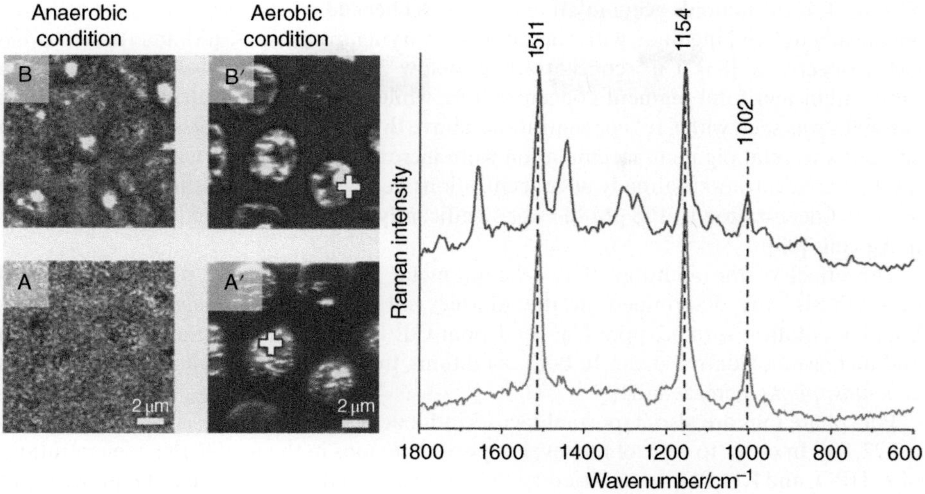

Figure 13.4 Representative images showing the distribution of carotenoids *in Rhodotholua mucilaginosa* (integration over the band at 1156 cm^{-1}, A and A′) and lipid bodies (2857 cm^{-1}, B and B′) grown in aerobic and anaerobic conditions. Single Raman spectrum (extracted from cross-marked points on the maps A′ and B′) showing features due to the mixture of lipids with carotenoids, and carotenoids (blue and red spectra, respectively). Adapted from Ref. [74] with permission from The Royal Society of Chemistry. (*See insert for color representation of the figure.*)

carotenoid accumulation (the maximal total carotenoid content of 17.245 mg dm^{-3}) that was evaluated as follows: $MgSO_4$ 0.12 g dm^{-3}, Na_2HPO_4 2.05 g dm^{-3}, $FeSO_4$ 0.03 g dm^{-3}, and Na_2CO_3 2.22 g dm^{-3} [75].

Hp responds to the presence of ferrous ions through enhanced production of astaxanthin [77]. The hyperaccumulation of carotenoids in *Hp* cells upon Fe^{2+} ions is the response to generation of hydroxyl radicals according to the Fenton reaction [59]. The supplementation of EDTA-chelated ferrous ions did not substantially affect the astaxanthin biosynthesis, as iron in this form did not undergo the Fenton reaction [78]. Previously, stimulation of astaxanthin synthesis by free radicals was observed for *Xd* yeast cells [79].

Addition of ferrous ions together with acetate enabled control of the cell cycle phase of the yeast cells. Generally, supplementation of acetate to the *Hp* culture induced formation of red cysts enriched in astaxanthin from green chlorophyll–rich biflagellated cells. Encystment was accompanied by a decrease in both protein and chlorophyll content. The addition of Fe^{2+} to acetate considerably accelerated formation of cyst and disappearance of cellular proteins, and drastically enhanced biosynthesis of astaxanthin [77].

The stimulatory or inhibitory effect of metal ions on carotenoids biosynthesis depends on the nature of a specific carotenogenesis enzyme. Several divalent cations (Ba^{2+}, Fe^{2+}, Mg^{2+}, Ca^{2+}, Zn^{2+}, and Co^{2+}) can act as chemical stimulants of carotenogenesis in *R. glutinis* cells [80]. Moreover, calcium, zinc, and ferrous cations resulted in both enhanced volumetric production (mg dm^{-1}) as well as cellular accumulation (mg g^{-1}) of carotenoids in *R. glutinis* mutants [81]. A carotenoid profile of *R. graminis* changes considerably under the influence of some trace elements: Fe^{3+}, Co^{2+}, Mn^{2+}, Al^{3+}, and Zn^{2+}. Two cations, Co^{2+} and Al^{3+}, exhibited a stimulatory effect on β- and γ-carotene production, while the accumulation of torulene and torularhodin was the highest under stimulation with Mn^{2+}, Al^{3+}, and Zn^{2+} [82].

The level of carotenoids accumulation in *Xd* was checked by culturing the yeast cells in a chemically defined medium, with Cu^{2+} and Fe^{2+} varying from 0 to 32 μM and from 0 to 108 μM, respectively [83]. Cu^{2+} concentrations below 3.2 μM progressively increased both astaxanthin and total pigment concentrations, while no significant effect on the studied variables was seen with Cu^{2+} concentrations above this value. Nevertheless, the astaxanthin content and total pigment accumulation were increased significantly with the increase of the Fe^{2+} concentration (already at concentrations below 1 μM), while the further increase of Fe^{2+} concentration to 108 μM did not significantly affect the production of astaxanthin in *Xd* cells [83].

The effect of the addition of two heavy metal ions (Cu^{2+} and Cd^{2+}) on carotenoid biosynthesis was determined in the marine red macroalga *Gracilaria tenuistipitata*. Supplementation with 0.2 ppm Cu^{2+} or 1 ppm Cd^{2+} resulted in decreased culture growth and increased oxidative stress. In both conditions, the content of lutein and β-carotene in *G. tenuistipitata* increased [84].

Phosphate ions are also important factors influencing carotenogenesis in microbial cells [17, 72, 83]. In order to control the level of phosphate ions in the media, the concentrations of K_2HPO_4 and KH_2PO_4 were varied. Astaxanthin accumulation and the cell number of *Hp* were checked in the three different phosphate concentrations: 0.85, 1.70, and 3.40 mM [72]. The overall effect of phosphate starving on *Hp* was similar to the effects observed in nitrogen-free cultures: phosphate starvation stimulated astaxanthin synthesis and inhibited chlorophyll formation in the algal cells. However, under phosphate starvation, the rate of astaxanthin accumulation was slower compared to in nitrogen-free conditions, and carotenoid content leveled off after 14 days [73]. Similarly, in *Xd* cells, an increase of the total pigment concentrations (4.0–4.6 mg dm^{-3}) as well as astaxanthin accumulation (1.7–2.3 mg dm^{-3}) upon a decrease of the phosphate concentration in the media (from 4.8 to 1.3 mM) was observed [85].

The effect of various citrate concentrations (0–58 mM) in the medium on *Xd* culture was also performed [85]. Citrate is one of the intermediates in the TCA (tricarboxylic acids) cycle, taking part in biosynthesis of the carbon skeleton of carotenoids and in lipids formation in microbial cells [5]. Low concentrations of citrate (up to 1.2 mM) revealed no effect on pigment accumulation, but supplementation of citrate at levels of 29 mM or higher was reported to increase the total carotenoid concentration in the yeast cells with parallel decreasing of proteins [85]. In contrast, administration of amino acids (glutamate, glutamine, aspartate, and asparagine) derived from TCA cycle intermediates resulted in increased growth of cells and decreased carotenoid production. In general, carotenoid accumulation depends on the quantities of reactive species generated during the TCA cycle. Supplementation of amino acids decreased the production of reactive oxygen species by lowering TCA cycle activity, causing a decrease of carotenoid production [86].

Increased salinity—induced, for instance, by the NaCl solution—can be an important exogenous stress factor stimulating microbial cells to enhanced carotenogenesis. Some of the yeast strains exhibited a significant increase in carotenoid production in response to the osmotic stress. *R. glutinis* and *R. mucilaginosa* produced 2.5-fold and sixfold more β-carotene after the addition of 10% NaCl at the beginning of the growth phase, respectively [87]. Also, in the strain of *Sporidiobolus salmonicolor*, the high level of β-carotene was obtained after the osmotic stress [87]. The highest yield of β-carotene per dry mass was obtained under mixed osmotic (NaCl) and oxidative (H_2O_2) stress factors. The β-carotene accumulation was over threefold higher when compared with control after incubation of the yeast culture with 2% of salt and 5 mmol dm^{-3} peroxide. Lycopene production during the stress experiments exhibited a very similar course to β-carotene changes [88].

A. agilis, a psychotropic bacteria isolated from Antarctic sea ice, can produce a series of geometrical isomers of the C_{50} carotenoid bacterioruberin; mono-, di-, and tetra-glycosylated derivatives of bacterioruberin; and a C_{50} hydrocarbon, tetraanhydrobacterioruberin. The overall pigment content decreased proportionally to the increased NaCl concentration, varying from 0 to 10% (w/v). However, no carotenoid production was observed in the medium containing 10% (w/v) NaCl [69].

13.7 Other chemical agents

Over 50 years ago, it was observed that addition of some nitrogen compounds enhances carotenoids production in *B. trispora* and *P. blakesleanus* [89, 90]. An inhibitor of lycopene cyclase (2-methylimidazole) at the 50 mg dm^{-3} level was found equally active as at higher concentrations (100 or 200 mg dm^{-3}). For concentrations in the range of 50–200 mg dm^{-3}, lycopene was produced nearly selectively (95% of total carotenoid content), whereas for a lower 2-methylimidazole concentration (10 mg dm^{-3}), carotenes were produced in the higher amount (15% of total carotenoid content) [91]. The influence of other inhibitors of lycopene cyclase, such as piperidine, triethylamine, pyridine, and creatinine, on carotenoid production was tested. The largest increases in the level of lycopene—about eightfold (270 mg dm^{-3}) and sixfold (198 mg dm^{-3})—were observed after stimulation of piperidine (in a dose of 500 ppm) and triethylamine (in a dose of 750 ppm), respectively. Most of the chemical compounds with a trimethylcyclohexyl ring (e.g., vitamin A, and α- and β-ionone) have been reported to enhance carotenoid accumulation in fungus cells [5]. Therefore, to obtain maximal stimulation of lycopene, vitamin A acetate at 1000 ppm was added to stimulate β-carotene production, and then piperidine at 500 ppm was added after 48 h. Under these conditions, 775±5 mg dm^{-3} of lycopene level was obtained quite selectively as the β-carotene was significantly lower (67±1 mg dm^{-3}) [92]. The concentration of β-carotene in *B. trispora* cells increased proportionally to vitamin A acetate concentration from 500 to 1000 ppm, and then decreased with the further concentration growth. The highest concentration of β-carotene (828±3 mg dm^{-3}) was obtained in a culture grown with vitamin A acetate at 1000 ppm [92]. A similar pattern of changes in the β-carotene production was observed: an increasing accumulation with rising concentrations of penicillin (from 500 to 1000 ppm) in *B. trispora* cells. Nevertheless, the received level of β-carotene was comparable with that of the control, when penicillin was added in the beginning of the experiment [92].

The effect of other nitrogen compounds such as diphenylamine and nicotine on carotenoids biosynthesis in *Xd* was studied. The oxidation of β-carotene was irreversibly inhibited by 10 μM of diphenylamine, and the dehydrogenation of phytoene was reversibly inhibited by 60 μM-diphenylamine. It was also found that 10 mM of nicotine inhibits the cyclization of lycopene, but after nicotine removal the initial carotenogenesis pathway was restored with a decrease in lycopene concentration and a subsequent accumulation of β-carotene [60].

13.8 pH

pH has an important influence on carotenoids formation, although usually it was considered as one of multiple tested compounds in the cultures of microorganisms. For example, pH as well as other factors affect cellular carotenogenesis in cultures of algae *Muriellopsis* cells. Maximum accumulation of lutein, violaxanthin, and β-carotene in the *Muriellopsis* culture was observed when cells were grown at pH 6.5, and it decreased markedly at lower and higher pH values. Nevertheless, the lutein level per cell showed maxima at pH 6 and 9, being five- to sevenfold higher than those at pH 6.5 [42]. Enhanced β-carotene accumulation at pH 6–7 and pH 7–8 values has also been reported for *B. trispora* [71] and for *Chlorococcum* sp. [61], respectively.

13.9 Multiple stress factors

The real problems in optimizing industrial-scale cultures of carotenoids is the fact that various discussed factors influencing carotenogenesis may have synergetic activity and act differently in different microorganisms. A complicated dependence between various factors results in the practical impossibility of establishing a single optimization scheme for various carotenoids producers. This is illustrated in this section based on the example of a single study describing optimization of a single carotenoid production in various microorganisms by manipulation of various factors [20]. Orasa *et al.* [20] reported that the optimal astaxanthin content in *Hp* was obtained in the conditions of a nitrogen-free medium if the initial pH of the medium was acidic (pH 4) and under light intensity of 350 mmol photons m^{-2} s^{-1}. For *N. wimmeri*, a better astaxanthin accumulation rate was obtained when 300 mM sodium acetate was used, while none of the conditions assayed (just three: initial acid pH, salinity stress, and nitrogen-free medium with sodium acetate) resulted in the increased astaxanthin production in *P. botryoides* [20]. Moreover, the optimal astaxanthin production was obtained after a different time period from that of the culture setup, and some crucial factors influencing the carotenogenesis (light and temperature) were kept constant [20]. As the number of factors influencing carotenogenesis is significant, testing their various combinations seems to be a time-consuming task. Therefore, development of complex statistical approaches is of basic importance in order to considerably increase carotenoid accumulation, particularly in the case of large-scale cultures.

13.10 Perspectives and conclusions

A number of factors discussed in this chapter—light, temperature, carbon and nitrogen sources, metal ions and salts, various chemical components, and even pH—affect the structure, content, and type of carotenoids in microbial cells. The combination of suitable stress-inducing stimuli considerably increases accumulation of carotenoids in industrial cultures of microbial cells. Knowledge about the influence of these factors is essential in light of growing demands for carotenoids production (the predicted market value of commercially used carotenoids is estimated to be nearly $1.4 billion in 2018 [1]) and increasing global ecological consciousness resulting in a need for natural products.

Only a few strains are being used in the current industrial production of carotenoids (e.g., *H. pluvialis*, *D. salina*, and chlorophycean microalgae for biosynthesis of astaxanthin, β-carotene, and lutein, respectively). To move forward, it is necessary to find new strains that efficiently respond to stress factors, have a high growing rate and low environmental demands, and produce a high content of desired carotenoids [3]. For example, a systematic study of 15 strains of chlorophycean microalgae has been investigated with emphasis on their carotenoid profiles. *Muriellopsis* sp., a strain with the shortest doubling time and the highest carotenoids production yield, has been indicated as the most prospective source for industrial biosynthesis of lutein [42]. Further systematic searches for low-cost new strains of algae or yeasts capable of efficient carotenogenesis are, therefore, essential.

Optimizing the conditions of cell growth and carotenogenesis of microorganisms is another key point in furthering the carotenoid biotechnology. As multiple factors control carotenoids production and their results are frequently synergistic, statistical methods are necessary to find the optimal combination of various factors. Previously, such statistical approaches were used to optimize a culture medium (carbon and nitrogen sources, trace elements, pH, and inorganic salts composition) for β-carotene and total carotenoid production by *B. trispora* [71] and *R. sphaeroids* [75], respectively. This kind of algorithm enables screening of the parameters and further designing of optimal conditions for microbial carotenoids production. Another strategy in the biosynthesis of carotenoids is genetic modification of microalgae cells [93]. Both these approaches can be further improved and used to plan large-scale cultures.

The recognized therapeutic value of carotenoids for the prevention and treatment of various diseases caused an enhanced need for these pigments. The carotenoid market requires increased carotenoids production from biological sources. Research directed toward optimizing the efficiency and selectivity of carotenogenesis in microbial organisms, parallel with studies aimed at assessing bioavailability and health effects of these naturally produced pigments, should be undertaken to improve production of carotenoids of designed properties.

Acknowledgments

This project was supported by the National Science Centre (DEC-2012/07/B/ST5/00889).

References

1. http://www.bccresearch.com/market-research/food-and-beverage/carotenoids-global-market-fod025d.html (last accessed July 1, 2015).
2. M. A. Borowitzka, "High-value products from microalgae: their development and commercialization," *J. Appl. Phycol.*, 2013, **25**, 743.
3. J. A. Del Campo, M. García-González, and M. G. Guerrero, "Outdoor cultivation of microalgae for carotenoid production: current state and perspectives," *Appl. Microbiol. Biotechnol.*, 2007, **74**, 1163.
4. L. C. Mata-Gómez, J. C. Montañez, A. Méndez-Zavala, and C. N. Aguilar, "Biotechnological production of carotenoids by yeasts: an overview," *Microb. Cell Factories*, 2014, **13**, 43.
5. P. Bhosale, "Environmental and cultural stimulants in the production of carotenoids from microorganisms," *Appl. Microbiol. Biotechnol.*, 2004, **63**, 351.
6. S. C. Orset and A. J. Young, "Exposure to low irradiances favors the synthesis of 9-cis beta, beta-carotene in *Dunaliella salina* (Teod.)," *J. Plant Physiol.*, 2000, **122**, 609.
7. A. Ben-Amotz, A. Katz, and M. Avron, "Isolation and characterization of a protein associated with carotene globules in the alga *Dunaliella bardawil*," *J. Phycol.*, 1982, **18**, 529.
8. A. Ben-Amotz, A. Lers, and M. Avron, "Stereoisomers of beta-carotene and phytoene in the alga *Dunaliella bardawil*," *Plant Physiol.*, 1988, **86**, 1286.
9. M. García-González, J. Moreno, J. C. Manzano, F. J. Florencio, and M. G. Guerrero, "Production of *Dunaliella salina* biomass rich in 9-cis-beta-carotene and lutein in a closed tubular photobioreactor," *J. Biotechnol.*, 2005, **115**, 81.

10. D. M. Deming, S. R. Teixeira, and J. W. Erdman, "All-trans beta-carotene appears to be more bioavailable than 9-cis or 13-cis beta-carotene in gerbils given single oral doses of each isomer," *J. Nutr.*, 2002, **132**, 2700.

11. A. Ben-Amotz and Y. Levy, "Bioavailability of a natural isomer mixture compared with synthetic all-trans beta-carotene in human serum," *Am. J. Clin. Nutr.*, 1996, **63**, 729.

12. H. Ohigashi, T. Osawa, J. Terao, S. Watanabe, and T. Yoshikawa (Eds.), *Food factors for cancer prevention*, Berlin: Springer, 1997, p. 548.

13. W. Stahl, W. Schwarz, and H. Sies, "Human serum concentrations of all-trans beta- and alpha-carotene but not 9-cis beta-carotene increase upon ingestion of a natural isomer mixture obtained from *Dunaliella salina* (Betatene)," *J. Nutr.*, 1993, **123**, 847.

14. L. Patrick, "Beta-carotene: the controversy continues," *Altern. Med. Rev.*, 2000, **5**, 530–45.

15. Y. Yong and Y.-K. Lee, "Do carotenoids play a photoprotective role in the cytoplasm of *Haematococcus lacustris* (Chlorophyta)," *Phycologia*, 1991, **30**, 257.

16. M. Kobayashi, T. Kakizono, N. Nishio, and S. Nagai, "Effect of light intensity, light quality, and illumination cycle on astaxanthin formation in a green alga, *Haematococcus pluvialis*," *J. Ferment. Bioeng.*, 1992, **74**, 61.

17. S. Boussiba, L. Fan, and A. Vonshak, "Enhancement and determination of astaxanthin accumulation in green alga *Haematococcus pluvialis*," *Methods Enzymol.*, 1992, **213**, 386.

18. C. Hagen, W. Braune, E. Birckner, and J. Nuske, "Functional aspects of secondary carotenoids in *Haematococcus lacustris* (Girod) Rostafinski," *New Phytol.*, 1993, **125**, 625.

19. C. Hagen, W. Braune, and L. O. Björn, "Functional aspects *of* secondary carotenoids in *Haematococcus lacustris*," *J. Phycol.*, 1994, **30**, 241.

20. M. Orosa, J. Valero, C. Herrero, and J. Abalde, "Comparison of the accumulation of astaxanthin in *Haematococcus pluvialis* and other green microalgae under N-starvation and high light conditions," *Biotechnol. Lett.*, 2001, **23**, 1079.

21. J. Steinbrenner and H. Linden, "Regulation of two carotenoid biosynthesis genes coding for phytoene synthase and carotenoid hydroxylase during stress-induced astaxanthin formation in the green alga *Haematococcus pluvialis*," *Plant Physiol.*, 2001, **125**, 810.

22. J. Steinbrenner and H. Linden, "Light induction of carotenoid biosynthesis genes in the green alga *Haematococcus pluvialis*: regulation by photosynthetic redox control," *Plant Mol. Biol.*, 2003, **52**, 343.

23. L. Fan, A. Vonshak, A. Zarka, and S. Boussiba, "Does astaxanthin protect *Haematococcus* against light damage?" *Z. Naturforsch., C: J. Biosci.*, 1997, **53**, 93.

24. Y. Lemoine and B. Schoefs, "Secondary ketocarotenoid astaxanthin biosynthesis in algae: a multifunctional response to stress," *Photosynth. Res.*, 2010, **106**, 155.

25. A. M. Collins, H. D. Jones, D. Han, Q. Hu, T. E. Beechem, and J. A. Timlin, "Carotenoid distribution in living cells of *Haematococcus pluvialis* (Chlorophyceae)," *PLOS ONE*, 2011, **6**, e24302.

26. B. T. Schoefs, N.-E. Rmiki, J. Rachadi, and Y. Lemoine, "Astaxanthin accumulation in *Haematococcus* requires a cytochrome P450 hydroxylase and an active synthesis of fatty acids," *FEBS Lett.*, 2001, **500**, 125.

27. F. Miao, D. Lu, Y. Li, and M. Zeng, "Characterization of astaxanthin esters in *Haematococcus pluvialis* by liquid chromatography-atmospheric pressure chemical ionization mass spectrometry," *Anal. Biochem.*, 2006, **352**, 176.

28. P. P. Lamers, C. C. van de Laak, P. S. Kaasenbrood, J. Lorier, M. Janssen, R. C. De Vos, R. J. Bino, and R. H. Wijffels, "Carotenoid and fatty acid metabolism in light-stressed *Dunaliella salina*," *Biotechnol. Bioeng.*, 2010, **106**, 638.

29. J. Mercke Odeberg, Å. Lignell, A. Pettersson, and P. Höglund, "Oral bioavailability of the antioxidant astaxanthin in humans is enhanced by incorporation of lipid based formulations," *Eur. J. Pharm. Sci.*, 2003, **19**, 299.

30. J. Bowen, C. Soutar, R. Serwata, S. Lagocki, D. White, S. Davies, and A. Young, "Utilization of (3S, 3′S)-astaxanthin acyl esters in pigmentation of rainbow trout (*Oncorhynchus mykiss*)," *Aquacult. Nutr.*, 2002, **8**, 59.

31. D. White, G. Page, J. Swaile, A. Moody, and S. Davies, "Effect of esterification on the absorption of astaxanthin in rainbow trout, *Oncorhynchus mykiss* (Walbaum)," *Aquacult. Res.*, 2002, **33**, 343.

32. G. I. Frengova and D. M. Beshkova, "Carotenoids from *Rhodotorula* and *Phaffia*: yeasts of biotechnological importance," *J. Ind. Microbiol. Biotechnol.*, 2009, **36**, 163.

33. P. S. Meyer and J. C. Du Preez, "Photo-regulated astaxanthin production by *Phaffia rhodozyma* mutants," *System. Appl. Microbiol.*, 1994, **17**, 24.

34. G. H. An and E. A. Johnson, "Influence of light on growth and pigmentation of the yeast *Phaffia rhodozyma*," *Antonie van Leeuwenhoek*, 1990, **57**, 191.

35. M. Vázquez, "Carotenoid profiles of *Xanthophyllomyces dendrorhous* strains," *Food Technol. Biotechnol.*, 2001, **39**, 123.

36. G. N. Coral-Hinostroza, T. Ytrestøyl, B. Ruyter, and B. Bjerkeng, "Plasma appearance of unesterified astaxanthin geometrical E/Z and optical R/S isomers in men given single doses of a mixture of optical 3 and 3'R/S isomers of astaxanthin fatty acyl diesters," *Comp. Biochem. Physiol., C: Comp. Pharmacol. Toxicol.*, 2004, **139**, 99.

37. M. Østerlie, B. Bjerkeng, and S. Liaaen-Jensen, "Plasma appearance and distribution of astaxanthin E/Z and R/S isomers in plasma lipoproteins of men after single dose administration of astaxanthin," *J. Nutr. Biochem.*, 2000, **11**, 482.

38. P. Foss, T. Storebakken, E. Austreng, and S. Liaaenjensen, "Carotenoids in diets for salmonids V," *Aquaculture*, 1987, **65**, 293.

39. M. Tada, "Methods for investigating photoregulated carotenogenesis," *Methods Enzymol.*, 1993, **214**, 269.

40. H. Sakaki, T. Nakanishi, A. Tada, W. Miki, and S. Komemushi, "Activation of torularhodin production by *Rhodotorula glutinis* using weak white light irradiation," *J. Biosci. Bioeng.*, 2001, **92**, 294.

41. P. Bhosale and R. Gadre, "Manipulation of temperature and illumination conditions for enhanced beta-carotene production by mutant 32 of *Rhodotorula glutinis*," *Lett. Appl. Microbiol.*, 2002, **34**, 349.

42. J. A. Del Campo, J. Moreno, H. Rodríguez, M. Angeles Vargas, J. N. Rivas, and M. G. Guerrero, "Carotenoid content of chlorophycean microalgae: factors determining lutein accumulation in *Muriellopsis* sp. (Chlorophyta)," *J. Biotechnol.*, 2000, **76**, 51.

43. E. Bar, M. Rise, M. Vishkautsan, and S. M. Arad, "Pigment and structural changes in *Chlorella zofingiensis* upon light and nitrogen stress," *J. Plant Physiol.*, 1995, **146**, 527.

44. T. Sakamoto and D. A. Bryant, "Temperature-regulated mRNA accumulation and stabilization for fatty acid desaturase genes in the cyanobacterium *Synechococcus* sp. strain PCC 7002," *Arch. Microbiol.*, 1997, **169**, 10.

45. F. Bohne and H. Linden, "Regulation of carotenoid biosynthesis genes in response to light in *Chlamydomonas reinhardtii*," *Biochim. Biophys. Acta*, 2002, **1579**, 26.

46. A. Sánchez Mirón, M.-C. Cerón García, F. García Camacho, E. Molina Grima, and Y. Chisti, "Growth and characterization of algal biomass," *Microb. Technol.*, 2002, **31**, 1015.

47. A. Shaish, A. Ben-Amotz, and M. Avron, "Production and selection of high α -carotene mutants of *Dunaliella bardawil*," *J. Phycol.*, 1991, **27**, 652.

48. J. Steinbrenner and G. Sandmann, "Transformation of the green alga *Haematococcus pluvialis* with a phytoene desaturase for accelerated astaxanthin biosynthesis," *Appl. Environ. Microbiol.*, 2006, **72**, 7477.

49. J. Myers and W. Kratz, "Relation between pigment content and photosynthetic characteristics in a blue-green algae," *J. Gen. Physiol.*, 1955, **39**, 11.

50. A. Ben-Amotz, "Effect of low temperature on the stereoisomer composition of B-carotene in the halotolerant alga *Dunaliella bardawil* (Chlorophyta)," *J. Phycol.*, 1996, **32**, 272.

51. S. Orset and A. J. Young, "Low temperatureinduced synthesis of α-carotene in the microalga *Dunaliella salina* (Chlorophyta)," *J. Phycol.*, 1999, **35**, 520.

52. C. Li, E. S. Ford, G. Zhao, L. S. Balluz, W. H. Giles, and S. Liu, "Serum α-carotene concentrations and risk of death among US Adults: the Third National Health and Nutrition Examination Survey Follow-up Study," *Arch. Intern. Med.*, 2011, **171**, 507.

53. J. M. Genkinger, E. A. Platz, S. C. Hoffman, G. W. Comstock, and K. J. Helzlsouer, "Fruit, vegetable, and antioxidant intake and all-cause, cancer, and cardiovascular disease mortality in a community-dwelling population in Washington County, Maryland," *Am. J. Epidemiol.*, 2004, **160**, 1223.

54. M. Hamer and Y. Chida, "Intake of fruit, vegetables, and antioxidants and risk of type 2 diabetes: systematic review and meta-analysis," *J. Hypertens.*, 2007, **25**, 2361.

55. P. Knekt, J. Ritz, M. A. Pereira, E. J. O'Reilly, K. Augustsson, G. E. Fraser, U. Goldbourt, B. L. Heitmann, G. Hallmans, and S. Liu, "Antioxidant vitamins and coronary heart disease risk: a pooled analysis of 9 cohorts," *Am. J. Clin. Nutr.*, 2004, **80**, 1508.

56. G. Bjelakovic, D. Nikolova, L. L. Gluud, R. G. Simonetti, and C. Gluud, "Mortality in randomized trials of antioxidant supplements for primary and secondary prevention: systematic review and meta-analysis," *JAMA*, 2007, **297**, 842.

57. G. Mosqueda-Cano and J. F. Gutiérrez-Corona, "Environmental and developmental regulation of carotenogenesis in the dimorphic fungus *Mucor rouxii*," *Curr. Microbiol.*, 1995, **31**, 141.

58. F. Shi, W. Zhan, Y. Li, and X. Wang, "Temperature influences β-carotene production in recombinant *Saccharomyces cerevisiae* expressing carotenogenic genes from *Phaffia rhodozyma*," *World J. Microbiol. Biotechnol.*, 2014, **30**, 125.

59. A. E. Tjahjono, Y. Hayama, T. Kakizono, Y. Terada, N. Nishio, and S. Nagai, "Hyperaccumulation of astaxanthin in a green alga *Haematococcus pluvialis* at elevated temperatures," *Biotechnol. Lett.*, 1994, **16**, 133.

60. L. M. Ducrey Sanpietro and M. R. Kula, "Studies of astaxanthin biosynthesis in *Xanthophyllomyces dendrorhous* (*Phaffia rhodozyma*): effect of inhibitors and low temperature," *Yeast*, 1998, **14**, 1007.

61. B.-H. Liu and Y.-K. Lee, "Secondary carotenoids formation by the green alga *Chlorococcum* sp.," *J. Appl. Phycol.*, 2000, **12**, 301.

62. Y. Durmaz, M. Donato, M. Monteiro, L. Gouveia, M. Nunes, T. G. Pereira, Ş. Gökpınar, and N. Bandarra, "Effect of temperature on a-tocopherol, fatty acid profile, and pigments of *Diacronema vlkianum* (Haptophyceae)," *Aquacult. Int.*, 2009, **17**, 391.

63. A. Kaczor and M. Baranska, "Structural changes of carotenoid astaxanthin in a single algal cell monitored in situ by Raman spectroscopy," *Anal. Chem.*, 2011, **83**, 7763.

64. J. A. Del Campo, J. Moreno, H. Rodríguez, M. Angeles Vargas, J. N. Rivas, and M. G. Guerrero, "Carotenoid content of chlorophycean microalgae: factors determining lutein accumulation in *Muriellopsis* sp. (Chlorophyta)," *J. Biotechnol.*, 2000, **76**, 51.

65. J. Sánchez, J. Fernández, F. Acién, A. Rueda, J. Pérez-Parra, and E. Molina, "Influence of culture conditions on the productivity and lutein content of the new strain *Scenedesmus almeriensis*," *Process Biochem.*, 2008, **43**, 398.

66. J. M. Fernández-Sevilla, F. A. Fernández, and E. M. Grima, "Biotechnological production of lutein and its applications," *Appl. Microbiol. Biotechnol.*, 2010, **86**, 27.

67. G. Frengova, E. Simova, and D. Beshkova, "Effect of temperature changes on the production of yeast pigments co-cultivated with lacto-acid bacteria in whey ultrafiltrate," *Biotechnol. Lett.*, 1995, **17**, 1001.

68. P. Buzzini and A. Martini, "Production of carotenoids by strains of *Rhodotorula glutinis* cultured in raw materials of agro-industrial origin," *Bioresourc. Technol.*, 2000, **71**, 41.

69. N. Fong, M. Burgess, K. Barrow, and D. Glenn, "Carotenoid accumulation in the psychrotrophic bacterium *Arthrobacter agilis* in response to thermal and salt stress," *Appl. Microbiol. Biotechnol.*, 2001, **56**, 750.

70. S. Hanada, A. Hiraishi, K. Shimada, and K. Matsuura, "Chloroflexus aggregans sp. nov., a filamentous phototrophic bacterium which forms dense cell aggregates by active gliding movement," *Int. J. Syst. Bacteriol.*, 1995, **45**, 676.

71. S. Choudhari and R. Singhal, "Media optimization for the production of beta-carotene by *Blakeslea trispora*: a statistical approach," *Bioresour. Technol.*, 2008, **99**, 722.

72. M. Harker, A. J. Tsavalos, and A. J. Young, "Factors responsible for astaxanthin formation," *Bioresour. Technol.*, 1996, **55**, 207.

73. S. Boussiba, W. Bing, J.-P. Yuan, A. Zarka, and F. Chen, "Changes in pigment profiles in the green algae *Haematococcus pluvialis* exposed to environmental stresses," *Biotechnol. Lett.*, 1999, **21**, 601.

74. M. Z. Pacia, K. Turnau, M. Baranska, and A. Kaczor, "Interplay between carotenoids, hemoproteins and the "life band" origin studied in live *Rhodotorula mucilaginosa* cells by means of Raman microimaging," *Analyst*, 2015, **140**, 1809.

75. D. Chen, Y. Han, and Z. Gu, "Application of statistical methodology to the optimization of fermentative medium for carotenoids production by *Rhodobacter sphaeroides*," *Process Biochem.*, 2006, **41**, 1773.

76. V. C. Culotta, S.-J. Lin, P. Schmidt, L. W. Klomp, R. L. B. Casareno, and J. Gitlin, "Intracellular pathways of copper trafficking in yeast and humans," *Adv. Exp. Med. Biol.*, 1999, **448**, 247–54.

77. M. Kobayashi, T. Kakizono, and S. Nagai, "Enhanced carotenoid biosynthesis by oxidative stress in acetate-induced cyst cells of a green unicellular alga, *Haematococcus pluvialis*," *Appl. Environ. Microbiol.*, 1993, **59**, 867.

78. M. A. Borowitzka, J. M. Huisman, and A. Osborn, "Culture of the astaxanthin-producing green alga *Haematococcus pluvialis*," *J. Appl. Phycol.*, 1991, **3**, 295.

79. W. A. Schroeder and E. A. Johnson, "Singlet oxygen and peroxyl radicals regulate carotenoid biosynthesis in *Phaffia rhodozyma*," *Int. J. Biol. Chem.*, 1995, **270**, 18374.

80. S. Komemushi, H. Sakaki, H. Yokoyama, and T. Fujita, "Effect of barium and other metals on the growth of D-lactic acid assimilating yeast *Rhodotorula glutinis* No 21," *J. Antibacter. Antifung. Agents*, 1994, **22**, 583.

81. P. Bhosale and R. Gadre, "Production of beta-carotene by a mutant of *Rhodotorula glutinis*," *Appl. Microbiol. Biotechnol.*, 2001, **55**, 423.

82. P. Buzzini, A. Martini, M. Gaetani, B. Turchetti, U. M. Pagnoni, and P. Davoli, "Optimization of carotenoid production by *Rhodotorula graminis* DBVPG 7021 as a function of trace element concentration by means of response surface analysis," *Enzyme Microb. Technol.*, 2005, **36**, 687.

83. L. Flores-Cotera and S. Sanchez, "Copper but not iron limitation increases astaxanthin production by *Phaffia rhodozyma* in a chemically defined medium," *Biotechnol. Lett.*, 2001, **23**, 793.

84. J. Collen, E. Pinto, M. Pedersen, and P. Colepicolo, "Induction of oxidative stress in the red macroalga *Gracilaria tenuistipitata* by pollutant metals," *Arch. Environ. Contam. Toxicol.*, 2003, **45**, 337.

85. L. Flores-Cotera, R. Martin, and S. Sanchez, "Citrate, a possible precursor of astaxanthin in *Phaffia rhodozyma*: influence of varying levels of ammonium, phosphate and citrate in a chemically defined medium," *Appl. Microbiol. Biotechnol.*, 2001, **55**, 341.

86. G. H. An, "Improved growth of the red yeast, *Phaffia rhodozyma* (*Xanthophyllomyces dendrorhous*), in the presence of tricarboxylic acid cycle intermediates," *Biotechnol. Lett.*, 2001, **23**, 1005.

87. I. Marova, E. Breierova, R. Koci, Z. Friedl, B. Slovak, and J. Pokorna, "Influence of exogenous stress factors on production of carotenoids by some strains of cartenogenic yeasts," *Ann. Microbiol.*, 2004, **54**, 73.

88. I. Marova, M. Carnecka, A. Halienova, E. Breierova, and R. Koci, "Production of carotenoid-/ergosterol-supplemented biomass by red yeast *Rhodotorula glutinis* grown under external stress," *Food Technol. Biotech.*, 2010, **48**, 56.

89. M. Elahi, C. O. Chichester, and K. L. Simpson, "Effect of CPTA and cycocel on the biosynthesis of carotenoids by *Phycomyces blakesleeanus* mutants," *Phytochemistry*, 1973, **12**, 1633.

90. L. Ninet, J. Renaut, and R. Tissier, "Activation of the biosynthesis of carotenoids by *Blakeslea trispora*," *Biotechnol. Bioeng.*, 1969, **11**, 1195.

91. K. Pegklidou, F. Mantzouridou, and M. Z. Tsimidou, "Lycopene production using *Blakeslea trispora* in the presence of 2-methyl imidazole: yield, selectivity, and safety aspects," *J. Agric. Food Chem.*, 2008, **56**, 4482.

92. S. M. Choudhari, L. Ananthanarayan, and R. S. Singhal, "Use of metabolic stimulators and inhibitors for enhanced production of beta-carotene and lycopene by *Blakeslea trispora* NRRL 2895 and 2896," *Bioresour. Technol.*, 2008, **99**, 3166.

93. T. L. Walker, S. Purton, and D. K. Becker, C. Collet, "Microalgae as bioreactors," *Plant Cell Rep.*, 2005, **24**, 629.

14 Syntheses with Carotenoids

Hans-Richard Sliwka and Vassilia Partali

Department of Chemistry, Norwegian University of Science and Technology, Trondheim, Norway

14.1 Introduction

Synthesize carotenoids—do not synthesize with carotenoids! This directive, established as a result of insubstantial yields and merciless decomposition, has been respected quite strictly [1]. Transgressing the rule is penalized by disregard. In a historical review on the "Development of carotenoid chemistry 1922–1991," reactions with N-bromosuccinimide (NBS), aniline, and thiophenol to Br-, N-, and S-carotenoids remained ignored [2, 3]. The summing-up speaker of a carotenoid conference intentionally omitted mentioning the authors' transformations to S, N, and Se carotenoids. The raison d'être of carotenoid chemists is still the synthesis of carotenoids. Previous synthetic-like procedures with carotenoids were predominantly carried out for structure elucidation [4]; *derivatization* was the employed term.

What exactly does the expression *syntheses with carotenoids* specify?

The implications become evident by two examples: (1) reaction of two different carotenoids with each other, that is, the esterification of carotenoid diacid bixin with carotenoid diol lutein to luteindibixinate **1**; and (2) reaction of a carotenoid with a noncarotenoid substance: Wittig olefination of C50:19 carotenedial with 2 mol of C15:3 phosphonium salt to extended zeaxanthin C80:27 **2** (Scheme 1) [5, 6]. (The linking bonds are marked with □ in the scheme.) These "syntheses with carotenoids" result in polyene compounds of (**1**) 28 discontinuous double bonds and (**2**) 27 conjugated double bonds, both **1** and **2** offering a high double-bond density of $18/nm^3$ and $20/nm^3$, respectively.

This chapter presents selected examples of "syntheses with carotenoids." Carotenoids are defined as polyenes of more double bonds (db) than retinoids (db = 5). Nevertheless, many syntheses with compounds of double bonds ≥6 were omitted, and references restricted to a few representative citations due to editorial reasons. Supplementary details

Carotenoids: Nutrition, Analysis and Technology, First Edition. Edited by Agnieszka Kaczor and Malgorzata Baranska.

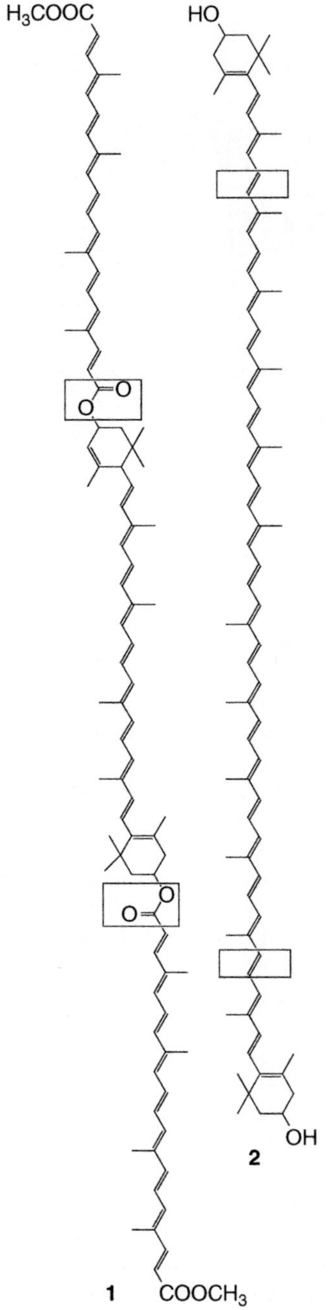

1 2

Scheme 1

may be retrieved in the article "Key to xenobiotic carotenoids" [7]. The authors hope that this fragmentary first survey on "syntheses with carotenoids" initiates more scientists to apply carotenoids in preparative organic chemistry.

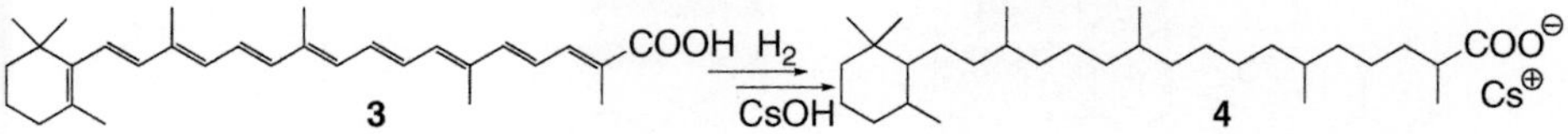

Scheme 2 Hydrogenation.

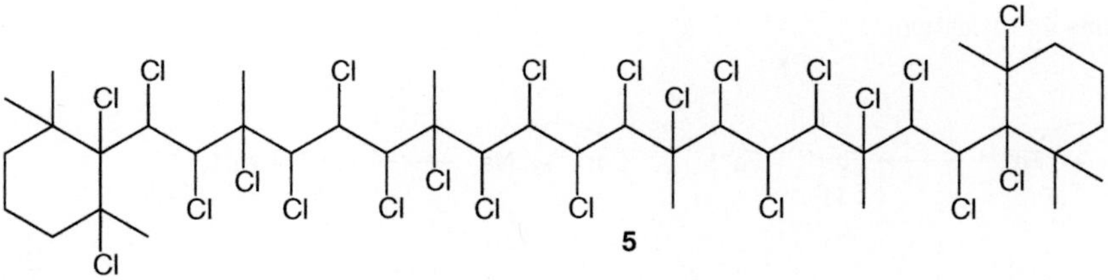

Scheme 3 Halogenation.

14.2 Reaction with double bonds

14.2.1 Hydrogenation

Hydrogenation of β,β-carotene with Raney nickel provided targeted products of 2, 4, and 6 C=C-bonds for antioxidant testing [8]. Perhydrogenation of lycopene-15,15′-^{3}H and β,β-carotene-15,15′-^{3}H allowed determining the coincidence of mass and radioactivity [9]. Hydrogenation of C30:9-carot**en**oic acid **3** afforded methyl branched C30:0-carot**an**oic acid, whose Cs salt **4** was required to ascertain the influence of unsaturation on surface and detergent properties (Scheme 2) [10]. Carot**an**oids occur in ancient sediments and petroleum [11]. Thus, β,β-carot**ane** and lycop**ane** are commercialized biomarkers [12].

14.2.2 Halogenation

ICl completed full halogenation of β,β-carotene C40:11 (**6**, $C_{40}H_{56}$) to $C_{40}H_{56}Cl_{22}$ **5** (Scheme 3) [13]. Prolonged reaction of tomato juice (lycopene) with bromine–water displays the rainbow colors by intermediary brominium ions until pale perbromolycop**ane** is observed [14]. When all –C=C– in carotenoids react with iodine, the acquired iodine index value indicates the number of double bonds [8, 13]. Colored iodine compounds occur in hexane, benzene, and diethyl ether. In chlorinated solvents, black ionic iodine complexes appeared absorbing in the near infrared [15].

14.2.3 Oxidation

Oxidation often degrades carotenoids to shorter fragments, regardless of the employed oxidation reagent [16]. Bubbling air ($^{3}O_2$) through a solution of β-carotene **6** led to 5,6-monoepoxide **7** besides many other products [17]; in analogy to retinoids polyepoxides such as **8** are expected, exposing carotenoids to reactive singlet oxygen $^{1}O_2$ [18]. Transient polyepoxide formation can be assumed when treating lycopene, lutein, and bixin with perbenzoic acid [13]. Industrial chemists devised an authentic preparative oxidation: zeaxanthin acetate **9** oxidized with sodium bromate to astaxanthin acetate **10** (Scheme 4) [19]. Astaxanthin esters are more stable and show a better bioavailability than astaxanthin when used in salmonid pigmentation.

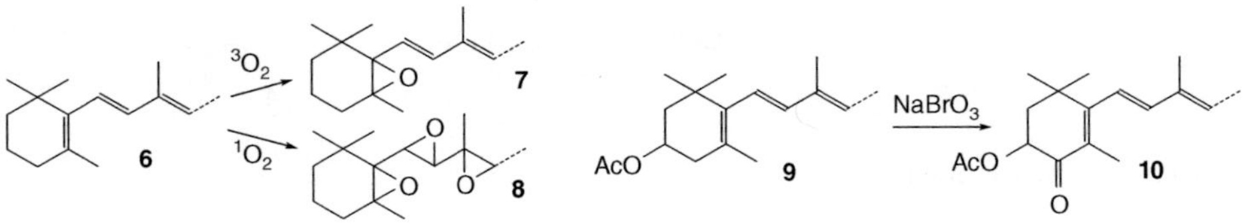

Scheme 4 Oxidation.

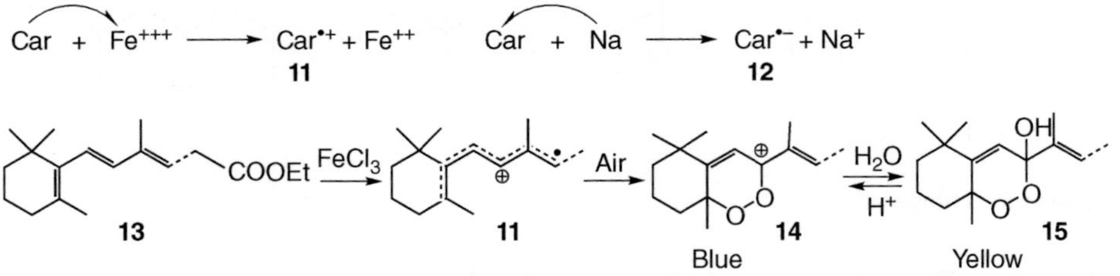

Scheme 5 Electron transfer reactions.

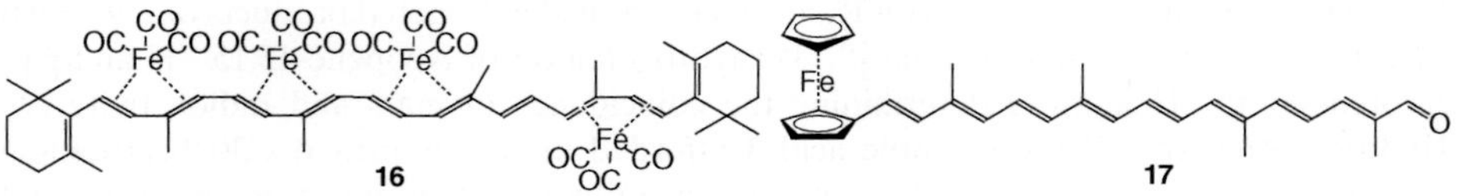

Scheme 6 Iron carbonyl carotenoids.

14.2.4 Electron transfer from and to carotenoids

Carotenoids convert to radical cations ($Car^{+\bullet}$ **11**) by transferring electrons to Fe^{3+}, Ti^{4+}, Ni^{2+}, Cu^{2+}, Ni^{2+}, I_2, BF_3, and $SnCl_3$ and to sensitizers (e.g., nitronaphthalene, tocopherol, and riboflavin) [20–24]. Carotenoids can also attract electrons (from radicals or from Na, K, Cs, Al–Hg, and BuLi under special experimental settings and from alkaline dimethyl sulfoxide [DMSO] at normal laboratory conditions) developing radical anions $Car^{-\bullet}$ **12** [25, 26]. Electrons can furthermore be imposed electrochemically on carotenoids or by ionizing rays (pulse radiolysis) [27, 28]. The dual function of dioxocarotenoids as electron donators and acceptors was quantitatively assessed [29]. Reactive $Car^{+\bullet}$ **11** or $Car^{-\bullet}$ **12** received no particular preparative interest, except $Car^{+\bullet}$ **11**; generated from C30-ester **13** with $FeCl_3$, cation radical **11** proceeded in air to easily interchangeable peroxide cation **14** (blue) and hydroxyl peroxide **15** (yellow) (Scheme 5) [30].

14.2.5 Iron carbonyl

Lycopene and β,β-carotene **6** add iron tricarbonyl affording iron carbonyl compounds with an elevated iron concentration (e.g., 20% Fe in **16**) [31]. The ferrocene moiety in push-pull polyene **17** (from ferrocenyl Wittig salt and C20:7 dialdehyde **21**) acts as electron donator (Scheme 6) [32].

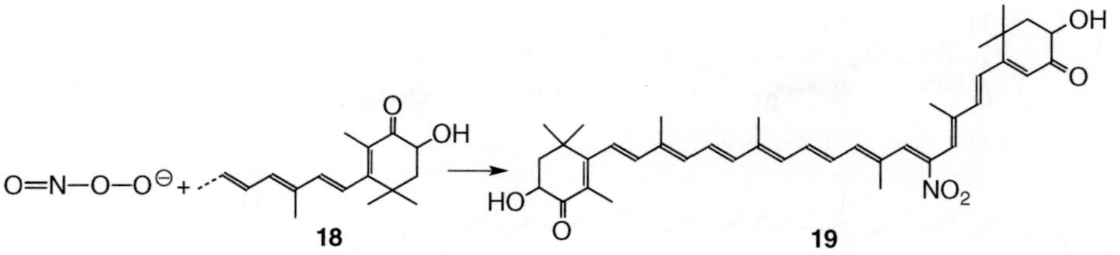

Scheme 7 Nitration.

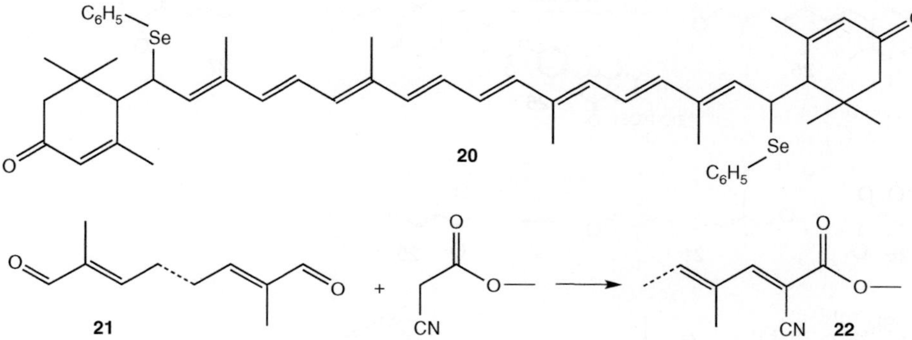

Scheme 8 In-chain carotenoids.

14.2.6 Nitration

Peroxynitrite directed a nitro group to the polyene chain of astaxanthin **18**. Similar to CF_3–, NO_2– turns adjacent double bonds to *cis*-configuration **19** (Scheme 7) [33,34].

14.2.7 In-chain modification

Benzene selenol and $ZnCl_2$ reacted with rhodoxanthin **49** (Scheme 12) to postulated diphenylselenide intermediate **20**; selenium was then expelled, providing ε,ε-carotene-3, 3'-dione [35]. Carotenals (e.g., C20:7 dialdehyde **21**) and carotenones subjected to Knoevenagel or Stobbe reactions delivered carotenoids with –COOH or –CN in-chain substituents (e.g., cyano carotenoic ester **22**) (Scheme 8) [36]. Several other in-chain substituted carotenoids are described [37]. Apparently, the preparative potential of the CN-group has so far been ignored. Syntheses with cross-conjugated carotenoids and an interesting diazacarotene [38] were probably not yet executed.

14.3 Transformation of substituents

14.3.1 –C=O → –C=C–

The reaction of carbonyl groups with phosphoranes represents the key sequence in polyene chain syntheses [39]. This classical procedure attained already in 1951 its limit with 19 conjugated double bonds [40]. An attempt in 1997 to surpass the traditional boundary by

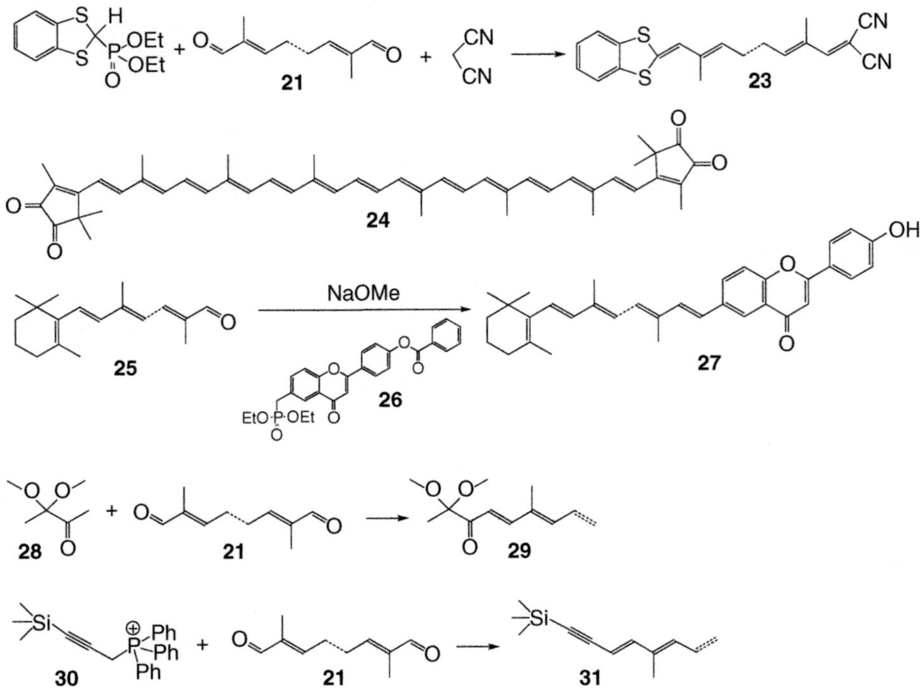

Scheme 9 –C=O → –C=C– transformations.

synthesizing a vinylogous β-carotene with 23 –C=C– bonds failed [41]. The failure to prepare carotenoic acid C50:17 confirmed additionally the customary threshold [10]. However, when C50:19 dialdehyde and C15:3 phosphonium salt assembled under microwave radiation, the new polyene record stretched to 27 –C=C– bonds in long zeaxanthin **2** (Scheme 1) [6]. Starting material C50:19 dialdehyde became available by successive elongation of carotenedials [6, 41]. Colored push-pull polyenes such as **23** were acquired from Wittig and Knoevenagel reactions of donor and acceptor moieties with dialdehydes, for example C20:7-crocetindial **21** [42]; aldehyde **21** is the crucial compound to extended violerythrin **24** (C48:15) [43]. C30-aldehyde **25** and flavonoid phosphorane **26** combined to create a dual carotenoid–flavonoid antioxidant **27** [44]. Aldol condensation of C20:7 dialdehyde **21** with dimethoxybutanone **28** effected C28:9 tetrone diacetale **29** exhibiting fluorescence (S_1–S_0) emission [45]. Ferrocenylphosphorane and C20-aldehyde **21** formed iron carotenoid **17** (Scheme 6) [32]. Trimethylsilyl alkyne phosphorane **30** coupled with C20-aldehyde **21** to siliconcarotenoid **31** (Scheme 9) [46].

C30-aldehyd **25** and other carotenals add a hydroxyl–methyl pentenone moiety when reacting with cyclocarbonate **32** to hydroxyketone **33** (Scheme 10) [47]. The outcome of a synthesis with Wittig salt C5:1 **34** and C20:7-pyran carotenoid **35** was pyran carotenoid C30:11 **36**, additionally elongated with two C5 units to C40:15 polyene pyran. Compound **36** deviates conjugation across the pyran ring [48]. Addition of acid to pyran carotenoid **36** afforded pyranium compound **37**, whose delocalized charge strongly increased absorption. Pyranium **37** exposes the structural elements of carotenoids and anthocyanidins [48]. A pyran carotenoid had been previously devised by reacting a 2*H*-pyran carbaldehyde with a C20:5 Wittig salt [49]. Conjugation meandered analogously in tetrafluorinated azulenodithiophene **38**, which

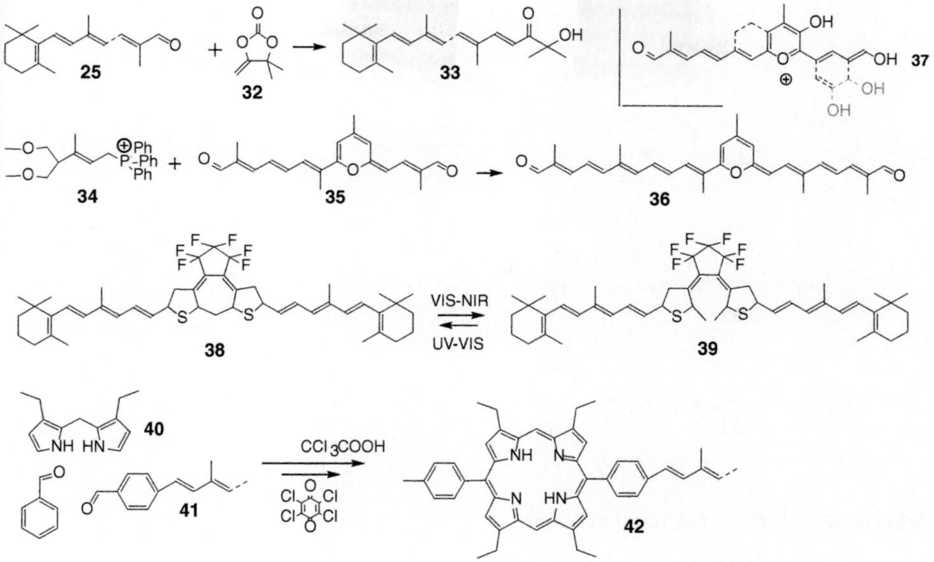

Scheme 10 –C=O → –C=C– transformations.

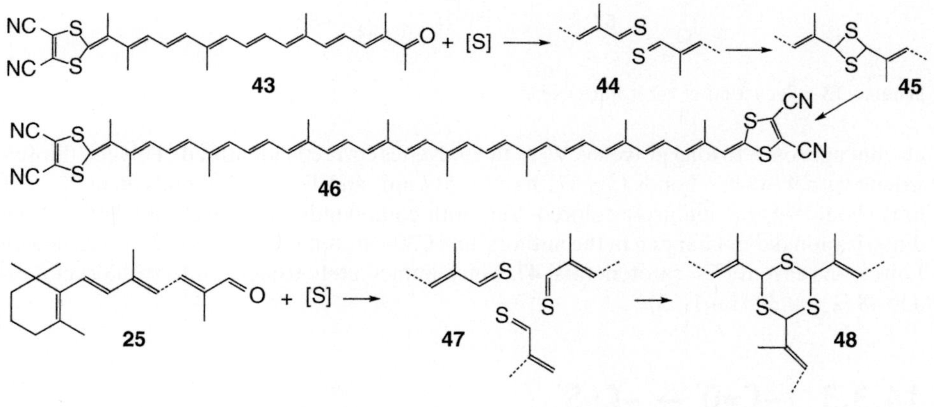

Scheme 11 –CH=O → –CH=S transformations.

opens under visible light (Vis)–near-infrared (NIR) irradiation to dithiophene **39** [50]. Dipyrrole **40** interfered with polyene benzaldehyde **41** to conformationally restricted carotenoporphyrine **42** (Scheme 10) [51]. Carotenoid–porphyrins are usually prepared with flexible ether (**75**), ester (**103**), or amide (**135**, **146**) linkages (Schemes 17, 24, 30, and 33).

14.3.2 -CH=O → CH=S

Lawesson reagent thiolated two molecules of aldehyde **43** (8 double bonds) to transient thial **44**, which cyclized to transitory dithiocyclobutane **45**; elimination of sulfur effected thiafulvalene **46** (17 –C=C– bonds) (Scheme 11) [52]. Thial dimerization would signify an

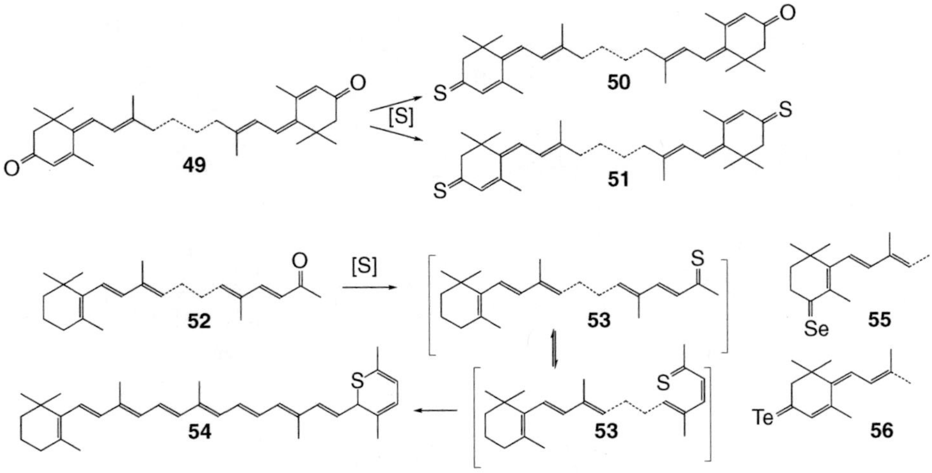

Scheme 12 –C=O → –C=S transformations.

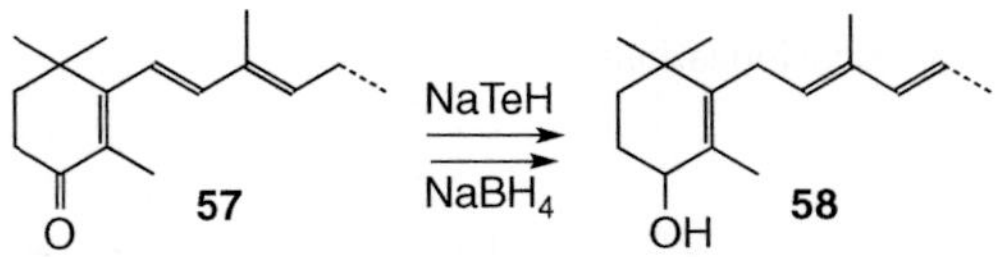

Scheme 13 Reduction of ketocarotenoids.

elegant approach to long polyenes. Were the polyenes correctly identified? Polyene thiofulvalene with 9 –C=C– bonds (λ = 471 nm, λ = 517 nm) and 17 –C=C– bonds **46** (λ_{max} = 551 nm) should appear intensely colored. Yet, both compounds were black in CH_2Cl_2. Thial dimerization did not happen in the authors' lab: C30-carotenal **25** (λ_{max} = 462 nm) gave with Lawesson reagent C30-carotenethial **47**, which immediately trimerized to trithiocyclohexane **48** (λ_{max} = 396 nm) [53].

14.3.3 –C=O → –C=S

Lawesson reagent changed rhodoxanthin **49** (echinenone and canthaxanthin **57**) to stable monothione **50** and unstable dithione **51** [53, 54]. Citranaxanthin **52** reorganized via postulated thione **53** to thiopyran **54** [53]. Hypothetical canthaxanthin selone **55** and rhodoxanthin tellone **56** preferentially operate as electron acceptors rather than electron donators (Scheme 12) [55].

14.3.4 –C=O → –C–OH

Carotenones and carotenals are routinely reduced with $LiAlH_4$ or $NaBH_4$ to carotenols; the progress of reduction can be followed visually [4]. Tellurium hydride in the presence of $NaBH_4$ hydrogenated the double bonds near the rings and the carbonyl groups in cantaxanthin **57** to xenobiotic diol **58** (Scheme 13) [56].

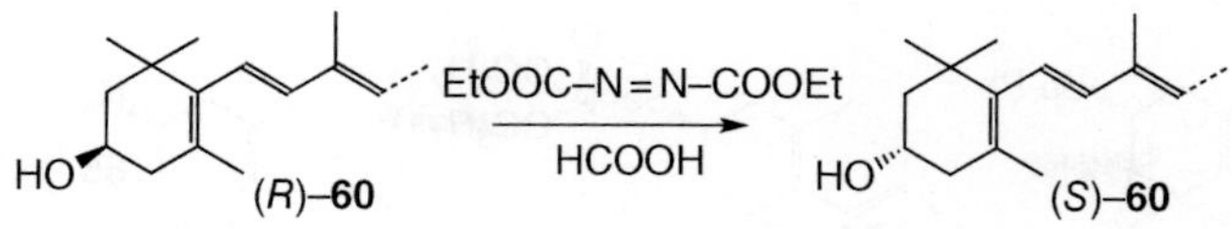

Scheme 14 Enantiomer inversion.

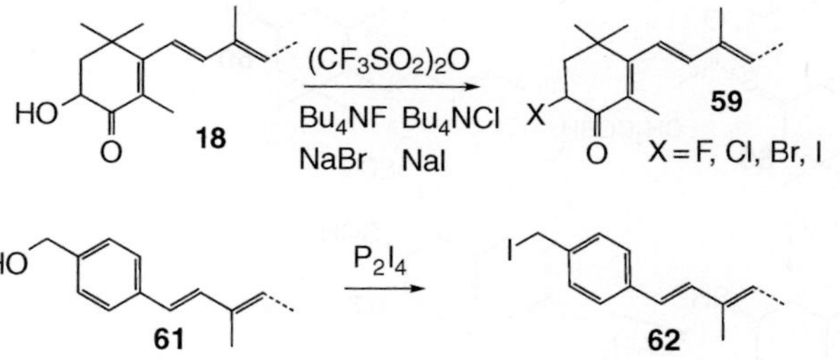

Scheme 15 Exchange of –OH with halogens.

14.3.5 Inversion of –OH

Zeaxanthin enantiomer (*R*)-**60** inverted to (*S*)-**60** in Mitsunobu reactions with diethylazodicarboxylate, formic acid, triphenylphosphine, followed by subsequent hydrolysis of the formiates (Scheme 14). This technique allows also a smooth approach to lutein and tunaxanthin diastereoisomers [57].

14.3.6 –OH → –F, –Cl, –Br, and –I

F, Cl, Br, and I interchanged the hydroxyl groups in astaxanthin **18**, leaving mono or dihalogen compounds **59** (Scheme 15) [58]. Astaxanthin bromide **72** operates as an intermediate in the synthesis of astaxanthin ether **73** (Scheme 17) [59]. Halogenated astaxanthin derivates were used in the study of carotenoproteins. A comparable –OH replacement with $CHCl_3$–HCl in zeaxanthin **60** and isozeaxanthin **70** afforded mono- and dichlorides [60]. Replacing –OH in benzylcarotenoid **61** with –I gave iodomethylphenyl carotenoid **62** (Scheme 15), employed in the construction of polyeneporphyrin ether **75** (Scheme 17) [61].

14.3.7 –OH → –SR, –SCN, –SH, –N_2, –NH_2, and –SeR

The Mitsunobu reaction of (*R*,*R*)-zeaxanthin **60** with benzene selenol, propylselenium phosphate, hydrazoic acid, thioacetic acid, and thiocyanic acid yielded (*S*)-phenylselenide **63**, (*S*)-selenium phosphate ester **64**, (*S*)-azide **65**, (*S*)-thioacetate **66**, and (*S*)-thiocyanate **67** (Scheme 16). Azide **65** upon reduction with NaTeH formed zeaxanthin (*S*)-mono and (*S*, *S*)-diamine **68**. Both thioacetate **66** and thiocyanate **67** gave (*S*)-thiol **69** [62–64]. The optical active N-, S-, and Se-carotenoids allowed examining the impact of substituents on the conformation of the cyclohexene β-end ring [65]. Allylic hydroxyl in lutein or isozeaxanthin **70** converted with thioacetic acid and $ZnCl_2$ to thioacetates (similar to **66**), which were hydrolyzed with KOH or reduced with $LiAlH_4$ to thiolutein (similar to **69**) [66]. Acetylcysteine replaced the hydroxyl group in isozeaxanthin **70**, providing sulfur carotenoid **71** [67].

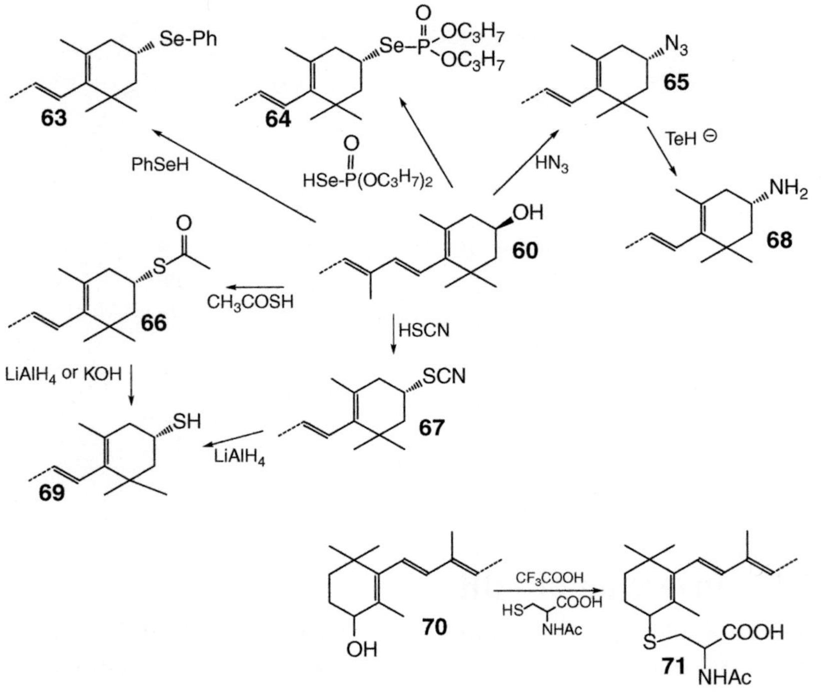

Scheme 16 Exchange of -OH with N, S, and Se substituents.

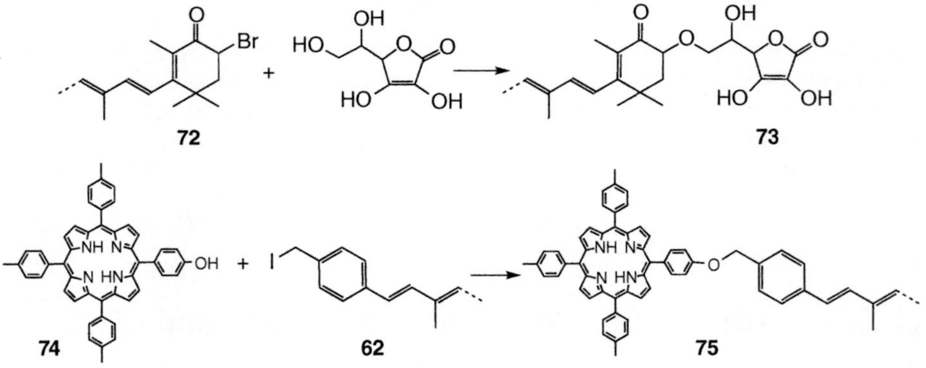

Scheme 17 Ether formation.

14.3.8 -OH → -OR

A C24-apocarotenoid combined with ethyl cellulose to a bixin–ethyl cellulose ether [68]. Astaxanthinbromide **72** and alcohols (e.g., vitamin C) produced ascorbic ether **73** [59]. Iodomethylphenyl carotenoid **62** (Scheme 15) connected with hydroxyphenyl porphyrin **74** to porphyrin carotenoid ether **75** (Scheme 17) [61].

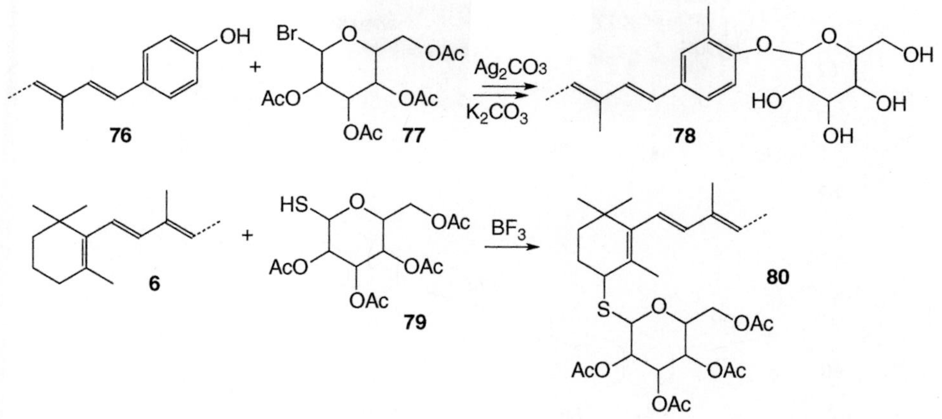

Scheme 18 Glycosidation of carotenoids.

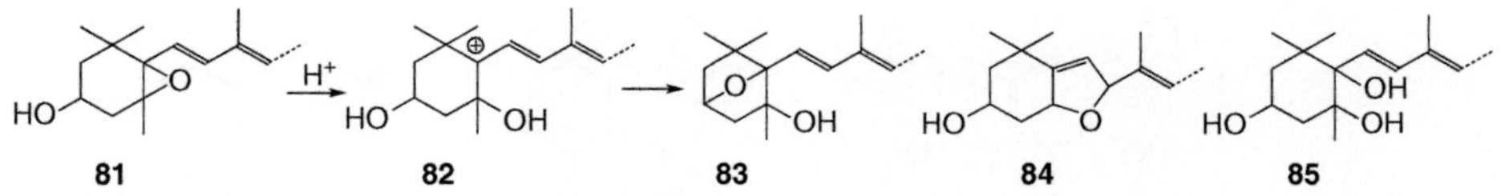

Scheme 19 Reactions with carotenoid epoxides.

14.3.9 -OH → glycosides

Carotenols were glycosylated with the intention of synthesizing some of the numerous natural occurring carotenoid glycosides [69, 70]. Acetylglucopyranosylbromid **77** adds to phenol carotenoid **76**, giving intermediary glucopyranosylbromid. Cleavage of the acetyl group progressed to hydrophilic glucose carotenoid **78**, which was then investigated for its aggregation properties (Scheme 18) [71]. Maltose was appended to astaxanthin **18**, engendering hydrophilicity [72]. Exposing carotenols or β,β-carotene **6** to boron trifluoride etherate led to cationic structures, which reacted with thioglucose **79** to thioglycoside **80** (Scheme 18) [73].

14.3.10 Reactions with carotenoid epoxides

Epoxide **81**, acidified to cation **82**, proceeded to oxabicyclo and furan compounds **83** and **84**, and triol **85** (Scheme 19) [74]. $AlCl_3$, $FeCl_3$, and $HgCl_2$ added to epoxides developed unstable colored complexes [75].

14.3.11 Reactions with halogen carotenoids

C18:7 diiodide **86** and dienylstannate **87** or dienylpinacol-boronate **88** delivered β,β-carotene **6**; other carotenoids were prepared similarly [76]. Dibromo-β,β-carotenoid **89**, exposed to alcohols, thiophenol, and aniline, provided ether **90**, sulfur carotenoid **91**, and nitrogen carotenoid **92** (Scheme 20) [2]. Halogen carotenoids enjoy no special considerations, although perhalogenated β,β-carotane diicosachloride $C_{40}H_{56}Cl_{22}$ **5** (Scheme 3) probably exhibits pesticide and disinfectant properties [13].

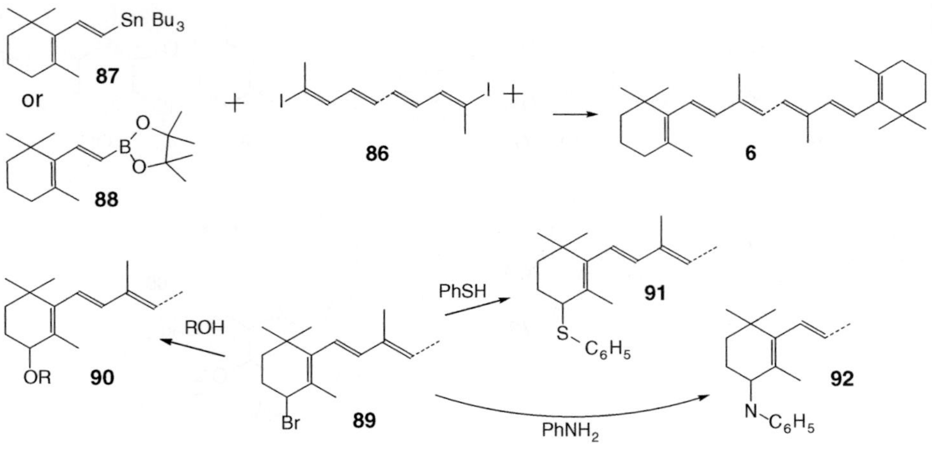

Scheme 20 Reactions with halogen carotenoids.

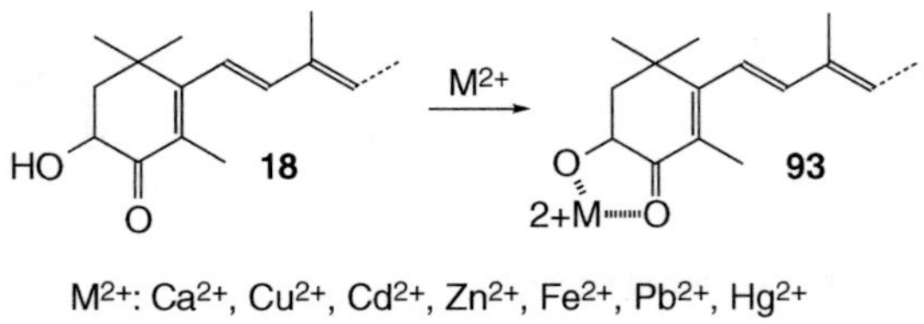

Scheme 21 Metal carotenoids.

14.3.12 Metal complexes with carotenols, carotenals, and carotenones

Astaxanthin **18** interferes with Ca^{2+}, Zn^{2+}, and Fe^{2+} to metal ion–astaxanthin complexes **93** (Scheme 21) [77]. Cu^{2+}, Pb^{2+}, Zn^{2+}, Cd^{2+}, and Hg^{2+} complexes are likewise anticipated with bathochromic shifted absorption [78].

14.4 Preparative derivatization

Oxime **94**, prepared from canthaxanthin **57**, appeared as precursor in the synthesis of hydrophilic oxime hydrochloride **95** (Scheme 22) [79]. A remarkable combination was envisioned by condensation of crocetin dialdehyde C20:7 **21** and tris(2-aminoethyl)-amine **96** to a macrocyclic tris-carotenoid hexaimine, which enclosed in a subsequent step two Cu(I) ions in dinuclear cryptate **97** [80]. Pyrrolidinium iodide **98** coupled with C30-aldehyde **25**, creating pyrrolidinium triiodide **99**, which is designed as radar-absorbing paint on military airplanes (Scheme 22) [81].

14.5 Syntheses with carotenoid acids and carotenols

The majority of "syntheses with carotenoids" are realized with carotenols and carotenoic acids.

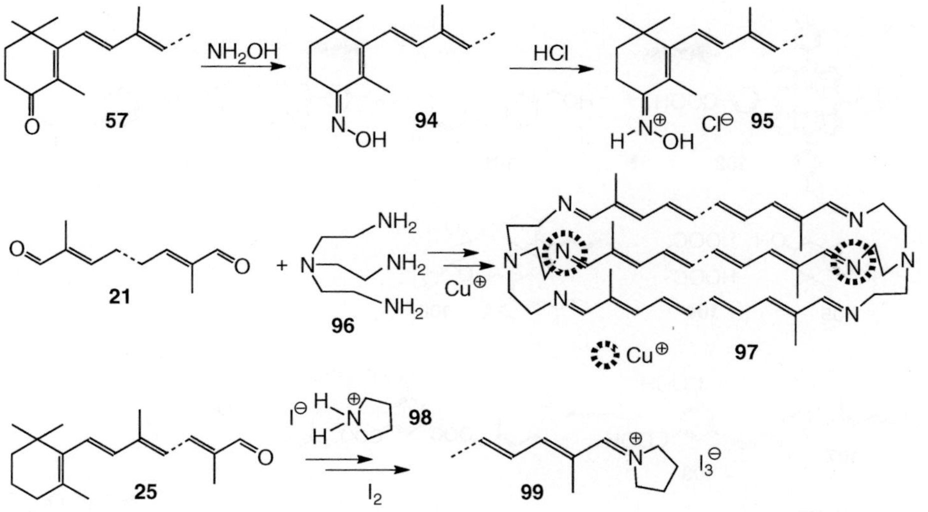

Scheme 22 Imine syntheses.

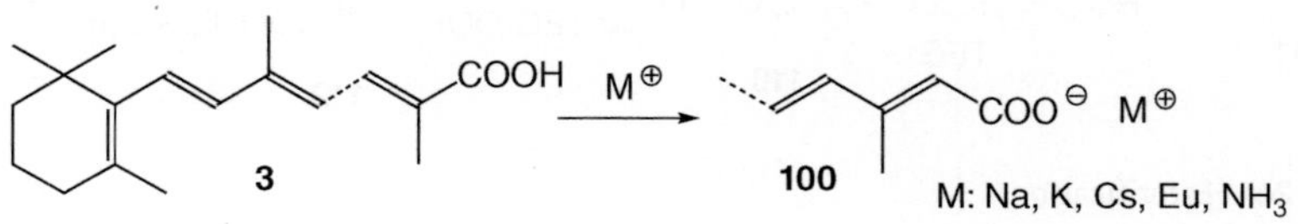

Scheme 23 Metal carboxylate formation.

14.5.1 -COOH → -COCl

Changing COOH to –COCl characterizes a genuine preparative method because carotenoid acid chlorides, such as **137** (Scheme 30), are exclusively applied as intermediates in the synthesis of glycosyl esters, carotenoid porphyrins, carotenoidglycerolipids, and diluteinbixinate **1** [5, 82, 83].

14.5.2 -COOH → COO– M⁺

Na, K, and Cs salts **100** from C30-acid **3** homologs (C22:6–C45:15) were required to determine surface tension and other surface properties. The shorter polyenes had no antenna function for fluorescence in Eu-carotenoates **100** (Scheme 23) [10, 24]. Ammonium salts have been obtained from crocin and amines [84]. Addition of NaOH to bixin results in amphiphilic Na_2–bixinate [85].

14.5.3 -COOH → COOR

Two dominant directions progressed in "syntheses with carotenoids":

1. Esterification of carotenols, for example astaxanthin **18**, and zeaxanthin **60** with acids
2. Ester formation of carotenoic acids, for example C30-acid **3**, crocetin, and bixin with alcohols.

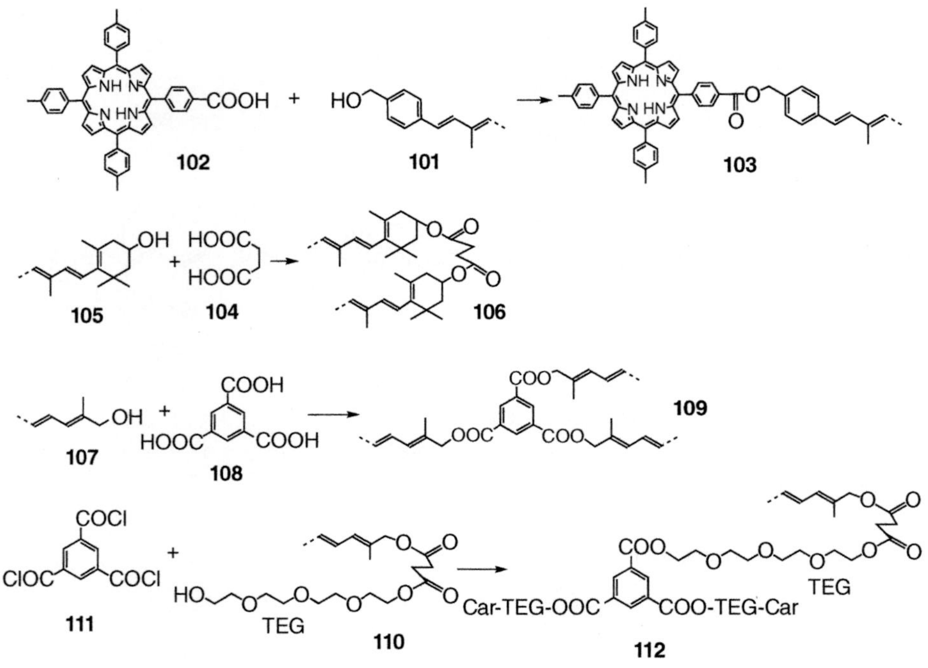

Scheme 24 Esterification.

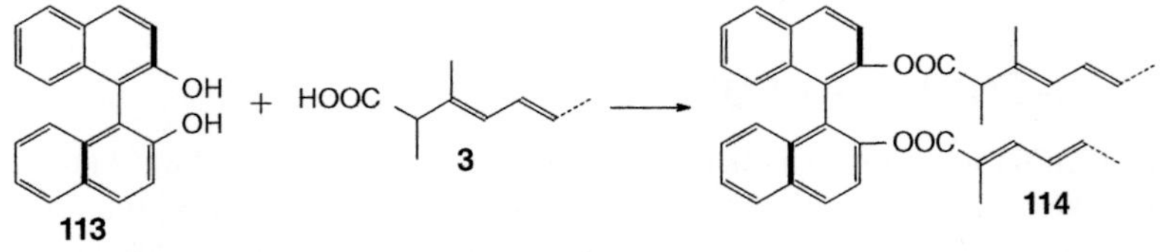

Scheme 25 Polyene binaphtholester.

Dilutein bixinate **1** illustrates a carotenol–carotenoic acid reaction (Scheme 1) [5]. Carotenoid esters from lutein and zeaxanthin **60** with bulky acids were prepared as derivatives facilitating crystallization [86]. Benzylcarotenol **101** proceeded with porphyrin acid **102** to carotenoid–porphyrin ester **103** [87, 88]. Succinic acid **104** served as a linker in connecting two molecules of cryptoxanthin **105** in succinate ester **106** [89]. Three carotenoids accumulated in ester **109** by reacting β-8′-apocarotenol **107** with benzene-1,3,5-tricarboxylic acid **108**; similarly, tetraethylene glycol (TEG) delivered with C30-monosuccinate the TEG ester **110**, again esterified with benzene-1,3,5-triacetic acid chloride **111** to carotenoid–TEG ester **112** (Scheme 24) [90]. Other carotenoid combinations failed, attesting that the outcome of apparently simple carotenol–acid esterifications cannot be predicted [91].

Binaphthol **113** and C30-acid **3** can be combined to form binaphtholester **114** (Scheme 25). Various conformations are expected; unfortunately, the chains did not overlay to induce exciton coupling (Figure 14.1, Color Supplement) [92].

Lipase esterification of *rac.* zeaxanthin **60** with palmitic acid proceeded selectively to *R,R*-zeaxanthin dipalmitate **115** with 50% ee, validating the possibility of enzymatic resolution of

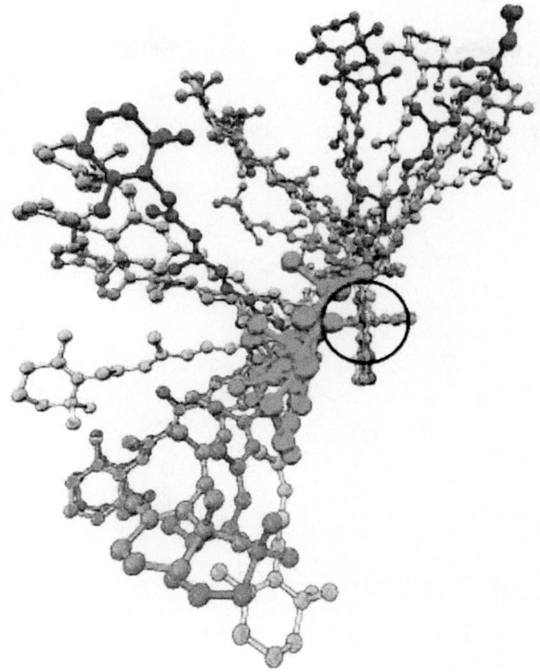

Figure 14.1 Polyene chain arrangement in binaphtholester **114** [92, 93]. Reproduced with permission of Zsolt Bikadi, Virtua Drug Ltd. (*See insert for color representation of the figure.*)

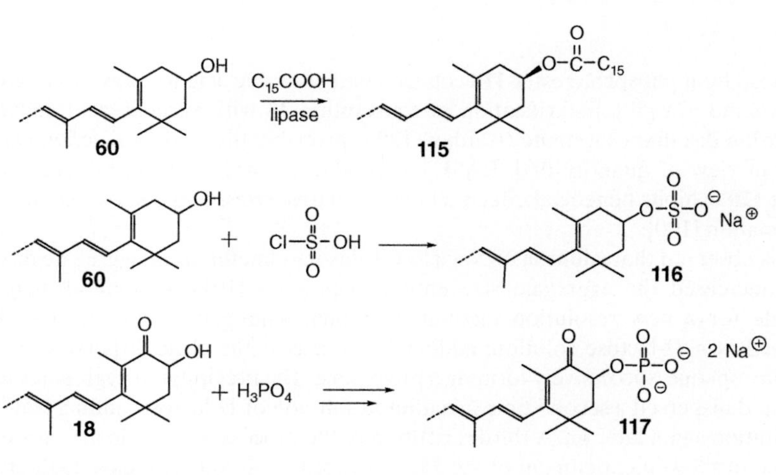

Scheme 26 Esterification.

carotenoid enantiomers [95]. 3*R*,3'*R*-Zeaxanthin ***R*-60** with formic acid under Mitsunobu conditions provided formiates of reversed configuration; hydrolysis gave 3*S*,3'*S*-zeaxanthin ***S*-60** (Scheme 14) [57]. Carotenols (e.g., zeaxanthin **60**) with chlorosulfonic acid converted to carotenoid sulfates **116**, which were afterward isolated from a marine sponge [96, 97]. Disodium diphosphate ester **117**, synthesized from astaxanthin **18**, emerged as a hydrophilic carotenoid derivate (Scheme 26) [98].

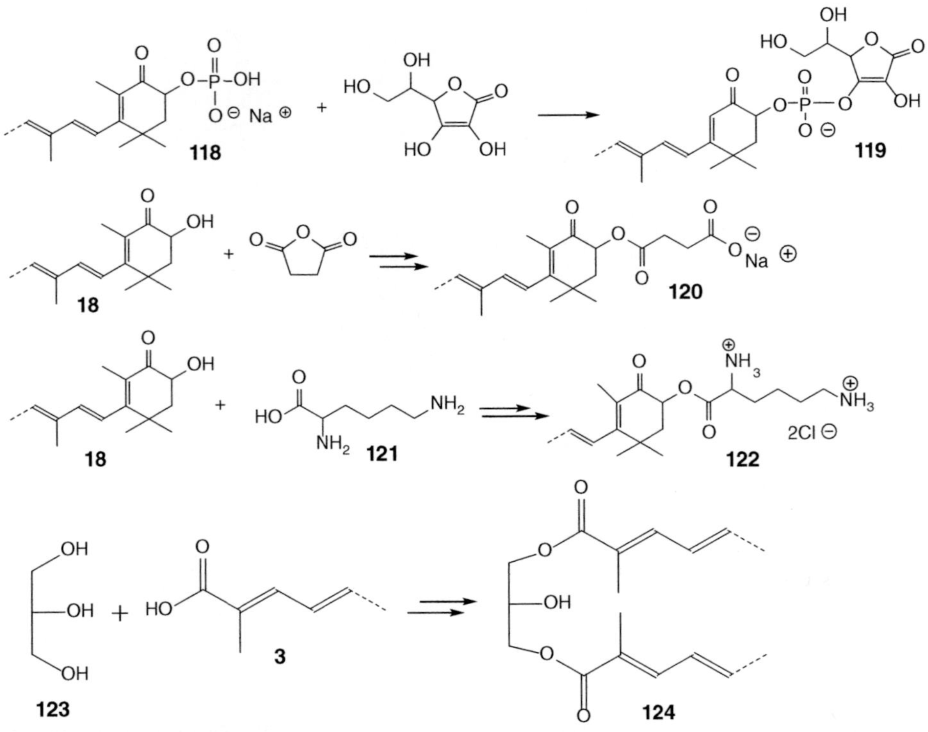

Scheme 27 Esterification.

Monosodium phosphate ester **118** converts with ascorbic acid to astaxanthin–ascorbate **119** (Scheme 27) [59]. Esterification of astaxanthin **18** with succinic acid anhydride to astaxanthin disodium succinate (Cardax) **120** is probably the leading reaction with carotenoids in view of quantity [99]. BASF has produced Cardax **120** in kilogram amounts. Cardax **120** exhibits beneficial effects against oxidative stress and diseases conditioned by inflammation [100].

It was observed that addition of NaCl to Cardax nanometer-sized aggregate dispersions slowly increased the aggregate size until precipitation [101]. This trend assigned the rationale for a new resolution method: fractional aggregation. *Rac*. Cardax **120** was dispersed in a *D*-lactose solution; adding NaCl caused the clear dispersion to become gradually opaque, successively forming a precipitate. The precipitated aggregates were collected and dispersed a second time in a diluted solution of *D*-lactose; adding NaCl caused precipitation again later on. A third repetition of the process resulted in aggregates whose CD spectra showed enrichment of the 3*S*,3′*S*-Cardax enantiomer (Figure 14.2) [102].

Astaxanthin disuccinate is the basis for a multitude of esters (e.g., with tartaric acid and resveratrol) [98, 103]. Astaxanthin **18** and lysine **121** delivered astaxanthin–lysine tetrachloride **122**, a true water-soluble competitor of crocin (Scheme 27) [104, 105]. The former Hawaii Biotech company, producer of Cardax **120** and many other astaxanhin esters, certainly merits the distinction "most prolific synthesizer with carotenoids." Fucoxanthin and fucoxanthinol were as well esterified directly or via succinates [106]. Zeaxanthin **60** and lutein, joined by ester bonds to pharmacophoric molecules (e.g., etoposide and vincristine), cure macular and

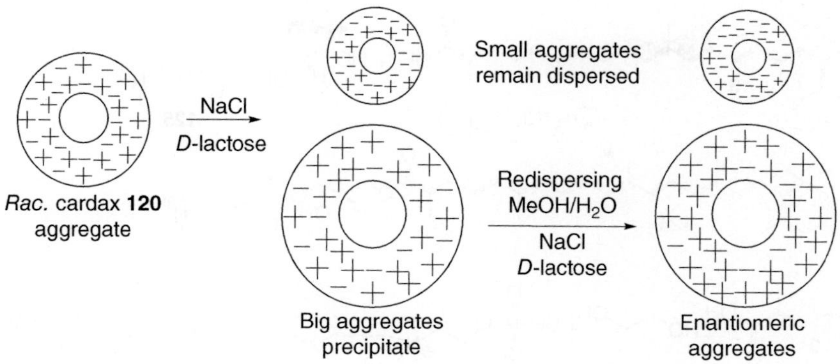

Figure 14.2 Fractional aggregation. Sliwka et al. 2007. Reproduced with permission of John Wiley & Sons.

retinal diseases [107]. Alkanols (C3:0–C16:0), alkenols (C3:1–C16:1), and cycloalcohols (C5–C8) with C30-acid **3** formed esters that are used advantageously as food colors [108]. Astaxanthin, when esterified with ferulic acid, is a better $^1O_2$-quencher [109]. Astaxanthin alkanoates with mono acids C1:0–C32:0 or diacids C2:0–C4:0 serve as fuel additives [110]. Carotenoids for gasoline or military aircraft paints (e.g., **99**) (Scheme 22) definitely represent very atypical carotenoid applications. In contrast, carotenoids are archetypical membrane stabilizers, and, consequently, carotenoids were enclosed in liposomes [111, 112]. Instead of confining carotenoids in liposomes, genuine carotenoid liposomes can be formulated from carotenoid lipids. Enzymatic esterification of C30-acid **3** with glycerol **123** resulted in the most unsaturated glycerolipid **124** [113].

Unsaturated acids starting from C10:1 (β-cyclogeranic acid) crossing C20:5 (retinoic acid) and C40:13 acid (torularhodin) to C45:15 are available naturally, commercially, or synthetically [24] for the preparation of polyene lipids, polyene aggregates, and polyene liposomes [114]. The manufacture of low conjugated polyenoic fatty compounds from nonconjugated fats by isomerization with iridium or rhodium catalysts results in a mixture of fats that are difficult to purify [115]. Well-defined polyene lipids become accessible with the mentioned carotenoic acids [101, 116]. Thus, C30-acid **3** and (*R*)-glycerophospho-choline **125** delivered polyene (*R*)-phospholipid **126**, consisting of optical active *P*-octamer aggregation units (Scheme 28 and Figure 14.3) [94].

A series of cationic polyene glycol phospholipids (e.g., **127**) revealed gene carrier properties [117–120]. C30-carotenoic acid choline esters (e.g., **128**) are equally effective gene carriers [121]. Dual antioxidant combinations are derived from glycerol **123**, C30-acid **3**, trolox **130**, or BHT [122, 123]. Triantioxidant molecule **131** was created by esterification of glycerol **123** with C30-acid **3**, 7-selenacaprylic acid **129**, and trolox **130** [83].

14.5.4 –COOR → –COOH

The apparent simple hydrolysis of carotenoid esters can, at times, fail; as a result, alternative means are indicated (enzymatic hydrolysis, and KOH in isobutanol at 85 °C) [122]. Ineffective hydrolysis of C30-ester **13T** to radioactive [10′-^{3}H]-C30-acid **3T** under standard conditions [4] became especially irritating (Scheme 29) [124]. Disaccharide ester crocin was unintentionally "fungilized" in the laboratory of the authors to diacid crocetin (C20:7) by the airborne fungus *Cladosporium cladosporioides* [125].

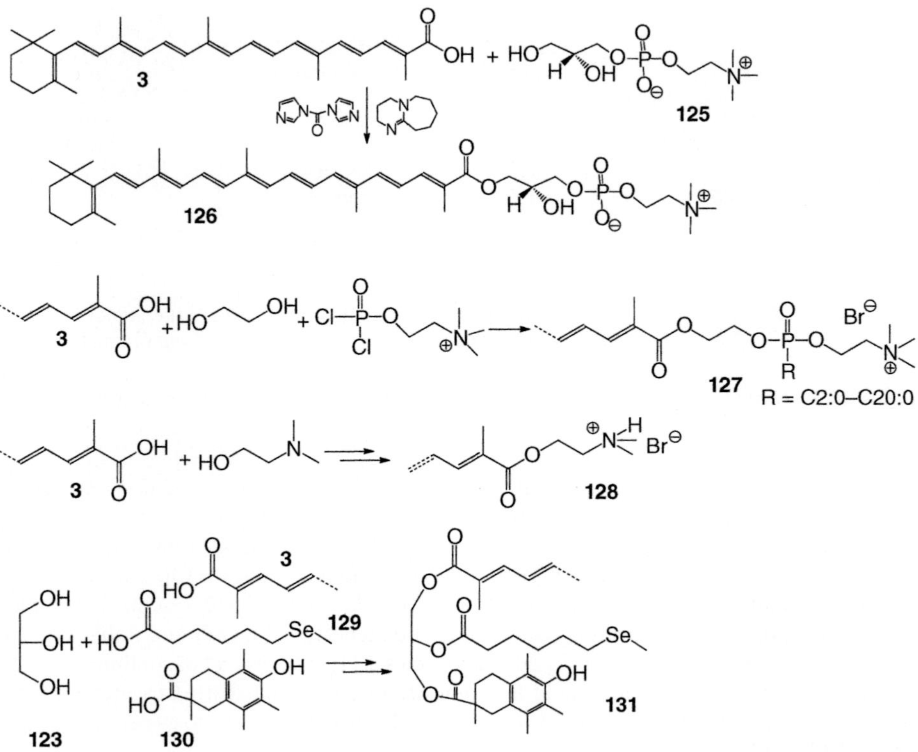

Scheme 28 Esterification.

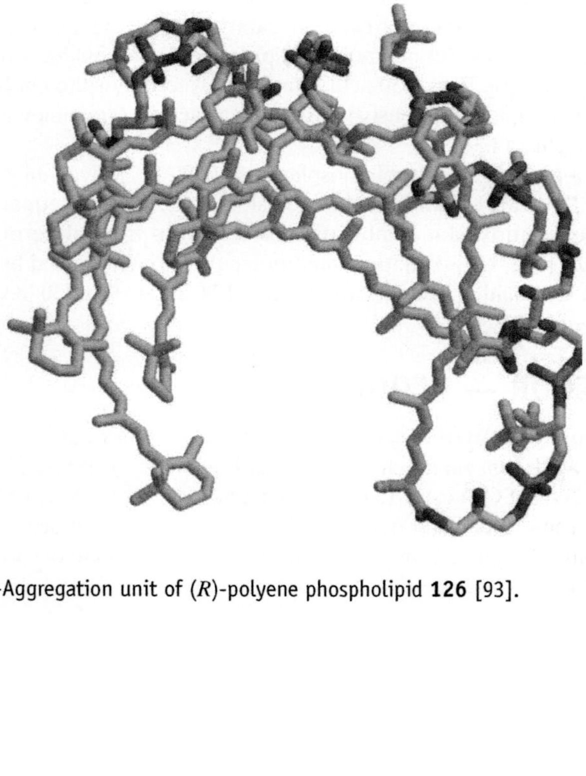

Figure 14.3 (*P*)-Aggregation unit of (*R*)-polyene phospholipid **126** [93].

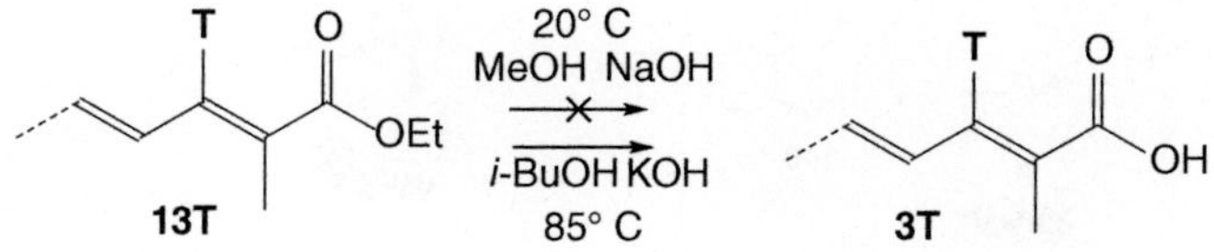

Scheme 29 Ester hydrolysis.

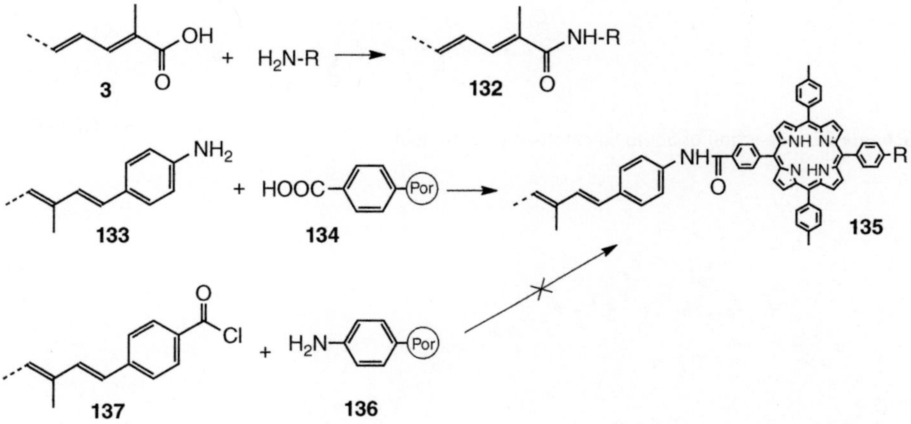

Scheme 30 Amide formation.

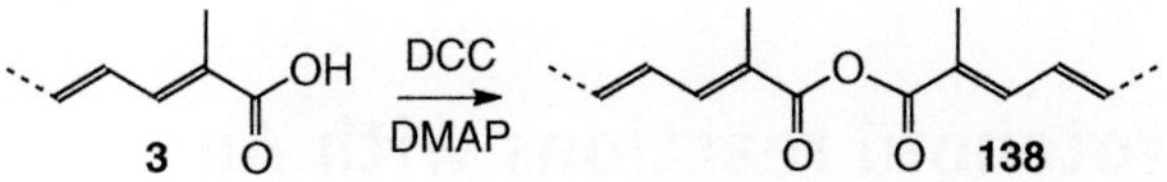

Scheme 31 Carotenoid acid anhydride.

14.5.5 -COOH → -CONH$_2$

Carotenoid acids (e.g., C30-acid **3**) easily react with amines, and several types of carotenoid amides **132** have been reported (Scheme 30) [126, 127]. Astaxanthin disuccinate also formed amides with amines and amino acids [98, 128]. Aminophenylcarotenoid **133** connects to porphyrin acid **134**, mimicking a photosynthetic center **135** [129]. Inversely, porphyrin amine **136** did not react with carotenoic acid chloride **137** to carotenoid porphyrins similar to **135** [130].

14.5.6 -COOH → -CO-O-OC- (carotenoid anhydrides)

Acid anhydride **138** inadvertently appeared as the main product in esterification reactions of C30-acid **3** with dicylohexylcarbodiimide (DCC) and dimethylaminopyridine (DMAP) (Scheme 31) [92].

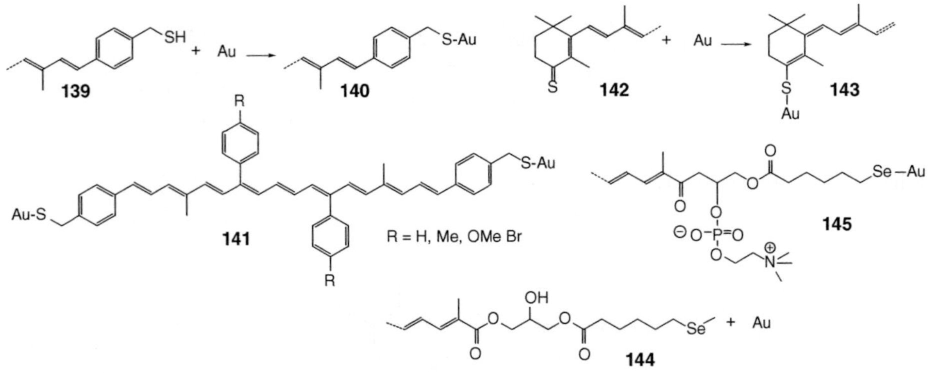

Scheme 32 Reaction of S and Se carotenoids with gold.

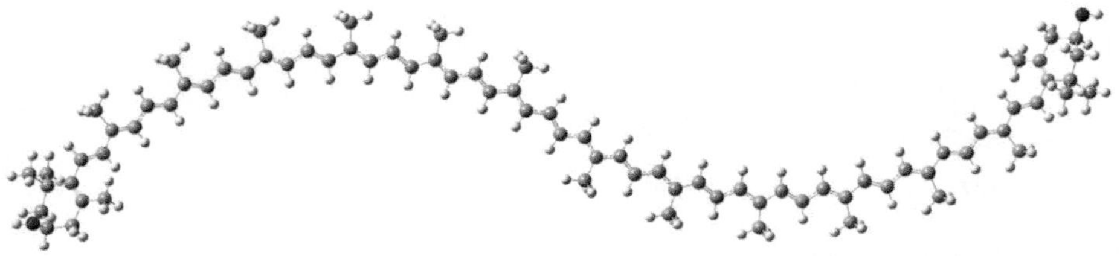

Figure 14.4 Distortion of elongated zeaxanthin **2** (C80:27; Scheme 1) [6].

14.6 Carotenoid reactions with Au

Benzylthiol carotenoid **139** self-attached on gold electrodes via an Au-thiolate bond **140**. The device convincingly confirmed the relevance of carotenoids as molecular wires [131]. In the same way, benzylthiol carotenoid **141** with two substituted in-chain benzene rings assembled on gold. The choice of the substituents allowed tuning conductivity [132]. Nonetheless, the occurrence of an isolating CH_2– group between the polyene chain, sulfur, and gold counteracts conductance. Applying carotenoid thiones (e.g., **142**) could increase conductivity by a conjugated polyene chain connection to the gold electrode (Au enthiolate **143**; Scheme 32) [53, 133]. Carotenoid thiones could possibly facilitate wire studies with even more isolating CH_2-units [134]. Nonetheless, the projected wire property of carotenoids is limited. Linear extension of carotenoid cables is precluded by considerable distortion, exemplified with long zeaxanthin **2** (Figure 14.4) [6].

Carotenoid lipids **144** and **145** assemble on gold surfaces and gold nanoparticles of a predefined size via a 7-selenaoctanoic group [135, 136]. The linking to gold occurs with a selenoate bond by dissociative absorption, expelling $-CH_3$ adjacent to Se [137].

Carotenoids converted to conductive materials by treatment with Lewis acids or alkali metals (e.g., rhodoxanthin **49** with FSO_3H, and canthaxanthin **57** with K in naphthalene) [138].

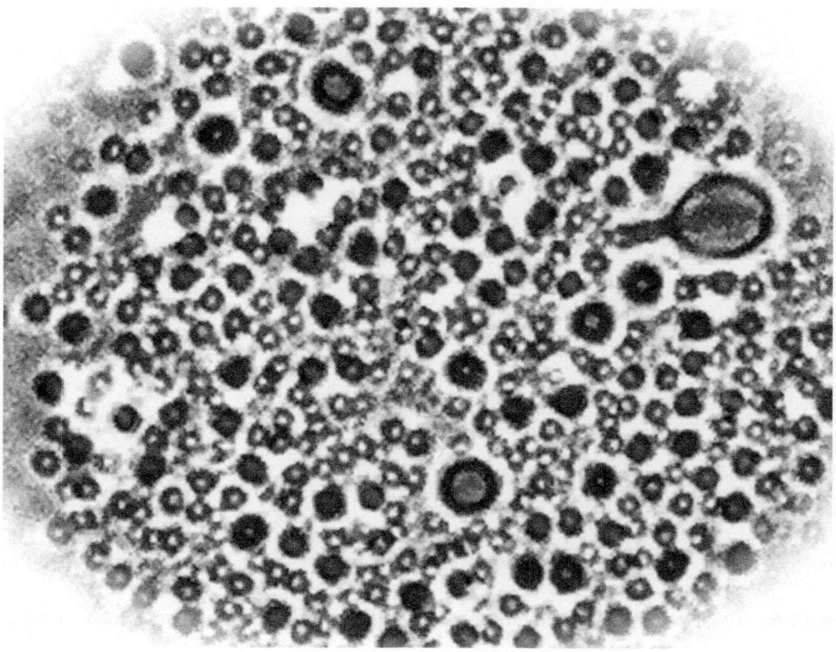

Figure 14.5 Vesicles (1–1.5 mm) of phospholipid **127** [117]. Reproduced with permission from Elsevier. (*See insert for color representation of the figure.*)

14.7 Valuation and conclusion

Several syntheses with carotenoids merit veritable admiration, such as the manufacture of molecular wires and of light-harvesting molecules. Carotenoid–porphyrin–fullerene derivatives represent definitely the most imaginative compounds synthesized with carotenoids [129]. The numerous efforts in increasing the hydrophilicity of carotenoids are valued for bioavailability and food color applications [90, 114]. The demand for modified carotenoids may rise in photochemistry, medicine, and light-harvesting research. Large-scale syntheses with carotenoids to pharmaceuticals are in negotiation. The physiological role of lipid enantiomers is generally ignored because glycerolipids lack optical activity. Consequently, the occurrence of a prevalent lipid enantiomer is so far not ascertained, in contrast to *L*-amino acids and *D*-sugars. Polyene glycerophospholipids (e.g., **126**) (Scheme 28) are likewise optically inactive in monomolecular solutions; however, in water, enantiomeric aggregation generates detectable optical activity (Figure 14.3) [94]. Gene-carrier phospholipids based on C30-acid **3** enable direct visual tracking of cellular localization; xenobiotic fluorescence tags become obsolete (Figures 14.5 and 14.6, Color Supplement) [117, 139]. The visual tracing ability of carotenoid derivatives is definitely underestimated.

The practical limitations of "syntheses with carotenoids" are evident. Syntheses with carotenoids require sufficient supply. Eleven carotenoids are marketed in kilograms or tonnes: β-carotene **6**, C30-ester **13**, astaxanthin **18**, C30-aldehyde **25**, citranaxanthin **52**, canthaxanthin **57**, zeaxanthin **60**, lutein, and lycopene [140], as well as bixin and crocetin (which are accessible after purification of commercial raw products) [85, 141]. Likewise available are mixed esters of astaxanthin and lutein. Carotenoid manufacturers offer in

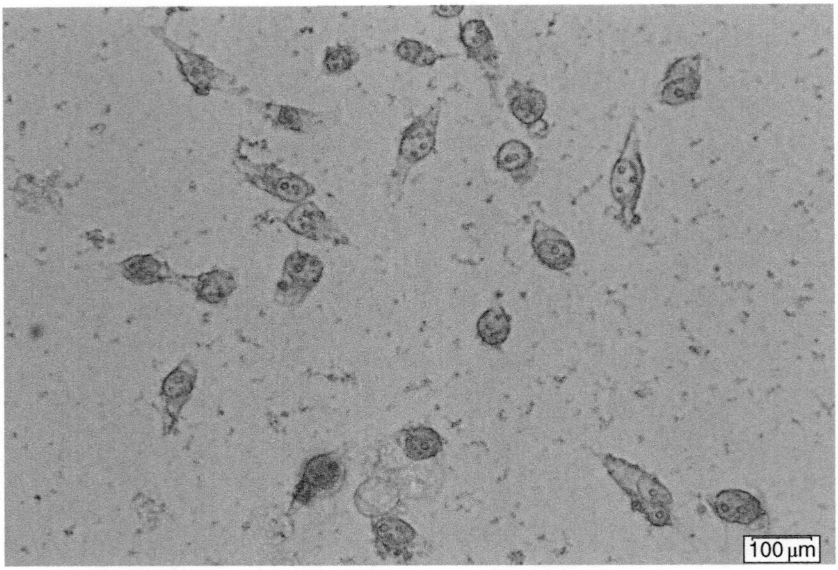

Figure 14.6 Visual tracking of **127** in cancer cells [139]. (*See insert for color representation of the figure.*)

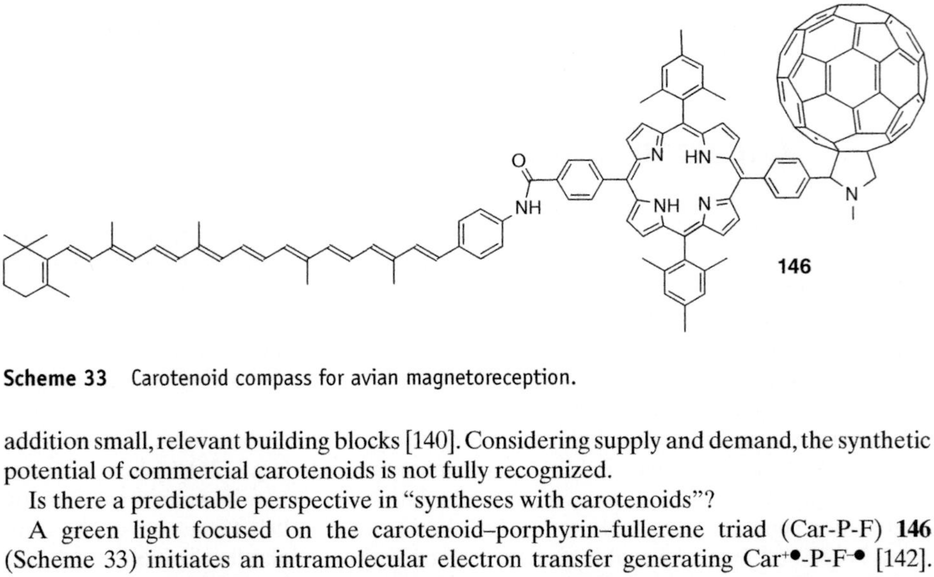

146

Scheme 33 Carotenoid compass for avian magnetoreception.

addition small, relevant building blocks [140]. Considering supply and demand, the synthetic potential of commercial carotenoids is not fully recognized.

Is there a predictable perspective in "syntheses with carotenoids"?

A green light focused on the carotenoid–porphyrin–fullerene triad (Car-P-F) **146** (Scheme 33) initiates an intramolecular electron transfer generating $Car^{+\bullet}$-P-$F^{-\bullet}$ [142]. The biradical is sensitive to the earth's weak magnetic field and may set the waypoints toward pioneering directions in "syntheses with carotenoids."

Acknowledgments

Many of the presented syntheses with carotenoids have been performed with supplies from compassionate industrial chemists. The authors gratefully recognize (chronologically) H. Mayer, B. Schulz, H. Ernst, and B. Schäfer for their significant support and, in addition, thank B. Schäfer for proofreading.

References

1. E. Widmer, T. Lukác, K. Bernhard, and R. Zell, "Technical procedures for the synthesis of carotenoids and related compounds from 6-oxo-isophorone 5: synthesis of astacene," *Helv. Chim. Acta.*, **65**, 671–83 (1982).
2. C. Martin and P. Karrer, "Carotinoidsynthesen 26. Einführung von Mercapto-Gruppen und Anilido-Gruppen in das β-Carotin," *Helv. Chim. Acta*, **42**, 464–6 (1959).
3. Eugster CH. The development of carotenoid chemistry as reflected in Helvetica Chimica Acta 1922-1991, *Helv. Chim. Acta*, **75**, 941–94 (1992).
4. Liaaen-Jensen S. Isolation, reactions," in O. Isler (ed.). *Carotenoids*, Basel: Birkhäuser, 1971, pp. 61–188.
5. L. W. Levy, R. H. Binnington, and A. S. Tabatznik, "Novel carotenoid esters," US2002/169334.
6. M. Zeeshan, H. R. Sliwka, V. Partali, and A. Martinez, "The longest polyene," *Org. Lett.*, **14**, 5496–8 (2012).
7. H. R. Sliwka and V. Partali, "Key to xenobiotic carotenoids," *Molecules*, **17**, 2877–928 (2012).
8. G. Gorbach and P. Hochbahn, "Stufenweise Hydrierung von Carotin," *Monatshefte*, **87**, 231–3 (1956).
9. S. C. Kushwaha, C. Subbaray, and J. W. Porter, "Conversion of lycopene-15,15′-3H to cyclic carotenes by soluble extracts of higher plant plastids," *J. Biol. Chem.*, **244**, 3635–42 (1969).
10. A. Zaidi, "Polyenoic acids and their alkali and europium salts," PhD thesis, Norwegian University of Science and Technology, Trondheim, Norway, 2014.
11. J. S. Sinninghe Damsté and M. P. Koopmans, "The fate of carotenoids in sediments: an overview," *Pure Appl. Chem.*, **69**, 2067–74 (1997).
12. Chiron AS, Trondheim, Norway.
13. R. Pummerer, L. Rebmann, and W. Reidel, "Über die Bestimmung des Sättigungszustandes von Polyenen mittels Chlorjods und Benzoepersäure," *Ber. dtsch. Chem. Ges.*, **62**, 1411–8 (1929).
14. M. E. MacBeath and A. L. Richardson, "Tomato juice rainbow: a colorful and instructive demonstration," *J. Chem. Edu.*, **63**, 1092–4 (1986).
15. B. F. Lutnaes, J. Krane, and S. Liaaen-Jensen, "On the structure of carotenoid iodine complexes," *Org. Biomol. Chem.*, **2**, 2821–8 (2004).
16. M. Carail and C. Caris-Veyrat, "Carotenoid oxidation products: from villain to saviour?" *Pure Appl. Chem.*, **78**, 1493–503 (2006).
17. K. Tsukida, M. Yokota, and K. Ikeuchi, "Epoxycarotenoids 11: air-oxidation of all-trans β-carotene," *Bitamin.*, **33**, 179–84 (1966).
18. I. Washington, S. Jockusch, Y. Itagaki, N. J. Turro, and K. Nakanishi, "Superoxidation of bisretinoids," *Angew. Chem.*, **44**, 7097–100 (2005).
19. M. D. Torres Cardona, G. Rodriguez, and G. C. Schloemer, "Method for producing esterified astaxanthin from esterified zeaxanthin," Prodemex S.A., Mexico, WO2004/039991.
20. L. A. Kispert, A. L. Focsan, and T. A. Konovalova TA, "Applications of ESR spectroscopy to understanding carotenoid radicals," in J. T. Landrum (ed.), *Carotenoids: physical, chemical, and biological functions and properties*, Boca Raton: CRC Press, 2010, pp. 159–88.
21. K. R. Naqvi, T. B. Melø, H. R. Sliwka, S. B. B. Mohamad, and V. Partali, "Photochemical and photophysical behaviour of vitamin E: interaction of its long-lived transient photoproducts with carotenoids," *Photochem. Photobiol. Sci.*, **2**, 381–5 (2003).

22. H. R. Sliwka, T. B. Melø, B. J. Foss, *et al.*, "Electron- and energy-transfer properties of hydrophilic carotenoids," *Chem. Eur. J.*, **13**, 4458–66 (2007).

23. G. Kildahl-Andersen, T. A. Konovalova, A. L. Focsan, L. D. Kispert, T. Anthonsen, and S. Liaaen-Jensen, "Comparative studies on radical cation formation from carotenoids and retinoids," *Tetrahedron Lett.*, **48**, 8196–9 (2007).

24. A. Zaidi, H. Li, H. R. Sliwka, V. Partali, H. Ernst, and T. B. Melø, "Energy and electron transfer reactions of polyenic acids with variable chain lengths," *Tetrahedron*, **69**, 219–27 (2013).

25. F. Ignatious and C. Mathis, "Thermal aging of tetraalkyl ammonium doped polyacetylenes," *Macromolecules*, **23**, 70–7 (1990).

26. C. L. Øpstad, H. R. Sliwka, and V. Partali, "Facile electron uptake by carotenoids under mild, non-radiative conditions: formation of carotenoid anions," *Eur. J. Org. Chem.*, 4637–41 (2010).

27. A. El-Agamey, R. Edge, S. Navaratnam, E. J. Land, and T. G. Truscott," Carotenoid radical anions and their protonated derivatives," *Org. Lett.*, **8**, 4255–8 (2006).

28. V. G. Mairanovsky, A. A. Engovatov, N. T. Ioffe, and G. I. Samokhvalov, "Electron-donor and electron-acceptor properties of carotenoids: electrochemical study of carotenes," *J. Electroanal. Chem.*, **66**, 123–37 (1975).

29. M. Zeeshan, H. R. Sliwka, V. Partali, and A. Martinez, "Electron uptake by classical electron donators: astaxanthin and carotenoid aldehydes," *Tetrahedron Lett.*, **53**, 4522–5 (2012).

30. H. Li, E. Rebmann, C. L. Øpstad, R. Schmid, H. R. Sliwka, and V. Partali, "Synthesis of a highly unsaturated, stable hydroxy peroxide: a yellow-blue color-changing carotenoid oxidation product with leuco dye properties," *Eur. J. Org. Chem.*, 4630–6 (2010).

31. M. Ichikawa, M. Tsutsui, and F. Vohwinke, "Iron carbonyl complexes of β-carotene and lycopene," *Z. Naturforschg. B*, **22**, 376–9 (1967).

32. F. Effenberger and H. Schlosser, "Synthesen endständig substitutierter, konjugierter Polyene," *Synthesis*, 1085–94 (1990).

33. R. Yoshioka, T. Hayakawa, K. Ishizuka, *et al.*, "Nitration reactions of astaxanthin and β-carotene by peroxynitrite," *Tetrahedron Lett.*, **47**, 3637–40 (2006).

34. D. Hoischen, L. U. Colmenares, I. Koukhareva, M. Ho, and R. S. H. Liu, "9-CF_3 and 13-CF_3-β-carotene, canthaxanthin and related carotenoids: synthesis, characterization and electrochemical data," *J. Fluorine Chem.*, **97**, 165–71 (1999).

35. H. R. Sliwka and S. Liaaen-Jensen, "Selenium carotenoids 2. Synthesis of ε, ε-carotene-3,3'-dione from rhodoxanthin," *Acta Chem. Scand.*, **49**, 856–7 (1995).

36. H. Ikeda, T. Sakai, and Y. Kawabe, "Organic nonlinear optical material," Idemitsu Kosan Co Ltd., 1990, JP2002534.

37. A. J. Aasen and S. Liaaen-Jensen, "Bacterial carotenoids 24. Carotenoids of thiorhodaceae 7. Cross-conjugated carotenals," *Acta Chem. Scand.*, **21**, 2185–204 (1967).

38. T. Miki and Y. Hara, "Studies on ethylenic compounds 3. Hydrazone-type derivatives of vitamin A aldehyde," *Chem. Pharm. Bull.*, **10**, 922–6 (1962).

39. R. Alvarez, B. Vaz, H. Gronemeyer, and A. R. de Lera, "Functions, therapeutic applications, and synthesis of retinoids and carotenoids," *Chem. Rev.*, **114**, 1–125 (2014).

40. P. Karrer and C. H. Eugster, "Carotinoidsynthesen 8. Synthese des Dodecapreno-β-Carotins," *Helv. Chim. Acta*, **34**, 1805–14 (1951).

41. G. Broszeit, F. Diepenbrock, O. Graf, *et al.*, "Vinylogous β-carotenes: generation, storage, and delocalization of charge in carotenoids," *Liebigs Ann. Recl.*, 2205–13 (1997).

42. M. Blanchard-Desce, I. Ledoux, J. M. Lehn, J. Malthête, and J. Zyss, "Push-pull polyenes and carotenoids: synthesis and non-linear optical properties," *J. Chem. Soc. Chem. Commun.*, 737–9 (1988).

43. F. Stenhorst, "Synthese und Spektroskopie tieffarbiger 2,2'-Dinorcarotinoide," PhD thesis, University of Düsseldorf, 1996.

44. S. Beutner, S. Frixel, H. Ernst, *et al.*, "Carotenylflavonoids, a novel group of potent, dual-functional antioxidants," *Arkivoc*, 279–95 (2007).

45. H. Bettermann, M. Bienioschek, H. Ippendorf, and H. D. Martin, "Dual fluorescence of diapocarotenoids," *J. Lumin.*, **55**, 63–70 (1993).

46. F. Effenberger and M. Wezstein, "Synthesis of aryl-terminated polyenaldehydes and polyenetriethoxysilanes for preparation of self-assembled monolayers on silicon surfaces," *Synthesis*, 1368–76 (2001).

47. A. Brüngger, H. Gründler, and W. Simon, "β-Keto alcohols and the process for the manufacture thereof," Roche Vitamins Inc., US1997/5648550.

48. C. L. Øpstad, H. R. Sliwka, and V. Partali, "New colours for carotenoids: synthesis of pyran polyenes," *Eur. J. Org. Chem.*, 435–9 (2010).

49. G. L. Olson, "Intermediate compounds for the preparation of polyene aldehydes," Hoffman-La Roche, Nutley, US1976/3997529.

50. A. T. Bens, D. Frewert, K. Kodatis, C. Kryschi, H. D. Martin, and H. P. Trommsdorff, "Coupling of chromophores: carotenoids and photoactive diarylethenes: photoreactivity versus radiationless deactivation," *Eur. J. Org. Chem.*, 2333–8 (1998).

51. A. Osuka, H. Yamada, and K. Maruyama, "Synthesis of conformationally restricted carotenoid-linked porphyrins," *Chem. Lett.*, 1905–8 (1990).

52. G. Märkl, N. Aschenbrenner, A. Baur, C. Rastorfer, and P. Kreitmeier, "Synthese von Polymethintetrathiafulvalenen durch Dimerisierung von ω-(1,3-Dithiol-2-ylidene) polyenalen mit dem Lawesson Reagens: Carotinoide und supracarotinoide Tetrathiafulvalene," *Helv. Chim. Acta*, **86**, 2589–609 (2003).

53. E. M. Sandru, J. Sielk, and J. Burghaus, *et al.*, "Thiocarbonyl polyenes: monomers, trimers, and thiopyrans," *Tetrahedron Lett.*, **53**, 6822–5 (2012).

54. H. R. Sliwka and S. Liaaen-Jensen, "Synthetic sulfur carotenoids 3. Carotenoid thiones-first preparation and spectroscopic properties," *Acta Chem. Scand.*, **48**, 679–83 (1994).

55. A. Martinez, "Keto, thione, selone, and tellone carotenoids: changing antioxidants to antireductants," *Can. J. Chem.*, **91**, 621–7 (2013).

56. H. R. Sliwka and S. Liaaen-Jensen, "Selective hydrogenation of carotenones 2. Reduction of rhodoxanthin to lutein and zeaxanthin, and of canthaxanthin to a dihydro-retro-carotenediol by tellurium hydride," *Acta Chem. Scand.*, **50**, 637–9 (1996).

57. H. R. Sliwka and S. Liaaen-Jensen, "Partial syntheses of diastereomeric carotenols," *Acta Chem. Scand. B*, **41**, 518–25 (1987).

58. J. Liu, N. L. Shelton, and R. S. H. Liu, "Study of α-crustacyanin utilizing halogenated canthaxanthins," *Org. Lett.*, **4**, 2521–4 (2002).

59. S. E. Lockwood, S. O'Malley, D. G. Watumull, L. M. Hix, H. Jackson, and G. Nadolski, "Pharmaceutical compositions including carotenoid ether analogs or derivatives for the inhibition and amelioration of disease," US2005/65096.

60. H. Pfander and U. Leuenberger, "Chlorinated carotenoids from $CHCl_3$–HCl-reaction," *Chimia*, **30**, 71–3 (1976).

61. D. Gust, T. A. Moore, R. V. Bensasson, *et al.*, "Stereodynamics of intramolecular triplet energy-transfer in carotenoporphyrins," *J. Am. Chem Soc.*, **107**, 3631–40 (1985).

62. H. R. Sliwka and S. Liaaen-Jensen, "Synthetic sulfur carotenoids 2. Optically-active carotenoid thiols," *Tetrahedron-Asym.*, **4**, 361–8 (1993).

63. H. R. Sliwka and S. Liaaen-Jensen, "Synthetic nitrogen carotenoids: optically-active carotenoid amines," *Tetrahedron-Asym.*, **4**, 2377–82 (1993).

64. H. R. Sliwka, "Selenium carotenoids 3. First synthesis of optically active carotenoid phosphates," *Acta Chem. Scand.*, **51**, 345–7 (1997).

65. H. R. Sliwka, "Conformation and circular dichroism of β, β-carotene derivatives with nitrogen-, sulfur-, and selenium-containing substituents," *Helv. Chim. Acta*, **82**, 161–9 (1999).

66. H. R. Sliwka and S. Liaaen-Jensen, "Synthetic sulfur carotenoids: 3'-thiolutein," *Acta Chem. Scand.*, **44**, 61–6 (1990).

67. A. Zand, A. Agócs, J. Deli, and V. Nagy, "Synthesis of carotenoid–cysteine conjugates," *Acta Biochim. Pol.*, **59**, 149–50 (2012).

68. G. Olatunji and S. Oladoye, "Synthesis and characterization of bixin–ethyl cellulose derivatives," *Cell Chem. Technol.*, **38**, 3–9 (2004).

69. V. M. Dembitsky, "Astonishing diversity of natural surfactants 3. Carotenoid glycosides and isoprenoid glycolipids," *Lipids*, **40**, 535–57 (2005).

70. M. Hanaura, A. Agócs, K. Böddi, J. Deli, and V. Nagy, "New methods for the synthesis of carotenoid glycosides," *Tetrahedron Lett.*, **55**, 3625–7 (2014).

71. S. Herweg, "Untersuchung und Entwicklung von Methoden zur Synthese glykosidischer Carotinoide," PhD thesis, University of Düsseldorf, 2008.

72. S. E. Lockwood, S. O'Malley, D. Watumull, L. M. Hix, H. Jackson, and G. Nadolski, "Carotenoid ether analogs or derivatives for controlling connexin 43 expression," US2005/148517.

73. V. Nagy, A. Agócs, E. Turcsi, and J. Deli, "Experiments on the synthesis of carotenoid glycosides," *Tetrahedron Lett.*, **51**, 2020–2 (2010).

74. V. Nagy, A. Agócs, E. Turcsi, and J. Deli, "Isolation and purification of acid-labile carotenoid 5,6-epoxides on modified silica gels," *Phytochem. Anal.*, **20**, 143–8 (2009).

75. D. Osianu, E. Nicoara, and C. Bodea, "In chain-epoxides of carotenoids 7. Astacene 9,10- and 11,12-epoxides," *Rev. Roum. Chim.*, **22**, 1085–8 (1980).

76. N. Fontán, B. Vaz, R. Alvarez, and A. R. de Lera, "A conjunctive diiodoheptaene for the synthesis of C-2-symmetric carotenoids," *Chem. Commun.*, **49**, 2694–6 (2013).

77. N. E. Polyakov, A. L. Focsan, and M. K. Bowman, and L. D. Kispert, "Free radical formation in novel carotenoid metal ion complexes of astaxanthin," *J. Phys. Chem. B*, **114**, 16968–77 (2010).

78. E. Hernández-Marin, A. Barbosa, and A. Martínez, "The metal cation chelating capacity of astaxanthin. Does this have any influence on antiradical activity?" *Molecules*, **17**, 1039–54 (2012).

79. J. Willibald, S. Rennebaum, S. Breukers, *et al.*, "Hydrophilic carotenoids: facile syntheses of carotenoid oxime hydrochlorides as long-chain, highly unsaturated cationic (bola)-amphiphiles," *Chem. Phys. Lipids*, **161**, 32–7 (2009).

80. J. M. Lehn, J. P. Vigneron, I. Bkouche-Waksman, J. Guilhem, and C. Pascard, "Carocryptands—tris-carotenoid macrobicyclic ligands: synthesis, crystal-structure, and dinuclear copper(I) complexes," *Helv. Chim. Acta*, **75**, 1069–77 (1992).

81. D. L. Coffen, E. Ho, C. Nocka, *et al.*, "Synthesis and evaluation of retinal Schiff-base salts and related-compounds as radar absorbing agents," *J. Prakt. Chem.*, **335**, 135–42 (1993).

82. H. Pfander, "Synthesis of carotenoid glycosylesters and other carotenoids," *Pure Appl. Chem.*, **51**, 565–80 (1979).

83. T. Naalsund, K. E. Malterud, V. Partali, and H. R. Sliwka, "Synthesis of a triantioxidant compound: combination of β-apo-8'-carotenoic acid, selenacapryloic acid and trolox in a triglyceride," *Chem. Phys. Lipids*, **112**, 59–65 (2001).

84. Y. Yang, H. Zhu, H. Ji, *et al.,* "Process for preparation of crocetin organic amine salts," JiangsuTiansheng Pharmaceutical Co. Ltd., CN103183603, 2013.

85. S. Breukers, C. L. Øpstad, H. R. Sliwka, and V. Partali, "Hydrophilic carotenoids: surface properties and aggregation behavior of the potassium salt of the highly unsaturated diacid norbixin," *Helv. Chim. Acta*, **92**, 1741–7 (2009).

86. A. Linden, B. Bürgi, and C. H. Eugster, "Confirmation of the structures of lutein and zeaxanthin," *Helv. Chim. Acta*, **87**, 1254–69 (2004).

87. G. Dirks, A. L. Moore, T. A. Moore, and D. Gust, "Light-absorption and energy-transfer in polyene-porphyrin esters," *Photochem. Photobiol.*, **32**, 277–80 (1980).

88. S. Shinoda and H. Tsukube, "Carotenoid-pyropheophorbide dyads: synthetic approaches to biological functions of carotenoids in photosynthesis systems," *Recent Res. Dev. Org. Chem.*, **2**, 429–39 (1998).

89. M. Háda, V. Nagy, A. Takátsy, J. Deli, and A. Agócs, "Dicarotenoid esters of bivalent acids," *Tetrahedron Lett.*, **49**, 3524–6 (2008).

90. M. Háda, V. Nagy, J. Deli, and A. Agócs, "Hydrophilic carotenoids: recent progress," *Molecules*, **17**, 5003–12 (2012).

91. M. Háda, V. Nagy, G. Gulyás-Fekete, J. Deli, and A. Agócs, "Towards carotenoid dendrimers: carotenoid diesters and triesters with aromatic cores," *Helv. Chim. Acta*, **93**, 1149–55 (2010).

92. C. L. Øpstad, unpublished results.

93. The molecule structure was calculated by Z. Bikadi, Virtua Drug Ltd., Budapest, Hungary.

94. B. J. Foss, H. R. Sliwka, V. Partali, *et al.,* "Optically active oligomer units in aggregates of a highly unsaturated, optically inactive carotenoid phospholipid," *Chem. Eur. J.*, **11**, 4103–8 (2010).

95. V. Partali, H. R. Sliwka, T. Anthonsen, and S. Liaaen-Jensen, "Enzymatic resolution of zeaxanthin," *Biocatalysis*, **6**, 145–9 (1992).

96. T. Ramdahl and S. Liaaen-Jensen, "Carotenoid sulfates 1. Partial syntheses of lycoxanthin sulfate and zeaxanthin disulfate," *Acta Chem. Scand. B*, **34**, 773–4 (1980).

97. S. Hertzberg, T. Ramdahl, J. E. Johansen, and S. Liaaen-Jensen, "Carotenoid sulfates 2. Structural elucidation of bastaxanthin," *Acta Chem. Scand. B*, **37**, 267–79 (1983).

98. S. F. Lockwood and G. Nadolski, "Water-dispersible carotenoids, including analogs and derivatives," US2007/15735.

99. D. A. Frey, E. W. Kataisto, J. L. Ekmanis, S. O'Malley, and S. F. Lockwood, "The efficient synthesis of disodium disuccinate astaxanthin (Cardax)," *Org. Process Res. Dev.*, **8**, 796–801 (2004).

100. S. F. Lockwood and G. J. Gross, "Disodium disuccinate astaxanthin (Cardax (TM)): antioxidant and antinflammatory cardioprotection," *Cardiovasc. Drug Rev.*, **23**, 199–216 (2005).

101. B. J. Foss, H. R. Sliwka, V. Partali, *et al.,* "Hydrophilic carotenoids: surface properties and aggregation behavior of a highly unsaturated carotenoid lysophospholipid," *Chem. Phys. Lipids.*, **134**, 85–96 (2005).

102. M. Zeeshan, "Synthesis and properties of long chain polyenes—synthesis and properties of cationic and anionic polyene lipids," Norwegian University of Science and Technology, Trondheim, Norway, PhD thesis, 2012.

103. S. E. Lockwood, S. O'Malley, D. G. Watumull, L. M. Hix, H. Jackson, and G. Nadolski, "Structural carotenoid analogs for the inhibition and amelioration of disease," WO2004/011423.

104. H. L. Jackson, A. J. Cardounel, J. L. Zweier, and S. E. Lockwood, "Synthesis, characterization, and direct aqueous superoxide anion scavenging of a highly water-dispersible astaxanthin-amino acid conjugate," *Bioorg. Med. Chem. Lett.*, **14**, 3985–91 (2004).

105. S. Nalum Naess, H. R. Sliwka, V. Partali, *et al.,* "Hydrophilic carotenoids: surface properties and aggregation of an astaxanthin-lysine conjugate, a rigid, long-chain, highly unsaturated and highly water-soluble tetracationic bolaamphiphile" *Chem. Phys. Lipids*, **148**, 63–9 (2007).

106. Y. Li and Q. Liu, "Preparation of carotenoid derivatives and their applications," Beijing Gingko Group Biological Technology, US2012/0220580.

107. D. M. Marcus and C. K. Chu, "Methods and compositions for treatment of macular and retinal disease," US2007/0259843.

108. J. Schierle, W. Simon, and W. Steinberg, Roche Vitamins AG, EP2001/1186245.

109. T. B. R. Papa, V. D. Pinho, E. S. P. do Nascimento, *et al.,* "Astaxanthin diferulate as a bifunctional antioxidant," *Free Radic. Res.*, **49**, 102–11 (2015).

110. M. Hugentobler, S. Ruf, B. Wuestenberg, "Novel use of carotenoid (ester)s," US2011/119995.

111. A. Milon, G. Wolff, G. Ourisson, and Y. Nakatani, "Organization of carotenoid-phospholipid bilayer systems: incorporation of zeaxanthin, astaxanthin, and their C50 homologs into dimyristoylphosphatidylcholine vesicles," *Helv. Chim. Acta*, **69**, 12–24 (1986).

112. W. I. Gruszecki, "Carotenoids in lipid membranes," in J. T. Landrum (ed.), *Carotenoids: physical, chemical, and biological funtions and properties*, Boca Raton, FL: CRC Press, 2010, pp. 19–30.

113. V. Partali, L. Kvittingen, H. R. Sliwka, and T. Anthonsen, "Stable, highly unsaturated glycerides: enzymatic synthesis with a carotenoic acid," *Angew. Chem. Int. Ed.*, **35**, 329–30 (1996).

114. H. R. Sliwka, V. Partali, and S. E. Lockwood, "Hydrophilic carotenoids: carotenoid aggregates," in J. T. Landrum (ed.), *Carotenoids: physical, chemical, and biological functions and properties*, Boca Raton, FL: CRC Press, 2010, pp. 31–58.

115. A. Basu, S. Bhaduri, and T. G. K. Kasar, "Process for the manufacture of conjugated polyenoic fatty compounds," EP1985/0160544.

116. B. J. Foss, S. Nalum Naess, H. R. Sliwka, and V. Partali, "Stable and highly water-dispersible, highly unsaturated carotenoid phospholipids: surface properties and aggregate size," *Angew. Chem. Int. Ed.*, **42**, 5237–40 (2003).

117. C. L. Øpstad, H. R. Sliwka, V. Partali, *et al.,* "Synthesis, self-assembling and gene delivery potential of a novel highly unsaturated, conjugated cationic phospholipid," *Chem. Phys. Lipids*, **170**, 65–73 (2013).

118. C. L. Øpstad, M. Zeeshan, A. Zaidi, *et al.,* "Novel cationic polyene glycol phospholipids as DNA transfer reagents: lack of a structure-activity relationship due to uncontrolled self-assembling processes," *Chem. Phys. Lipids*, **183**, 117–36 (2014).

119. L. J. Popplewell, A. Abu-Dayya, T. Khanna T, *et al.,* "Novel cationic carotenoid lipids as delivery vectors of antisense oligonucleotides for exon skipping in Duchenne muscular dystrophy," *Molecules*, **17**, 1138–48 (2012).

120. S. Machado, S. Calado, D. Bitoque, *et al.,* "Cationic polyene phospholipids as DNA carriers for ocular gene therapy," *BioMed. Res. Int.*, http://dx.doi.org/ 10.1155/2014/703253 (2014).

121. M. D. Pungente, E. Jubeli, C. L. Øpstad, *et al.,* "Synthesis and preliminary investigations of the siRNA delivery potential of novel, single-chain rigid cationic carotenoid lipids," *Molecules*, **17**, 3484–500 (2012).

122. E. Larsen, J. Abendroth, V. Partali, B. Schulz, H. R. Sliwka, and E. G. K. Quartey, "Combination of vitamin E with a carotenoid: alpha-tocopherol and trolox linked to β-apo-8'-carotenoic acid," *Chem. Eur. J.*, **4**, 113–7 (1998).

123. E. Karagiannidou, T. R. Størseth, H. R. Sliwka, V. Partali, K. E. Malterud, and M. Tsimidou, "Synthesis of two modified carotenoids and their behavior during light exposure," *Eur. J. Lipid Sci. Technol.*, **105**, 419–26 (2003).

124. P. V. Reddy, M. Rabago-Smith, and B. Borhan, "Synthesis of all-*trans*-[10'-^{3}H]-8'-apo-β-carotenoic acid," *J. Labelled Compd. Radiopharm.*, **45**, 79–89 (2002).

125. T. Bjørk, "*Syntese av crocin-derivater*," Master's thesis, Department of Chemistry, Norwegian University of Science and Technology, Trondheim, 2008.

126. Q. Quinkert, K. R. Schmieder, G. Durner, K. Hache, A. Stegk, and D. H. R. Barton, "Light-induced reactions 12. Convenient synthesis of dimethylcrocetin," *Chem. Ber.*, **110**, 3582–614 (1977).

127. J. H. Fuhrhop, M. Krull, A. Schulz, and D. Möbius, "Bolaform amphiphiles with a rigid hydrophobic bixin core in surface monolayers and lipid-membranes," *Langmuir*, **6**, 497–505 (1990).

128. B. J. Foss, G. Nadolski, and S. F. Lockwood, "Synthesis of carotenoid analogs or derivatives with improved antioxidant characteristics," US2009/99061.

129. T. A. Moore, A. L. Moore, and D. Gust, "The design and synthesis of artificial photosynthetic antennas, reaction centres and membranes," *Philos. T. Roy. Soc. B*, **357**, 1481–98 (2002).

130. B. Incekara-Fleck, "Synthese von neuen Carotinoporphyrinmodellsystemen zur Untersuchung von Energietransferprozessen," PhD thesis, University of Düsseldorf, 2002.

131. G. K. Ramachandran, J. K. Tomfohr, J. Li, *et al.*, "Electron transport properties of a carotene molecule in a metal-(single molecule)-metal junction," *J. Phys. Chem. B*, **107**, 6162–9 (2003).

132. Y. A. Zhao, S. Lindsay, S. Jeon, *et al.*, "Combined effect of polar substituents on the electronic flows in the carotenoid molecular wires," *Chem. Eur. J.*, **19**, 10832–5 (2013).

133. A. Ion, V. Partali, H. R. Sliwka, and F. G. Banica, "Electrochemistry of a carotenoid self-assembled monolayer," *Electrochem. Commun.*, **4**, 674–8 (2002).

134. N. Krings, H. H. Strehblow, J. Kohnert, and H. D. Martin, "Investigations on the monolayer structure of thiol SAMs and the influence of conjugated π-bonds on the electronic molecular conductivity," *Electrochim. Acta*, **49**, 167–74 (2003).

135. B. J. Foss, A. Ion, V. Partali, H. R. Sliwka, and F. G. Banica, "Electrochemical and EQCM investigation of a selenium derivatized carotenoid in the self-assembled state at a gold electrode," *J. Electroanal. Chem.*, **593**, 15–28 (2006).

136. E. G. Sandru, "Polyene nanoparticles," Trondheim: Norwegian University of Science and Technology, PhD thesis, 2013.

137. B. J. Foss, A. Ion, V. Partali, H. R. Sliwka, and F. G. Banica, "O-1-[6-(methylselanyl)-hexanoyl]glycerol as an anchor for self-assembly of biological compounds at the gold surface," *Coll. Czech Chem. Commun.*, **69**, 1971–96 (2004).

138. F. Feichtmayr, H. Naarmann, J. Paust, and K. Penzien, "Preparation of electrically conductive carotenoids," BASF SE, US1982/4336201.

139. E. Jubeli, L. Raju, N. Abdul Khalique, *et al.*, "Polyene-based cationic lipids as visually traceable siRNA transfer reagents," *Eur. J. Pharm. Biopharm.*, **89**, 280–9 (2015).

140. H. Ernst, "Recent advances in industrial carotenoid synthesis," *Pure Appl. Chem.*, **74**, 2213–26 (2002).

141. S. Nalum Naess, A. Elgsaeter, B. J. Foss, *et al.*, "Hydrophilic carotenoids: Surface properties and aggregation of crocin as a biosurfactant," *Helv. Chim. Acta*, **89**, 45–53 (2006).

142. K. Maeda, K. B. Henbest, F. Cintolesi, *et al.*, "Chemical compass model of avian magnetoreception," *Nature*, **453**, 387–90 (2008).

Index

Note: Page numbers in *italics* denote figures (when outside text page ranges)

Carotenoids: Nutrition, Analysis and Technology, First Edition. Edited by Agnieszka Kaczor and Malgorzata Baranska.

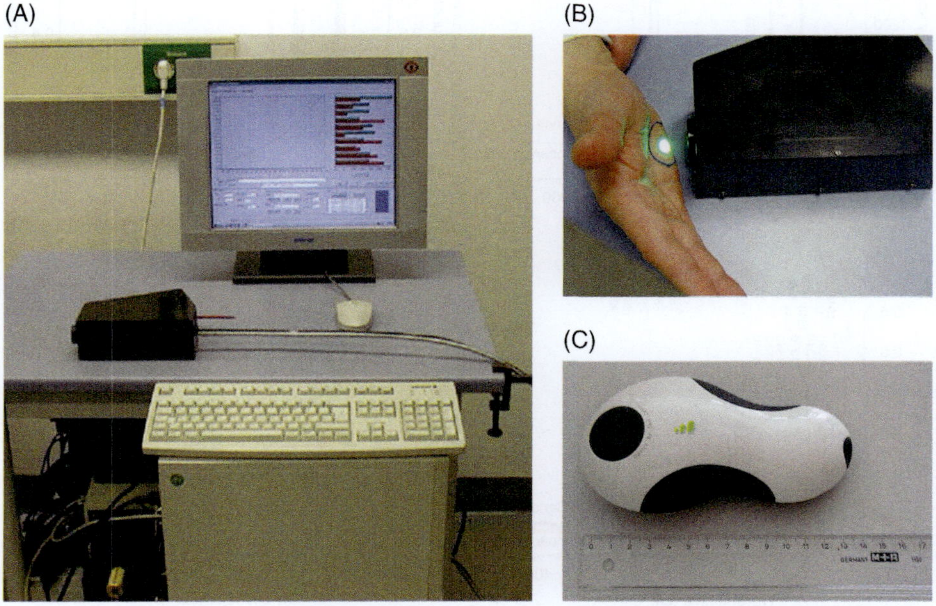

Figure 2.1 (A, B) Raman resonance spectrometer developed at the CCP; and (C) a biozoom® skin scanner based on reflectance spectroscopy for the detection of carotenoids in human skin.

Carotenoids: Nutrition, Analysis and Technology, First Edition. Edited by Agnieszka Kaczor and Malgorzata Baranska.

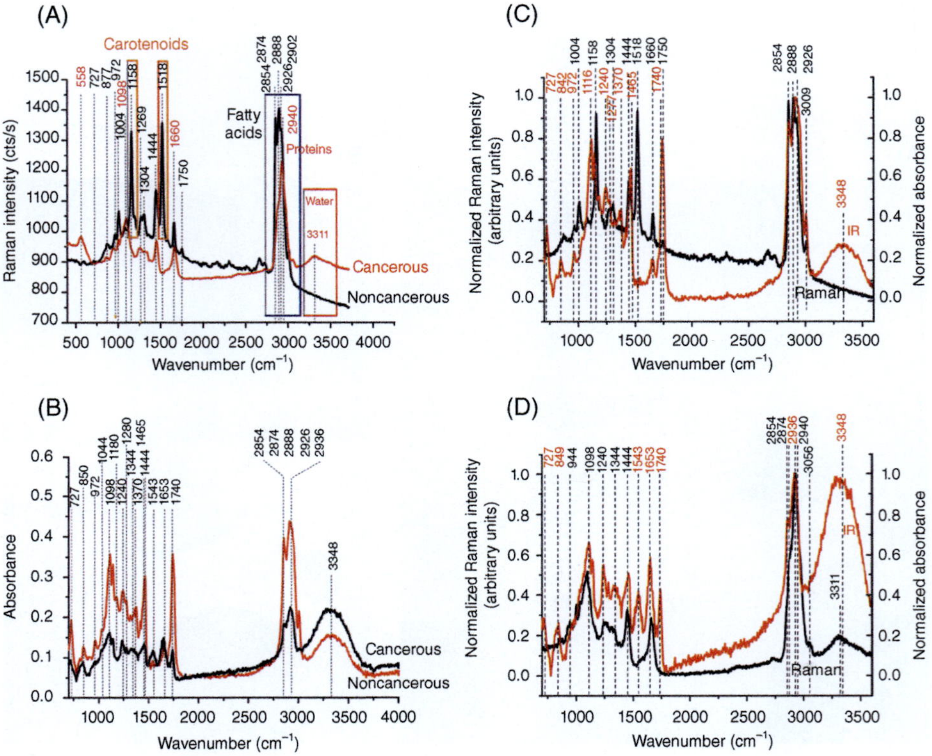

Figure 3.2 The average Raman and infrared (IR) spectra for the noncancerous and cancerous breast tissues (infiltrating ductal carcinoma). (A) Raman spectra of patient P81; (B) IR spectra of patient P83; (C) Raman spectrum for the noncancerous normal breast tissues of patient P81, and IR spectrum for the noncancerous normal breast tissues of patient P83; and (D) Raman spectrum for the cancerous breast tissues of patient P81, and IR spectrum for the cancerous breast tissues of patient P83. Figure reprinted upon Creative Commons Attribution License (http://creativecommons.org/licenses/by/2.0) from Ref. [37].

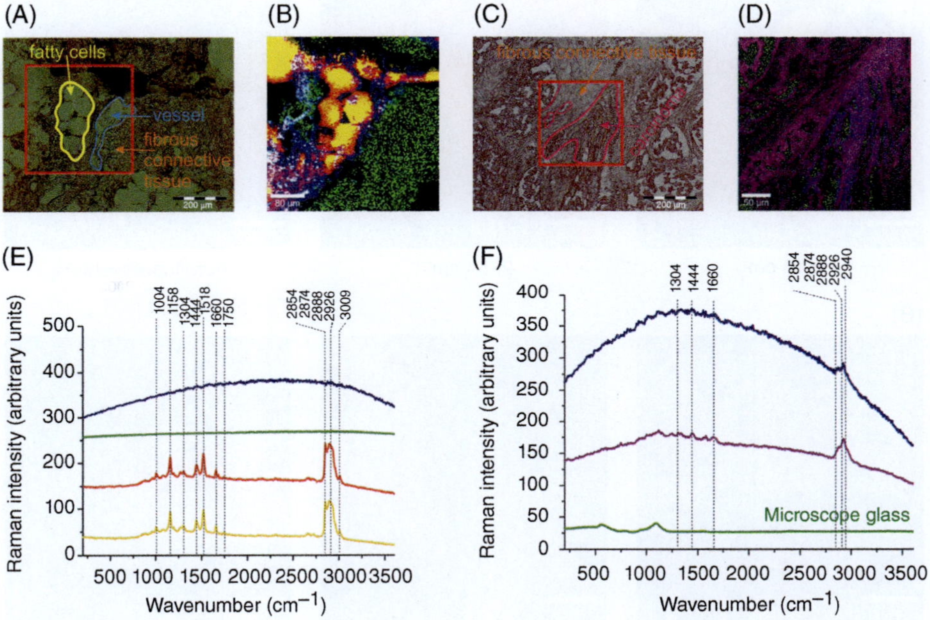

Figure 3.3 Raman image and spectra of the noncancerous and cancerous breast tissue of patient P81. Noncancerous breast tissue: (A) Microscope image (B) Raman image (400 × 400 µm) from the region marked in (A); and (C) Raman spectra (integration time: 0.05 s). Cancerous breast tissue: (D) Microscope image, (E) Raman image (300 × 300 µm) from the region marked in (D), and (F) Raman spectra (integration time: 0.036 s). The colors of the spectra correspond to the colors in the image. Mixed areas are displayed as mixed colors. Figure reprinted upon Creative Commons Attribution License (http://creativecommons.org/licenses/by/2.0) from Ref. [37].

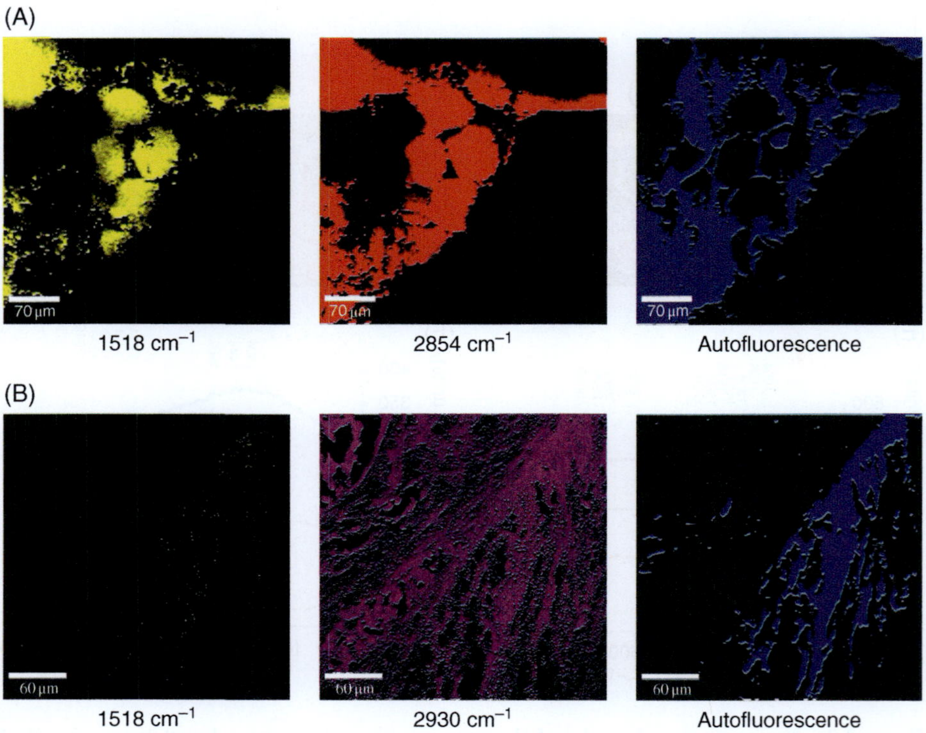

Figure 3.4 Raman images: (A) noncancerous and (B) cancerous breast tissue of patient P81. Filters: carotenoids (1518 cm^{-1}), monounsaturated fatty acids (2854 cm^{-1}), proteins (2930 cm^{-1}), and autofluorescence (1800 cm^{-1}). Figure reprinted upon Creative Commons Attribution License (http://creativecommons.org/licenses/by/2.0) from Ref. [37].

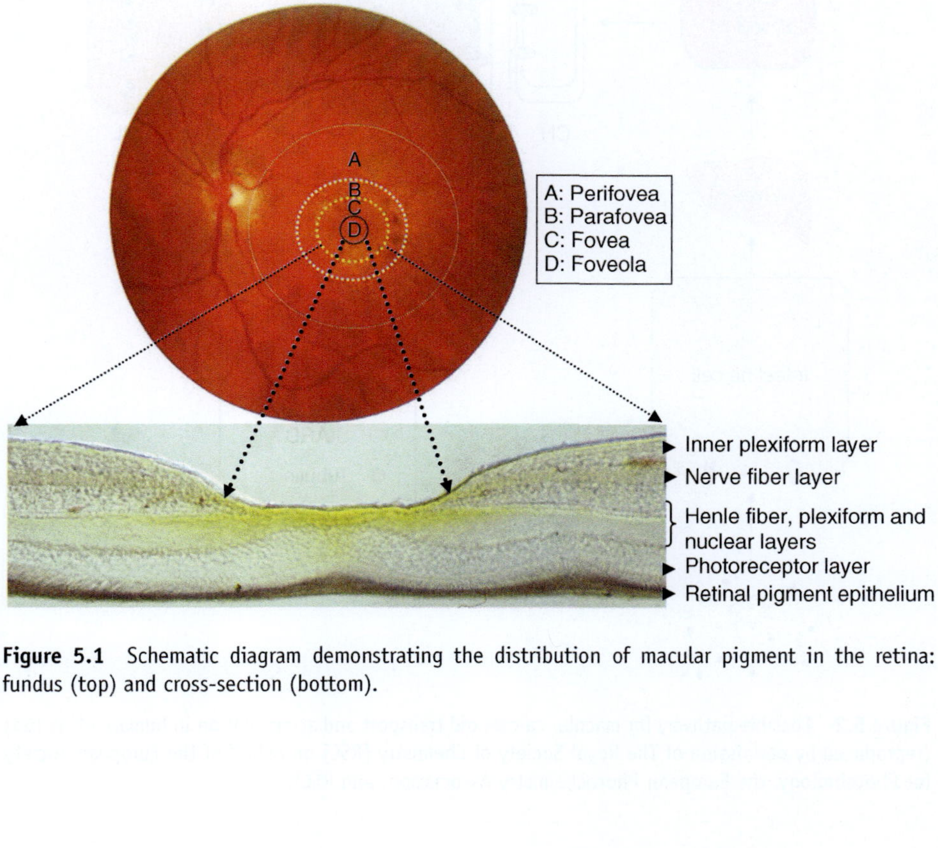

Figure 5.1 Schematic diagram demonstrating the distribution of macular pigment in the retina: fundus (top) and cross-section (bottom).

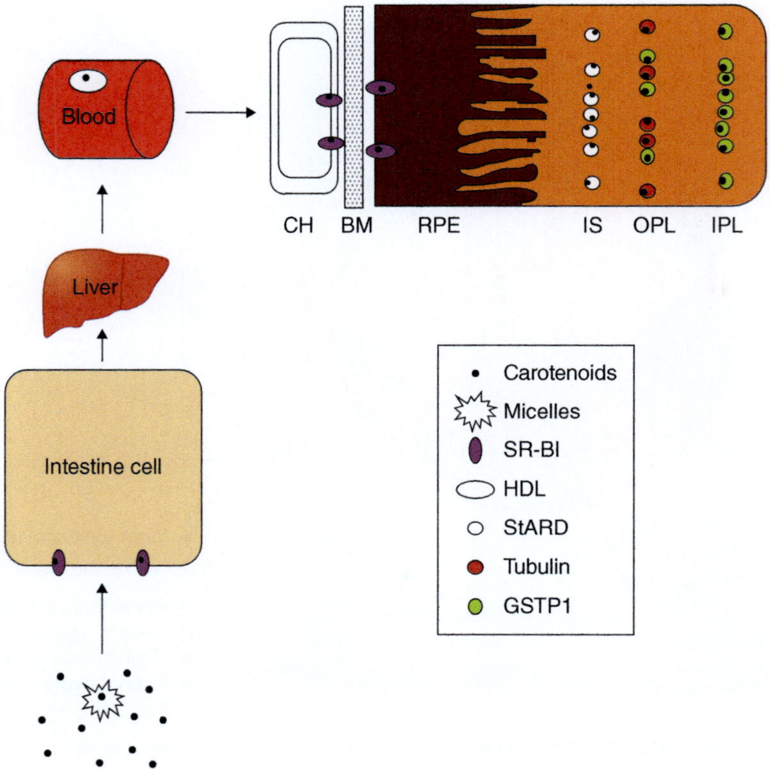

Figure 5.2 Possible pathway for macular carotenoid transport and accumulation in human retina [64] (reproduced by permission of The Royal Society of Chemistry [RSC] on behalf of the European Society for Photobiology, the European Photochemistry Association, and RSC).

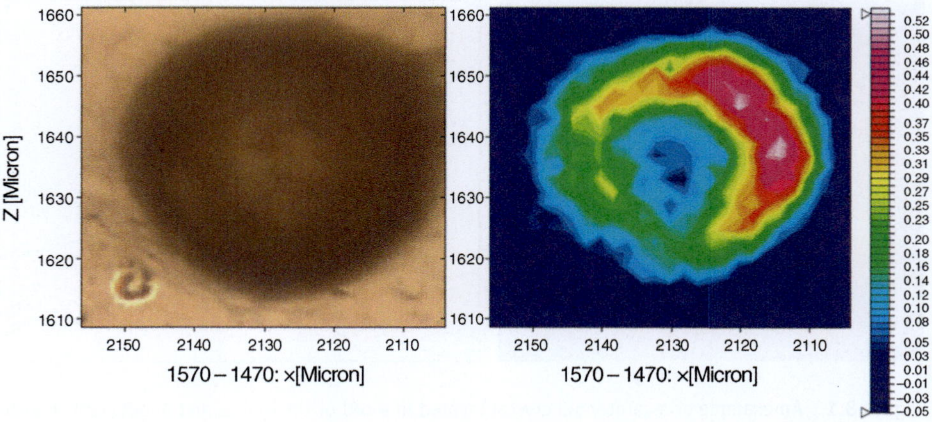

Figure 6.2 A visual image focused inside of the *Haematococcus pluvialis* cell with the collapsed cytoplasm (on the left, magnification 40×) and distribution of astaxanthin (AXT) in the sample (on the right) obtained by integration of the marker band at 1520 cm^{-1} (color code defined in the scale). The map was obtained by measuring 729 points (the distance between points on the x and z axes equals 2.0 μm). Reproduced from Ref. [93] with kind permission of Analyst Owner Societies.

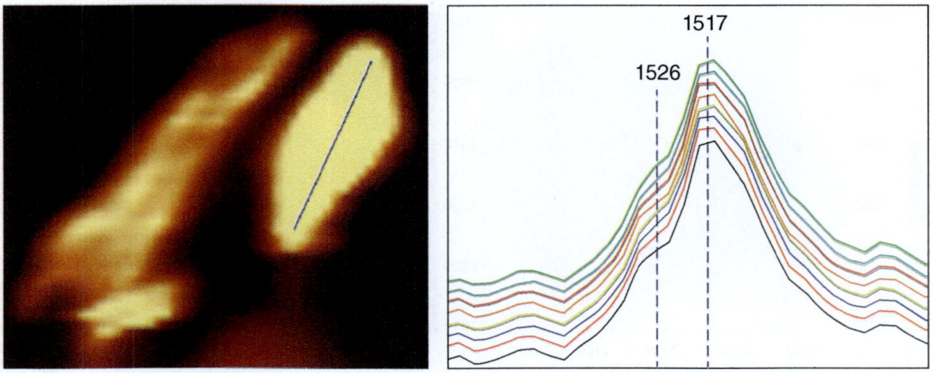

Figure 8.1 An example of a carotenoid crystal located in a cell of the high α and β root. Left: Raman map obtained by the integration of the ν_1 band. Right: Raman spectra (532 nm) in the range of the ν_1 band extracted every 0.2 μm along a marked line. Reprinted with permission from M. Roman, K. M. Marzec, E. Grzebelus, P. W. Simon, M. Baranska, and R. Baranski, "Composition and (in)homogeneity of carotenoid crystals in carrot cells revealed by high resolution Raman imaging," *Spectrochimica Acta Part A: Molecular and Biomolecular Spectroscopy*, **136**, 1395–1400 (2015) [7]. Copyright (2015) Elsevier.

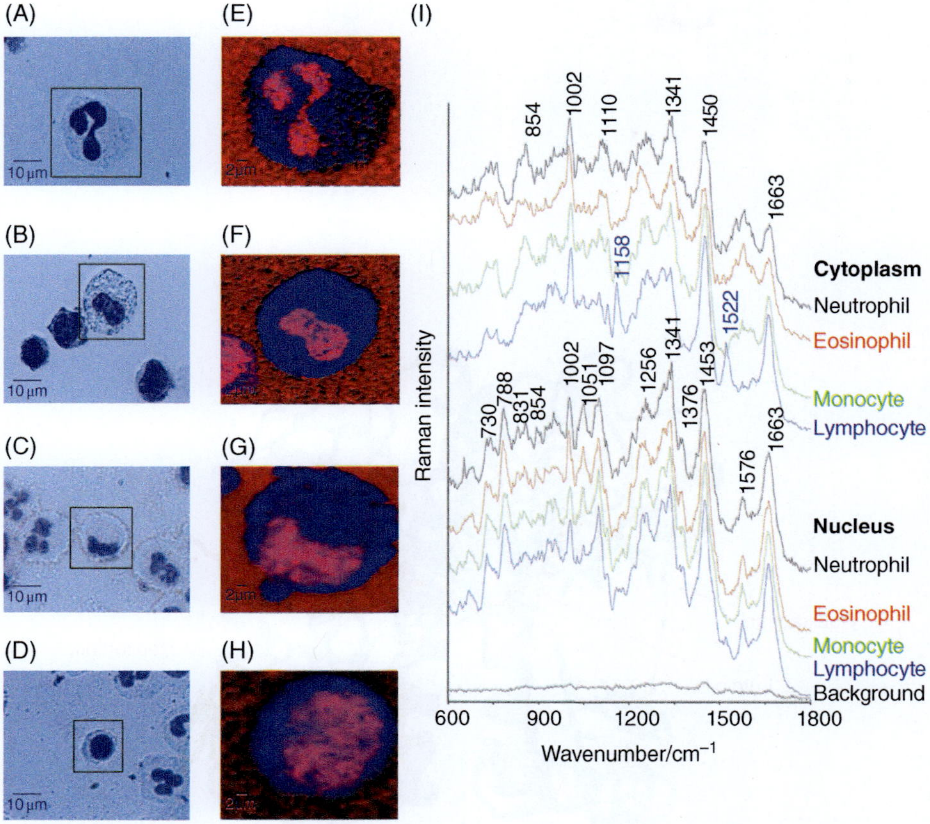

Figure 8.4 Morphological characteristics of the different leukocytes: neutrophil (A and E), eosinophil (B and F), monocyte (C and G), and lymphocyte (D and H). (A–D) White light images after Kimura staining; (E–H) false color Raman images of the same cell using the intensity at ~788 cm^{-1} to highlight the nucleus (pink) and the intensity of the CH stretching between 2800 and 3050 cm^{-1} to color code the overall cell area (blue). (I) Averaged Raman spectra of the cytoplasm, nucleus, and background region. Reprinted with permission from A. Ramoji, U. Neugebauer, T. Bocklitz, M. Foerster, M. Kiehntopf, M. Bauer, and J. Popp, "Toward a Spectroscopic Hemogram: Raman Spectroscopic Differentiation of the Two Most Abundant Leukocytes from Peripheral Blood," *Analytical Chemistry*, **84**, 5335–5342 (2012) [41]. Copyright (2012) American Chemical Society.

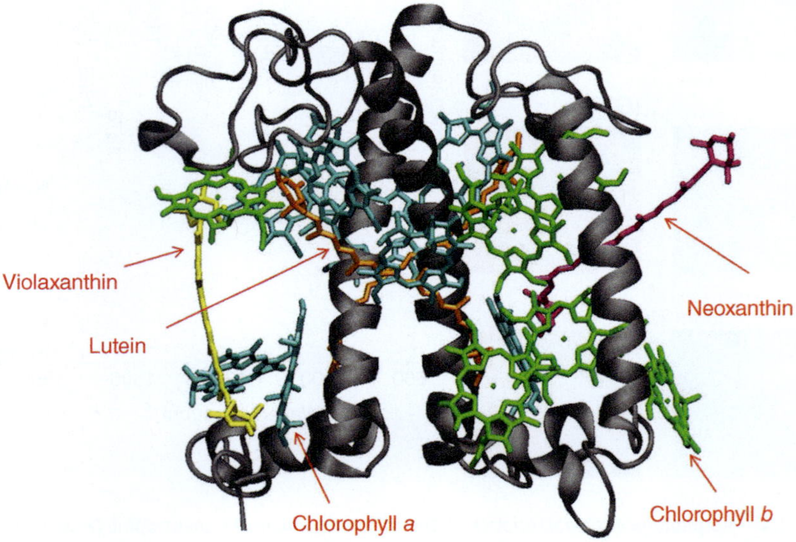

Figure 9.3 Model of the structure of the LHCII pigment–protein complex, based on the crystallographic data PDB: 2bhw.

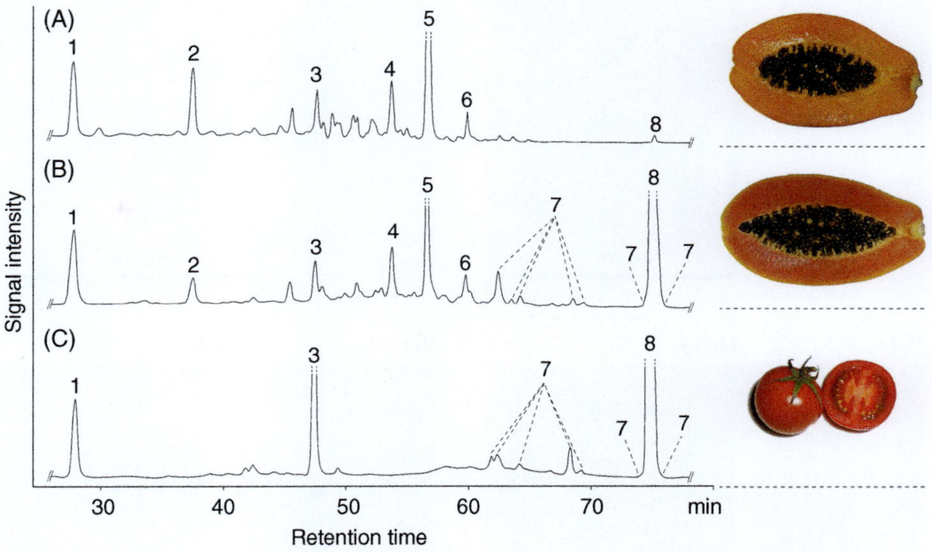

Figure 11.2 Separation of carotenoids and carotenoid esters from (A) yellow papaya, (B) red papaya, and (C) tomato fruit by high-performance liquid chromatography (HPLC) monitored at 450 nm. 1: β-Apo-8-carotenal (added as internal standard); 2: β-cryptoxanthin; 3: β-carotene; 4: β-cryptoxanthin caprate; 5: β-cryptoxanthin laurate; 6: β-cryptoxanthin myristate; 7: *Z*-lycopene isomers; and 8: all-*E*-lycopene. (Reproduced with permission from Schweiggert *et al.*, 2011 [22]. © Springer.)

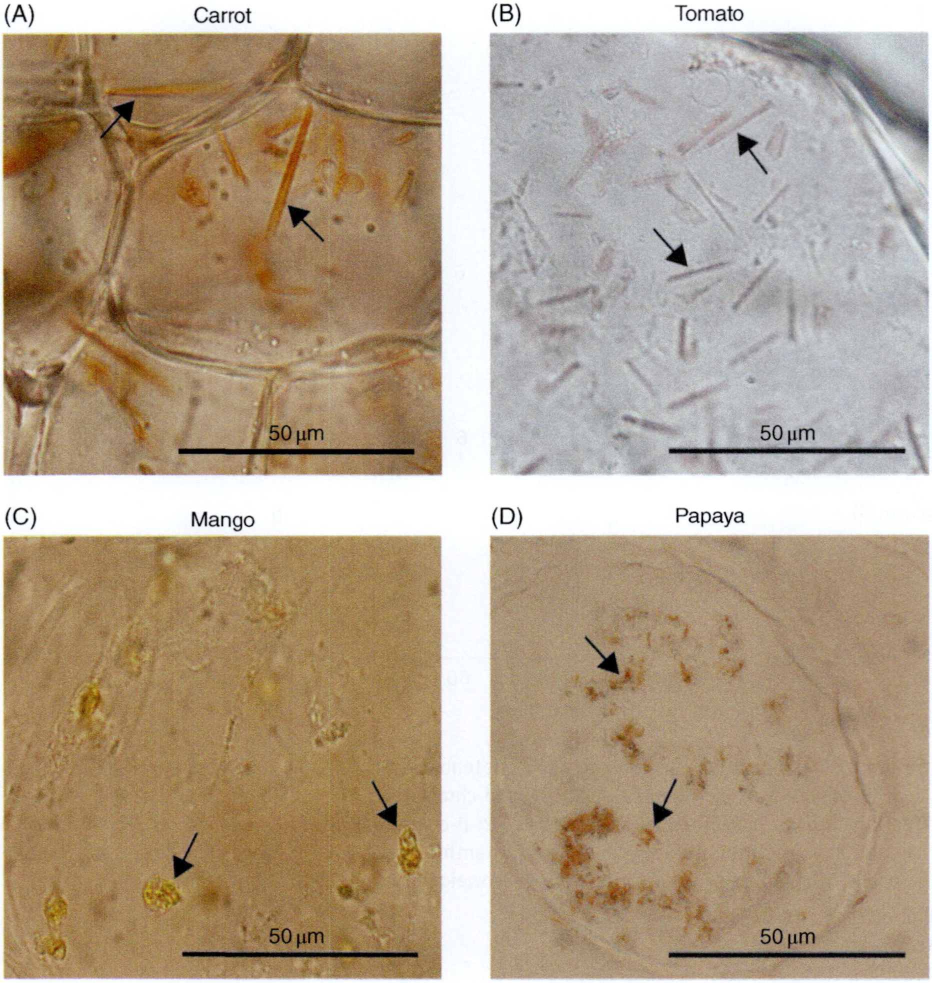

Figure 11.3 Light micrographs of carrot root and mango, papaya, and tomato fruits. The chromoplasts are marked with arrows. (Reproduced with permission from Schweiggert *et al.*, 2012 [24]. © Elsevier.)

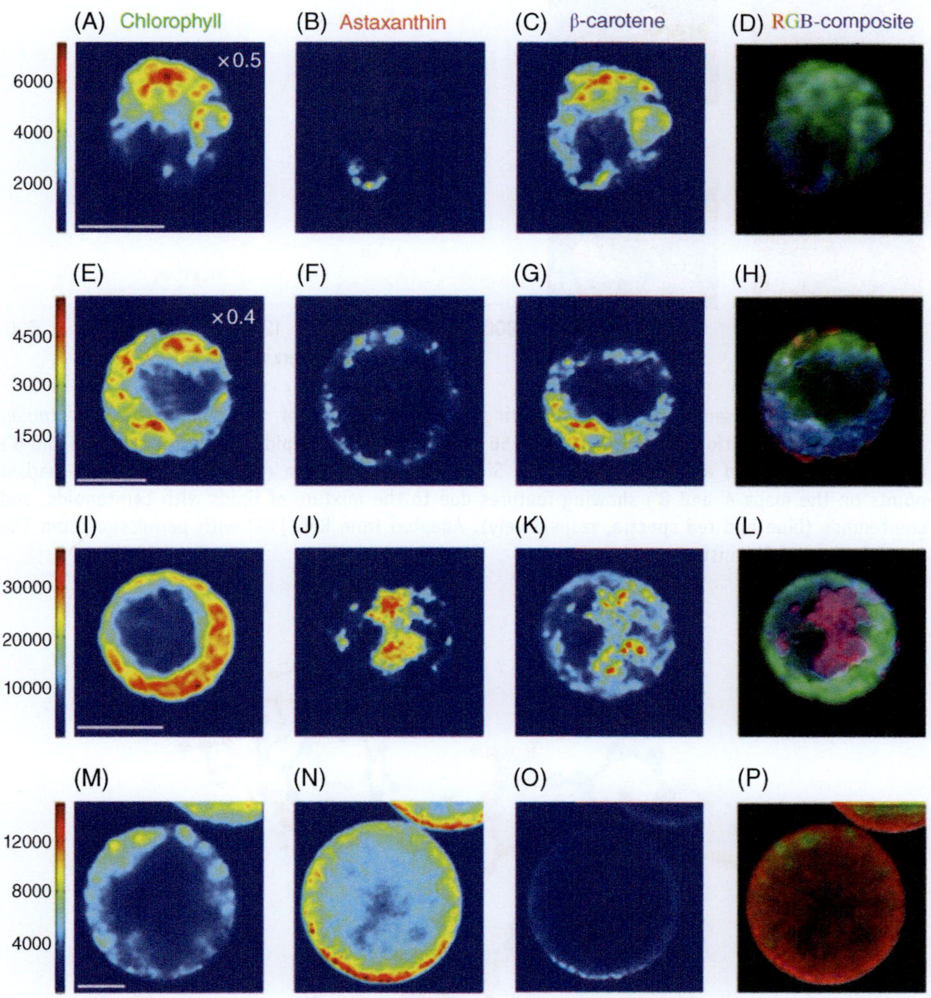

Figure 13.1 Multivariate curve resolution (MCR) concentration maps for spectral components representing chlorophyll, astaxanthin, and β-carotene. (A–D) Flagellated motile cell. (E–H) Palmella stage cell under noninductive conditions. (I–L) Palmelloid cell under inductive conditions for 24 hours; and (M–P) large red cyst (aplanospore). In all images, the scale bar represents 10 mm. Note that in (A) and (E), the intensity has been scaled by 0.5 and 0.4, respectively, for clarity. The intensity scales are not comparable across cell types as the acquisition parameters were optimized for each cell image; however, within a cell type, the intensities within the concentration map represent relative component concentrations. Composite RGB images are created by overlaying the individual concentration maps that have been pseudo-colored, as indicated in the image titles [25]. Figure reprinted upon Creative Commons Attribution License (CCAL).

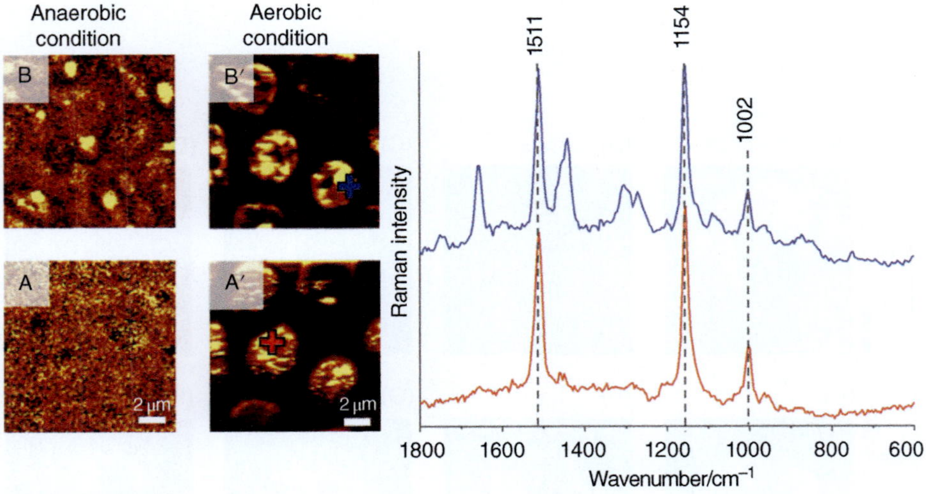

Figure 13.4 Representative images showing the distribution of carotenoids *in Rhodotholua mucilaginosa* (integration over the band at 1156 cm^{-1}, A and A′) and lipid bodies (2857 cm^{-1}, B and B′) grown in aerobic and anaerobic conditions. Single Raman spectrum (extracted from cross-marked points on the maps A′ and B′) showing features due to the mixture of lipids with carotenoids, and carotenoids (blue and red spectra, respectively). Adapted from Ref. [74] with permission from The Royal Society of Chemistry.

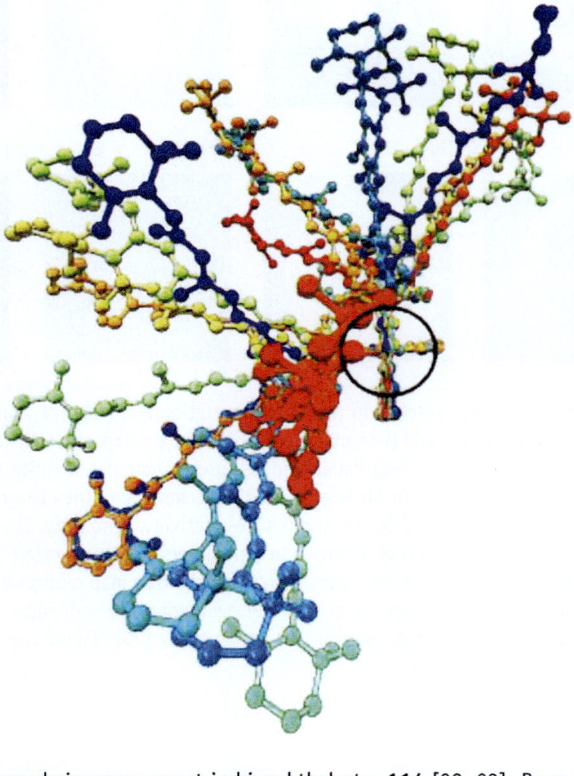

Figure 14.1 Polyene chain arrangement in binaphtholester **114** [92, 93]. Reproduced with permission of Zsolt Bikadi, Virtua Drug Ltd.

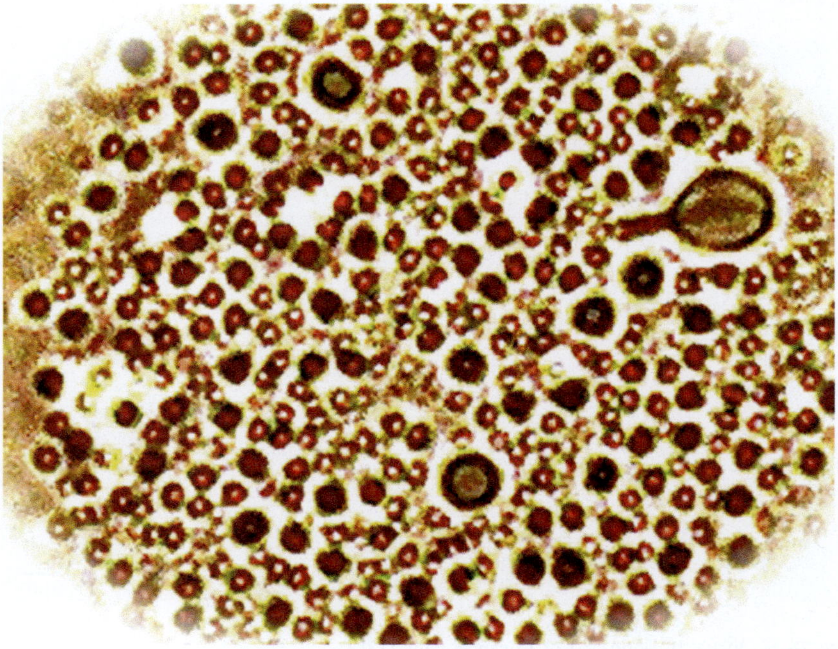

Figure 14.5 Vesicles (1–1.5 mm) of phospholipid **127** [117]. Reproduced with permission from Elsevier.

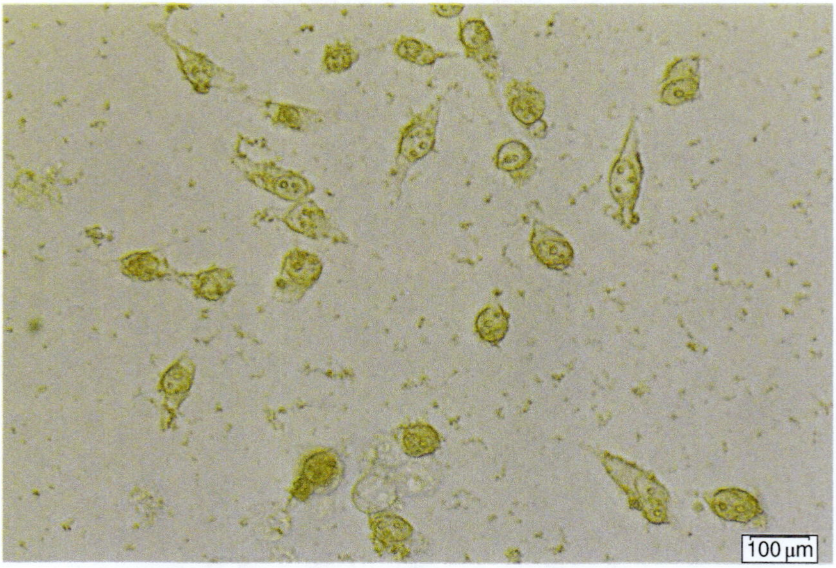

Figure 14.6 Visual tracking of **127** in cancer cells [139].

Printed and bound by CPI Group (UK) Ltd, Croydon, CR0 4YY

12/10/2026

14980521-0001